Modern Microbiology an

Modern Microbiology

and Pathology for Nurses

J. M. GIBSON

BA, MB, BS

BLACKWELL SCIENTIFIC PUBLICATIONS

OXFORD LONDON EDINBURGH MELBOURNE

© 1979 by Blackwell Scientific Publications
Osney Mead, Oxford, OX2 0EL
8 John Street, London, WC1N 2ES
9 Forrest Road, Edinburgh, EH1 2QH
P.O. Box 9, North Balwyn, Victoria, Australia

All rights reserved. No part of this publication may be reproduced, stored in a retrieval system, or transmitted, in any form or by any means, electronic, mechanical, photocopying, recording or otherwise without the prior permission of the copyright owner.

First published 1979

British Library
Cataloguing in Publication Data

Gibson J M
Modern microbiology and pathology for nurses
1. Pathology
I. Title
616.07'02'4613   RT65

ISBN 0-632-00449-5

Distributed in U.S.A. by
Blackwell Mosby Book Distributors
11830 Westline Industrial Drive
St. Louis, Missouri 63141
and in Canada by
Blackwell Mosby Book Distributors
86 Northline Road, Toronto
Ontario, M4B 3E5

Printed and bound in Great Britain by
Whitstable Litho Ltd., Whitstable, Kent

Contents

	Acknowledgments	vii
	Author's Note	viii
1	Infections	1
2	Bacteria, Part 1: Cocci and Gram-positive Bacilli	8
3	Bacteria, Part 2: Gram-negative Bacilli, Cocco-bacilli, Vibrios, Spirochetes, Rickettsiae, Fungi	17
4	Viruses	26
5	Parasites	35
6	Inflammation	46
7	Immunity, Hypersensitivity, Autoimmunity, Collagen Diseases	49
8	Disorders of Fluid and Electrolyte Balance	56
9	Degenerations	63
10	Neoplasms	66
11	Circulatory System	71
12	Respiratory System	81
13	Blood	93
14	Alimentary System	112
15	Pancreas, Liver, Biliary Tract	126
16	Urinary System	136
17	Skin	145
18	Metabolic and Deficiency Diseases	150
19	Nervous System	156
20	Pituitary, Adrenal and Thyroid Glands	167
21	Muscles, Joints, Bones and Parathyroid Glands	184

Contents

22	Male Genital System	195
23	Female Genital System; Breast	200
24	Pregnancy; Infertility	208
25	Inherited Diseases	211
26	Eye	214
27	Ear	218
	Index	220

Acknowledgements

The author wishes to thank for their help:
Dr John Gibson for compiling the Index and for assistance throughout the preparation of the manuscript;
Dr D. Donaldson, Consultant Chemical Pathologist, Redhill General Hospital, for kindly giving permission to use biochemical values from his own laboratory publications and data, some of which are quoted in this text;
Dr R. Earl, Consultant Haematologist, Redhill General Hospital, for discussions on the chapter on haematology and helpful suggestions.
Their contributions are gratefully acknowledged.

Author's Note

Normal values, normal results and examples of abnormal results are given for general guidance only. In any particular case reference should be made to values specified by the laboratory in which the test is performed.

Chapter 1 Infections

Infections are diseases which can be transmitted from one person to another or from animal to man. They are caused by various kinds of micro-organisms:
bacteria   viruses   rickettsiae
fungi   protozoa (see Chapter 5).
These organisms may attack the body as a whole or a particular part of it.

The stages of an infection

1. INCUBATION PERIOD

The incubation period is the period between a person becoming infected and developing symptoms. It is the time taken by the micro-organism to multiply to such a number that its harmful effects on the body become apparent. During this time the person may be infectious, capable of transmitting the micro-organism to another person, e.g. with a streptococcal or viral infection of the upper respiratory tract he can infect other people by talking, coughing, laughing and sneezing.

2. DISEASE PERIOD

During this period the patient is ill. The illness may be acute (lasting for days or weeks) or chronic (lasting for months or years). According to the type of infection he may discharge harmful organisms in:
expired air
discharge from nose, mouth, ear, eye
urine
faeces
discharge from ulcers, wounds, skin, internal organs.

3. RECOVERY PERIOD

Clinical recovery from some diseases ends the danger of infection. *Carriers* are people who excrete the micro-organism after recovery. They can be:
(a) *convalescent carriers:* they excrete the organism only during convalescence;
(b) *temporary carriers:* they excrete the organism for not more than a year;
(c) *chronic carriers:* they excrete the organism for more than a year; this can happen after typhoid fever.

Symptomless excretors (contact carriers) are people who acquire an infectious organism without apparently developing the disease. This can happen with:
poliomyelitis
staphylococcus aureus infection
diphtheria
streptococcal sore throat
dysentery
meningococcal meningitis
It is particularly liable to happen during an epidemic of a particular infection. Symptomless excretors can infect other people who can either develop the disease or become carriers themselves.

Transmission of Infection

Micro-organisms are spread:
1, from man to man;
2, from animal to man;
3, from other sources.

1. SPREAD FROM MAN TO MAN

(a) *Transplacental infection.* Some organisms can pass through the placenta from an infected mother to her child. These include rubella virus, smallpox virus and *Treponema pallidum,* the organism of syphilis.

(b) *Infection of the newly-born baby.* At birth a baby is sterile, but he quickly becomes infected with a number of organisms which in normal conditions do him no harm. These include:
(i) *E. coli* (sometimes called by its old name *B. coli*), which inhabit the intestine. They cause disease if they get out of their normal habitat, causing peritonitis if they get into the peritoneal cavity, and infection of the urinary tract if they get into it.
(ii) Various *staphylococci,* which live on the skin and sometimes cause boils and other infections of it.
(iii) Various *streptococci* and *pneumococci* which live in the nose and can cause infection if the mucous membrane there becomes diseased.

(c) *Later infections.* Man can infect man during the incubation period, during the disease period, and from a carrier state.

2. SPREAD FROM ANIMAL TO MAN

Many diseases can be transmitted from animal to man, e.g.:

Cows	tuberculosis, abortus fever – by milk, anthrax - from hides and bone-meal
Sheep	anthrax – from wool
Goats	Malta fever (a brucella infection) – from milk
Cats	cat-stratch fever – by scratching
Dogs	rabies – by biting
Rats	plague – via fleas; leptospirosis – via water
Mice	salmonella infections – from faeces
Ducks	salmonella infections – from faeces and eggs
Tortoises	salmonella infections – from faeces
Monkeys	several viral infections – by biting or via mosquitoes

3. SPREAD FROM OTHER SOURCES

Wounds can become infected by the organisms of tetanus and gas gangrene if infected soil or manure get into them.

Routes of Infection

1. RESPIRATORY TRACT

Many infectious diseases are transmitted by the respiratory tract. They include:

common cold	influenza
tuberculosis	diphtheria
whooping cough	measles
pneumonic plague	rubella (German measles)
meningococcal meningitis	
streptococcal sore throat and tonsillitis.	

They are spread by:
(a) kissing
(b) the use of infected cups, mugs, glasses, cutlery
(c) droplet infection. Droplets are particles of secretion, which may contain micro-organisms, expelled from the respiratory passages by loud talking, shouting, coughing and sneezing. A big sneeze can expel a million droplets. Droplets vary in size. Large ones travel less than a metre in the air before falling to the ground; small ones can shoot across a room. Small ones dry up while in the air and the dried secretion remains suspended for some hours before falling to the ground. If a person who coughs or sneezes has pathogenic organisms in his respiratory passages he is likely to infect any one within range.

2. DUST

Many infections are spread by dust and contact with infected surfaces. People with a respiratory tract infection can spread infection by:
(a) dried droplets in dust – on the floor, in bedclothes, clothes, furnishings;

(b) infecting the hands by touching or picking the nose, using a handkerchief;
(c) bedmaking, dusting, sweeping.

Some micro-organisms survive in dust for days or weeks if not exposed to direct sunlight, e.g.:
the micro-organisms of tuberculosis, smallpox, diphtheria
streptococci   staphylococci

3. INTESTINAL TRACT

Intestinal and other infections are produced by swallowing harmful micro-organisms, e.g.:
typhoid and paratyphoid fever   dysentery
cholera   abortus fever
tuberculosis

These organisms are spread by:
(a) faecal contamination of hands, by bedpans, nappies, clothes;
(b) infection of food by a carrier;
(c) infection of water-supply by a carrier or by a leaking lavatory or sewer.

4. INOCULATION

Inoculation is the transmission of a micro-organism through the skin or a mucous membrane.

(a) *Contact*. Some organisms can invade the body through the intact skin or a mucous membrane, e.g.:
the organisms of syphilis and gonorrhoea;
the organism of leprosy;
the organism causing boils, impetigo.

(b) *Infection of a wound*. Wounds and damaged surfaces (cuts, bruises, burns, surgical incisions, the uterus after childbirth) can be infected. Organisms which can infect various sites are:
the organisms of tetanus, gas gangrene, anthrax;
Staphylococcus aureus (of which there are resistant 'hospital' strains carried by nurses and doctors);
Streptococcus pyogenes (which is liable to infect the uterus after childbirth).

(c) *Infection*. (i) Medical injections: serum hepatitis virus can be transmitted by using needles and syringes which have been in contact with infected blood, or by transfusing infected blood.
(ii) Biting insects:
mosquitoes: malaria, yellow fever
fleas: plague
lice: typhus fever.

Pathogenicity

Pathogenicity is the ability of a micro-organism to cause disease. A *pathogen* is a micro-organism capable of causing disease. Not all micro-organisms are harmful. Some live on the skin or in the intestine without causing harm; some in the intestine can be beneficial to man as a source of certain vitamins.

Some organisms always cause the same disease, e.g. *Clostridium tetani* always causes tetanus.

Some organisms can cause different diseases, e.g. *Streptococcus pyogenes* can cause tonsillitis, scarlet fever, erysipelas, and puerperal fever.

Some organisms are harmless and even essential in one part of the body, but cause disease if they get into another part, e.g. *E. coli* lives in the bowel and causes diseases if it gets into the peritoneal cavity or urinary tract: however, some 'enteropathic' strains of *E. coli* cause gastroenteritis in infants.

Detection of Bacteria

Identification of bacteria can be direct or indirect.

Direct identification: bacteria are grown on suitable culture media, isolated and seen under the microscope.

Indirect identification: the presence and identity of bacteria are deduced from the results of tests in the blood ('serological methods'), biochemical tests, etc.

A *strain* of a micro-organism is one that shows a change from the basic type. Such a change is produced during the division of the organism into two and can occur either naturally or when it is being grown as a culture. One effect of this may be a modification of the virulence of the organism. The *virulence* is the degree of pathogenicity of an organism, the degree to which it can produce a disease. Some strains may have a high virulence, some a low virulence, some be non-pathogenic. The virulence of an organism can be reduced by growing it in conditions or on media it does not like, a method that is used when it is necessary to have a weak strain for use as a vaccine, which is administered to a person to prevent his getting a particular infection.

TOXINS

A toxin is the bacterial constituent or product which has a harmful effect on cells in the tissues. They are usually classified as:
exotoxins
endotoxins

(a) *Exotoxins.* Exotoxins are produced by living bacteria and pass out of the bacteria which produce them into the surrounding fluid. If the organisms dies and starts to degenerate, large amounts of exotoxin can escape. Exotoxins are protein substances and are antigens which stimulate an antibody reaction. Among the organisms that produce exotoxins are:

Corynebacterium   *C. diphtheriae* (which causes diphtheria);
Clostridium   *Cl. tetanus* (which causes tetanus);
Shigella   *Sh. dysenteriae* (which causes one kind of dysentery).

(b) *Endotoxins.* Endotoxins form an essential part of the organism and are liberated from it only when it dies. They are composed of a complex of polysaccharide-protein-lipid, and are relatively weak stimulators of antibodies. Among the organisms that produce endotoxins are:

Vibrio   *V. cholerae* (which causes cholera);
Escherichia   *E. coli* (which causes peritonitis and infections of the urinary tract).

Microbiological Identification

Micro-organisms are identified by appropriate methods, according to the nature of the material submitted for examination and the likely organisms. *Specimens* submitted for microbiological examination can be:
swabs from throat, mouth, wounds, rectum, vagina, ear, eye

CSF	blood	urine
faeces	skin	nails
pus	sputum	hairs

1. MICROSCOPIC EXAMINATION

The material submitted or specimens from a culture are placed on a slide and examined with a light microscope.

(a) *Wet preparations* are unstained preparations which are examined for the size and shape and in particular any movements of the micro-organism

(b) *Stained preparations* are preparations in which the micro-organisms are fixed to a slide by heating and then stained with an appropriate stain. The organisms are killed in the process and cannot therefore be examined for any motility they might have had in life.

Special microscopic methods

(i) *Dark ground microscopy.* This is a method for showing some thin organisms, which show up as bright objects against a black background, e.g. *Tr. pallidum,* which causes syphilis.
(ii) *Fluorescence microscopy.* Some dyes fluoresce when illuminated by ultra-violet light, and some bacteria can be identified in this way, e.g. *Myco. tuberculosis* when stained with auramine.
(iii) *Electron microscopy.* Most viruses are too small to be seen with a light microscope. An

electron microscope is used to examine both them and the internal structure of micro-organisms.

2. STAINING REACTIONS

Bacteria can be stained by various dyes and are classified according to the ways in which they stain.

(a) *Gram stain*. This is a violet stain by which bacteria are divided into those which are Gram positive and those which are Gram negative.

(i) *Gram positive bacteria* are those which stain violet with the stain and do not lose the colour when treated with acetone or alcohol. They include:
all cocci except the *gonococcus* and *meningococcus*;
bacilli of tetanus, diphtheria, tuberculosis, leprosy.

(ii) *Gram negative bacteria* are those which lose the violet stain when treated with acetone or alcohol and then stain pink with carbol fuchsin or neutral red. They include:
all bacilli except the Gram positive ones.

The Gram stain is related to biological differences in bacteria:

(i) Gram positive bacteria have a more clearly defined cell wall, which is more resistant to destruction. Gram negative bacteria have a less clearly defined wall and are more fragile.

(ii) Gram positive bacteria produce diffusible substances which can be filtered off and purified, e.g. antigens used in immunization.

(iii) Gram negative bacteria contain endotoxins which are released from them when their cell wall deteriorates.

(iv) Some Gram positive bacteria form spores. No Gram negative bacteria form spores.

(v) There are differences in sensitivity to antibiotics and disinfectants between Gram positive and Gram negative bacteria.

(b) *Ziehl-Neelsen stain*. Acid-fast bacilli are those which in this method stain a bright red with carbol fuchsin and cannot be decolourised by acetone or alcohol. They include:
bacilli of tuberculosis and leprosy.

3. CULTURE OF BACTERIA

A *culture* is a growth of a micro-organism. Bacteria are grown in media composed of chemical substances known to encourage the growth of the suspected organism or to inhibit the growth of unwanted ones, such as any likely to have contaminated the specimen.

The medium can be liquid or solid. The addition of 1 per cent of agar (a seaweed derivative) causes a fluid to set to a firm jelly, which provides a suitable surface on which to culture bacteria. Such media are called 'agars'.

The agar media are usually placed in Petri dishes, circular glass or plastic dishes with a lid. The material containing suspected bacteria is streaked across the surface of the medium, and the dish is then incubated at an appropriate temperature and inspected, usually after 18 hours. Colonies of organisms appear as white or coloured growths of varying and sometimes distinctive appearance. The growth of one type of organism may sometimes be seen to have inhibited the growth of another type of organism growing near it.

(a) *Nutrient agar*. This is a straw-coloured basic culture medium composed of peptone, meat extract, sodium chloride and agar.

(b) *Blood agar*. This is composed of nutrient agar to which blood has been added. The surface has a granular appearance. It is used to detect certain bacteria which have the property of destroying red blood cells and are hence called 'haemolytic'.

(c) *Chocolate agar*. This is so-called because of its dark brown colour due to the presence of blood heated to provide a nutritious medium for certain organisms. It does not contain chocolate.

(d) *MacConkey's medium*. This contains nutrient agar plus bile salts, and is light pink and transparent. It is used for the growth of bowel pathogens. The growth of non-bowel organisms is inhibited.

4. SEROLOGICAL METHODS

The presence and identity of bacteria are deduced from the results of testing blood by 'serological methods'. Antigen-antibody reactions (see Chapter 7) can be used, the common practice being to use known antisera to detect suspected antigens.

(a) *Precipitation.* When antigen and antibody in solution in suitable quantities combine, they come out of solution and form a visible precipitate. The test can be done in 3 ways:
(i) It is carried out in a tube in which the solid precipitate falls to the bottom.
(ii) It is carried out on a small scale in a capillary tube, a ring of precipitate forming at the interface where antigen and antibody meet.
(iii) It is carried out in a gel diffusion technique. Small holes are cut in agar plates and filled with antigen and antiserum; antigen and antibody diffuse towards each other through the medium and form white lines of precipitate where they meet.

(b) *Agglutination.* Cells or bacteria agglutinate (i.e. clump together) when an antibody combines with an antigen on their surface. The *qualitative test* is performed on a slide. The *quantitative test* is performed in a series of tubes, in which progressively higher dilutions of antiserum are added to a standard quantity of cell suspension. The 'titre' is the highest dilution of antiserum at which agglutination takes place.

The *Widal test* and the *Weil Felix reaction* are two types of agglutination test.

(c) *Complement fixation test.* This test can be used where an antigen-antibody reaction produces no visible result. Many antigen-antibody reactions require the presence of 'complement', a complex of substances, in order to occur. There is no visible reaction, but the 'complement' is fixed, i.e. is no longer available to take part in another antigen-antibody reaction. The serum in which complement may or may not have been fixed is then added to a system in which haemolysis occurs only if it has not been fixed. If there is no haemolysis, the complement was fixed and therefore the antibody was present; if there is haemolysis the complement was free (i.e. not used) and therefore antibody was not present.

The *Wassermann reaction* (W.R.) uses this principle to detect the antibodies of syphilis.

(d) *Toxin neutralization.* Antibodies can be detected by their action in blocking the effects of a toxin acting as an antigen, e.g. the Nagler reaction for *Clostridium perfringens*.

5. BIOCHEMICAL TESTS

Biochemical tests are used to detect the chemical activity of bacteria and to identify bacteria.

(a) *Fermentation of carbohydrates.* This means that bacteria form acid from carbohydrates or produce gas. The acid is detected by a change in colour with the use of an indicator and the gas by bubbles seen in a special tube.

A test of *lactose fermentation* is important in distinguishing bacteria which are pathogenic in the intestine and those which are not.

Other carbohydrate fermentation tests are used to distinguish pathogenic staphylococci from non-pathogenic staphylococci, and the *meningococcus* from the *gonococcus*.

(b) *Indole production.* Organisms are grown in a tube of peptone water, and then Ehrlich's rosindole reagent is added. A rose-pink colour occurs if indole is present. This distinguishes *E. Coli* from *Salmonella*.

(c) *Urea test.* Bacterial urease splits urea with the production of ammonia, a change detected by a change of colour in an indicator. The test distinguishes *Proteus* from other intestinal bacteria.

6. ANIMAL INOCULATIONS

Animal inoculations are used to identify organisms which produce the characteristic disease in the tissues of the animal used, and to test the virulence of the organism. Guinea pig inoculation is used to identify the organism that causes tuberculosis and to test the virulence of the organism that causes diphtheria.

Detection of Virus Diseases

Microscopy

1. LIGHT MICROSCOPY

Many viruses produce 'inclusion bodies' in the nucleus and cytoplasm of cells. These are rounded, oval or irregular masses and are thought to be either viral particles or degenerative changes in the cell.

2. ELECTRON MICROSCOPY

Virus particles can be seen and assigned to a group e.g. pox or herpes viruses.

Growth of viruses

Viruses can grow only in living cells. These may be:
(a) the whole animal
(b) the developing egg
(c) tissue culture.

(a) *Animals* are not used much except for identifying rabies and Coxsackie A, for both of which mice are used.

(b) *Eggs:* different viruses grow particularly well in different parts of the egg.
yolk sac: suitable for Rickettsia and Psittacosis, not for the true viruses
amniotic sac: for influenza and mumps (myxoviruses)
chorio-allantoic membrane: particularly useful for pox and herpes viruses

(c) *Tissue culture:* (i) *Primary cell culture:* this is prepared from monkey kidney, human embryo kidney or human amnion cell culture. These are used once.
(ii) *Continuous cell lines:* this is derived from malignant tumours and can be kept going indefinitely, e.g. 'HeLa' cell culture from human carcinoma of the cervix.
(iii) *Semi-continuous lines:* these last for 30-40 cultures, e.g. W138 from human embryo lung cells.

Detection of virus from tissue culture:
(i) *Cytopathic effect:* this is a characteristic appearance of cells due to degeneration produced by some viruses.
(ii) *Interference with cytopathic effect:* specific antibodies can block the cytopathic effect, giving indirect evidence of the presence of the virus.
(iii) *Haemadsorption:* some viruses produce haemagglutination, which causes red cells to stick to the surface of monkey tissue infected by the virus.

Serological methods

1. VIRUS NEUTRALIZATION

A virus is made non-infective (i.e. neutralized) when an antibody combines with the viral antigen. Virus and antibodies are inoculated into tissue culture or egg.

2. HAEMAGGLUTINATION INHIBITION

Specific antibodies prevent agglutination of red cells by viruses.

3. COMPLEMENT FIXATION TEST

See p. 6

Chapter 2   Bacteria, Part 1: Cocci and Gram-positive Bacilli

Bacteria are microscopic single-celled organisms which multiply by dividing into two. They are separated into classes according to their shape:
coccus: spherical
bacillus: straight rod
cocco-bacillus: half way between a coccus and a bacillus
vibrio: curved rod
spirochete: spiral.

STRUCTURE OF A BACTERIUM

(a) *Cell wall.* The cell wall is composed mainly of mucopeptides. It is a rigid structure which maintains the shape of the bacterium and allows various chemical substances to pass through it in both directions.

(b) *Protoplast.* This is the part of the organism enclosed within the cell wall. It is composed mainly of nucleic acid.

Some bacteria have additional features:
(i) *Capsule.* Some bacteria (e.g. the *pneumococcus*) are enclosed within a thick capsule. The capsule is resistant to phagocytosis by phagocytic cells.
(ii) *Flagellum.* Some bacteria (e.g. the typhoid bacillus) have flagella attached to the outside. With rapid undulating movements these flagella move the bacterium along.
(iii) *Spore.* A spore is a rounded or oval structure with a thick coat into which some bacteria (e.g. the tetanus bacillus) can convert themselves when conditions are bad for them. In it they remain inactive and resistant to drying, heating and disinfectants. When conditions improve for them, they convert themselves back into their former active state.

GROWTH OF BACTERIA

For bacteria to multiply certain requirements have to be satisfied. If bacteria do not get them, they die or turn into spores.
Water. Bacteria die or go into a state of suspended animation if they become too dry.
Organic matter. Medically important bacteria require organic matter as a source of the energy they produce for their ordinary metabolic activities.
Inorganic salts. Traces of phosphate, sulphate, magnesium, calcium, iron, zinc, copper, cobalt and molybdenum are necessary for certain enzyme systems within the bacterium and for the control of osmosis.
Gases. Carbon dioxide is necessary for their metabolic activities. *Aerobic organisms* are organisms which grow only in the presence of oxygen (e.g. the bacillus of tuberculosis). *Anaerobic organisms* are organisms which grow only in the absence of oxygen (e.g. *Clostridia*). Many organisms will tolerate both the presence and absence of oxygen.
pH. Most medically important bacteria grow best in a neutral or slightly alkaline medium (pH 7.2-7.6).
Temperature. Medically important bacteria grow best at body temperature, about 37°C.

GRAM-POSITIVE COCCI

Staphylococcus

Staphylococci are Gram-positive cocci which grow in grape-like clusters.

Staphylococcus aureus (Staphylococcus pyogenes) gets its name from the yellow colour of its colonies (although sometimes white, depigmented colonies grow). It is normally present in the anterior nares and on the skin of many people, being especially common in the perineal region. On these sites it can live harmlessly, but in other parts it is very dangerous. It is the commonest cause of pyogenic (pus-producing) infections in man. The strains of *Staph. aureus* found in hospitals are likely to be penicillin-resistant, as they have become able to produce penicillinase, which destroys penicillin; and they may have become resistant to other drugs. As the cause of 'hospital' staphylococcal infection *Staph. aureus* is responsible for:

over half the cases of sepsis in surgical wounds; in maternity units: breast abscesses in mothers, and sticky eyes and skin lesions in babies; several hundred deaths a year in Britain from staphylococcal infections caught in hospitals. It also causes:

boils	carbuncles
pustules	infections of wounds and burns
pemphigus neonatorum	
styes	acute osteomyelitis
mastitis	perinephric abscess

staphylococcal pneumonia
staphylococcal food poisoning (a form of food poisoning in which the toxin produced by the organism is in the food at the time it is eaten); staphylococcal enteritis due to the administration of antibiotics (the antibiotics kill the micor-organisms normally present in the intestine, organisms which with the acid of the gastric juice normally keep down the number of staphylococci there.)

Dispersal of *Staph. aureus* into the air is common. Men are more likely to shed them than women, and the skin of the perineal region is the main source.

Microscopy

Staphylococci are Gram-positive and grow in grape-like clusters.

Culture

Cultures grow on solid media, such as nutrient agar, as golden or white, rounded, shiny colonies. The colonies will grow in concentrations of sodium chloride which inhibit the growth of other organisms, and in this way it is possible to grow staphylococci from specimens (e.g. faeces) in which there are normally large numbers of other organisms.

Coagulase production

This is a test to distinguish pathogenic staphylococci from non-pathogenic ones. Pathogenic staphylococci produce a clot when incubated with human plasma, due to the production by them of coagulase, an enzyme.

Biochemical test

This is a test to distinguish pathogenic staphylococci from non-pathogenic ones. Pathogenic staphylococci ferment mannitol, a carbohydrate; non-pathogenic ones do not.

Phage-typing

This is a method of identifying different strains of a bacterium by the phages which infect it. A phage is a virus which infects the bacterium and can destroy it. Phage-typing is used to distinguish different strains of *Staph. aureus.*, and is an important method of tracing the source of infection in hospital outbreaks.

Streptococcus

Streptococci are Gram-positive cocci which grow in chains.

Streptococcus pyogenes is present in the throat of 5-10 per cent of healthy people. It causes:
acute tonsillitis (streptococcal sore throat);
scarlet fever (which is an acute tonsillitis with a rash produced by the action on a sensitive person of a toxin produced by the streptococcus);
erysipelas;
some cases of impetigo (in association with *Staph. aureus*);
puerperal sepsis;
streptococcal cellulitis and septicaemia.

A streptococcal infection can be followed three weeks later by:
acute proliferative glomerulonephritis;
rheumatic fever.

Streptococci are not found in the inflamed tissues in these two conditions, and it is thought that they are the result of autoimmunization.

Streptococcus faecalis is a normal inhabitant of the intestine and is sometimes called an 'enterococcus'. It causes:
urinary tract infections;
wound infections (especially after intestinal operations);
infective endocarditis (subacute bacterial endocarditis).

Streptococcus viridans, which gets its name from a greenish zone around its colonies, is normally present in the throat and mouth. It can get into the blood during dental operations and extractions and when people with severe pyorrhoea bite hard. Any organisms that get into the blood of healthy people are quickly destroyed, but in people with congenital heart disease or with heart valves damaged by rheumatic fever they can cause:
infective endocarditis (subacute bacterial endocarditis).

Anaerobic streptococci are streptococci which will form colonies only in the absence of oxygen. They are found normally in the vagina, intestine and upper respiratory tract. They are non-haemolytic. They are responsible for some cases of:

puerperal sepsis	lung abscess
wound infection	appendix abscess

Microscopy

Streptococci are all Gram-positive and tend to grow in chains, especially in liquid media.

Culture

Strep. pyogenes: grows on blood agar. Colonies are greyish white and show characteristic beta haemolysis (see below), a zone of clear, colourless medium surrounding the colony.
Strep. faecalis: grows on MacConkey's medium, containing bile salts. It may be alpha, beta or non-haemolytic (see below).
Strep. viridans: grows on blood agar. Colonies are surrounded by a greenish zone (hence the name *viridans*) of alpha haemolysis (see below).

Haemolysis

Alpha haemolysis: red cells are partly destroyed and haemoglobin converted into a green pigment.
Beta haemolysis: red cells are lysed and haemoglobin is decolourized. Streptococci showing beta haemolysis are known as 'haemolytic streptococci'.
Gamma haemolysis: means non-haemolytic.

Serological test

Strep. pyogenes produces a powerful antigen known as streptolysin

0. In cases of rheumatic fever and acute proliferative glomerulonephritis a high titre of anti-streptolysin antibody confirms that a streptococcal infection is a recent one.

Lancefield grouping

Streptococci can be classified according to the presence of specific carbohydrates. Lancefield groups are labelled alphabetically:
Strep. pyogenes forms Group A carbohydrates
Strep. faecalis forms Group B carbohydrates
Strep. viridans does not form these carbohydrates.

Streptococcus Pheumoniae (commonly called Pneumococcus)

The *pneumococcus* is a Gram-positive coccus which grows in pairs or short chains. It is surrounded by a thick capsule which protects it from phagocytosis (destruction and absorption by phagocytic cells). It is present in the throat of many healthy people. It causes:
lobar pneumonia
some cases of bronchopneumonia
meningitis, in adults.

Culture

On blood agar the *pneumococcus* grows as a smooth glistening colony, often showing a ring of degeneration so that the colony has a hollow surrounded by an outer ring. It has a zone of alpha haemolysis around it similar to that of *Str. viridans*.

Biochemical tests

Certain biochemical tests are used to distinguish it from similar organisms (especially *Str. viridans*); it ferments inulin (a carbohydrate), is dissolved by bile and bile salts, and is killed by optochin (a copper compound).

GRAM-NEGATIVE COCCI

Neisseria Meningitidis (commonly called Meningococcus)

The *meningococcus* (*Neisseria meningitidis*) is oval or bean-shaped. The cocci live in pairs, side by side. About 5 per cent of healthy people carry meningococci in their throats. The percentage of carriers rises sharply in epidemics of meningococcal meningitis.
 It causes:
meningococcal meningitis.

Microscopy

The cocci are Gram-negative and grow in pairs.

Culture

Cultures are grown from nasopharyngeal swabs, blood, CSF, pus. Growths on blood agar or chocolate agar are encouraged by being grown in a chamber containing carbon dioxide.

Biochemical tests

Meningococci and *gonococci* resemble one another, and tests using the fermentation of carbohydrates are used to distinguish them. The *meningococcus* ferments glucose and maltose, producing acid from them. The *gonococcus* ferments glucose only, producing acid.

NEISSERIA GONORRHOEA
(commonly called GONOCOCCUS)

The *gonococcus (Neisseria gonorrhoea)* is oval or bean-shaped. The cocci live in pairs, side by side, and resemble meningococci.
 It causes:
gonorrhoea;
gonococcal conjunctivitis in infants born to infected mothers.
It quickly dies outside the body.

Microscopy

They are Gram-negative diplococci and are frequently seen within polymorphs.

Cultures

Cultures grow well on chocolate agar. *Stuart's medium* is used to transport swabs to the laboratory; gonococci can stay alive in it.

Biochemical tests

Tests of the fermentation of carbohydrates are used to distinguish them from meningococci. See MENINGOCOCCUS.

GRAM-POSITIVE BACILLI

B. Anthracis

B. anthracis is a large square-ended bacillus surrounded by a capsule. In unfavourable conditions it turns itself into a spore. It causes: anthrax.
 B. anthracis occurs in animals, especially cattle and sheep, which excrete it into the soil where it can as a spore remain for years, turning itself back into a bacillus and infecting other animals that graze on the same land. In Britain anthrax is a rare disease in man, but it is an occupational hazard of farmers, vets and handlers of hides, wool and hair. It occurs in two forms: (a) pulmonary anthrax (woolsorter's disease), a severe form of bronchopneumonia, acquired by inhaling infected dust; and (b) cutaneous anthrax (malignant pustule), acquired through the skin. Both forms are dangerous and can be followed by a fatal septicaemia.

Microscopy

The organisms are Gram-positive and being large, square-ended rods have a distinctive appearance.

Cultures

Cultures can be grown from pus or blood. They grow on ordinary media and the cultures look like hairs.

Clostridia

Clostridia are small, Gram-positive, anaerobic bacilli and bear spores. Some live normally in the intestine. All the pathogenic varieties produce exotoxins. They include:
Clostridium tetani
Clostridium perfringens
Clostridium botulinum

Clostridium Tetani

Cl. tetani causes:
tetanus.
 The spore grows at one end of the bacillus and gives it a drumstick appearance. It is present in the intestine of horses and other animals. It occurs commonly in land that has been manured, sometimes in the dust of hospitals, houses and streets, occasionally in surgical catgut (made from sheep intestine) and in

human faeces. It is liable to be the cause of infection in:
dirty, deep or extensive wounds in which anaerobic conditions exist;
septic abortion;
rarely, surgical wounds, when dressings, glove powder, etc., have not been adequately sterilized.

Infection can be prevented by immunization.

The clinical features of tetanus are due to a toxin produced by the organism. The toxin passes along motor nerve fibres to enter nerve-cells in the brain and spinal cord, where it increases the excitability of motor nerve-cells by interfering with the transmission at the synapses of nerves. The masseter muscles are especially affected, with the production of lock-jaw.

> It is often impossible to isolate this organism, and the diagnosis has usually to be made on clinical grounds.

Microscopy

It is a Gram-positive bacillus with a characteristic drum-stick appearance in the spore state.

Culture

It is cultured on blood agar and produces haemolysis. It is a motile organism and if inoculated onto the bottom of a slope of agar it swarms up the slope.

Biochemical test

It does not ferment any carbohydrate.

Toxin production

When injected into mice and guinea pigs a filtrate of the toxin produces paralysis and convulsions. The effects are neutralized by an injection of antitoxin.

Clostridium Perfringens

Cl. perfringens (Cl. Welchi) is a Gram-positive bacillus enclosed within a capsule. It is normally present in a human faeces. It causes.
gas gangrene
one kind of food poisoning.

(a) *Gas gangrene*. This infection is liable to occur in wounds where there is a lot of dead tissue and contamination by soil. The organisms multiply in dead tissues and produce a toxin which kills off cells and produces bubbles of gas. The infection is particularly likely to occur in:
severe injuries of soft tissues
compound fractures
septic abortion.

(b) *Food poisoning*. Food poisoning by this organism is due to the ingestion of large numbers of live organisms and not to the toxin. The organism is resistant to heat and can survive boiling, and is likely to be present in left-over, made-up, reheated meat dishes.

Gas gangrene type

Microscopy

It is a large non-motile capsulated bacillus. Its spores are oval, subterminal and do not bulge beyond the edge of the rod.

Culture

On blood agar alpha haemolysis occurs around grey colonies.

Biochemical test

Nagler reaction: on Nagler medium (human serum or egg yolk) a zone of opalescence appears around the colonies due to the action of a toxin produced by the organism. The reaction is inhibited by the specific antitoxin, and this provides another confirmation of the organism.

2. Food poisoning type

Culture

On blood agar the colonies are similar in appearance to the gas gangrene type, but there is no haemolysis.

Heat

The organisms are very heat-resistant and the spores can survive boiling.

Clostridium Botulinum

Cl. botulinum is a bacillus found in soil. It produces a toxin which when present in food produces a severe kind of food-poisoning. Botulism is rare in Britain. It can occur in home-preserved vegetables, but as the toxin is destroyed by boiling for ten minutes it does not occur in properly cooked food. The toxin is a neurotoxin which produces paralysis of the ocular, pharyngeal and laryngeal muscles and is frequently fatal.

Microscopy

The organism is motile. The spores are oval, subterminal and bulging.

Culture

Cultures grown in anaerobic conditions are large, grey and irregular. On blood agar haemolysis occurs around them.

Exotoxin identification

The toxin can be identified from food or intestinal contents.

Animal inoculation

Injected into a guinea pig the toxin produces difficult breathing, paralysis and death.

Corynebacterium Diphtheriae

C. diphtheriae is a Gram-positive, non-sporing, non-encapsulated bacillus. It causes: diphtheria.

Diphtheria begins as an acute inflammation of the upper respiratory tract, usually on the tonsils and fauces, sometimes in the nose, pharynx or larynx. The inflamed area ulcerates and the ulcerated area becomes covered with a thick, tenacious, white membrane formed of dead cells, fibrin, polymorphs and bacteria. The bacillus produces a powerful toxin which affects the heart, nerves, kidneys and adrenal glands. The disease can be prevented by immunization and is rare in countries where children are immunized against it.

Throat swab

The organism can be identified by film and culture.

Microscopy

The organisms are slightly curved and as they divide various shapes of V's and Z's appear, with the film as a whole looking like Chinese characters.

Culture

The organisms form dark, slate-grey colonies in about 48 hours on tellurite medium, a blood or chocolate agar with potassium tellurite, which inhibits the growth of most other bacteria.

Toxin production

Toxin production is demonstrated on an Elek plate treated with specific antitoxin, with white lines of toxin-antitoxin precipitate appearing.

MYCOBACTERIA

Mycobacteria are acid-fast, non-sporing and non-motile bacilli. The medically important mycobacteria are:
Myco. tuberculosis
Myco. leprae.

Mycobacterium Tuberculosis

Myco. tuberculosis (B. tuberculosis, Koch's bacillus) is a thin bacillus. It causes:
tuberculosis.

Two types of the bacillus cause disease in man:
human type
bovine type.

Both types look the same, but they grow differently on media and have different effects on some animals. They produce identical lesions in the tissues of the body.

A *tubercle* is the basic lesion. It consists of fibroblasts, lymphocytes, giant cells, modified histiocytes and a central area of necrosis. *Caseation* is the term given to the typical necrosis of tuberculosis with a cheesy, acellular material. *Satellite tubercles* are secondary tubercles which form around the primary tubercle. If the disease is progressing, the tubercles run together to form larger tuberculous masses, which caseate and form abscesses. If healing is taking place, fibrous tissue forms around the tuberculous masses, enclosing them in a fibrous capsule. With further healing the fibrous tissue can calcify.

The *human type* is spread by droplet infection or by the inhalation of infected dust. It causes:
pulmonary tuberculosis.

Spread to other tissues causes:
tuberculosis of bones and joints;
tuberculous meningitis;
tuberculosis of kidney, etc.

The *bovine type* is caused by drinking milk from infected cows. It has ceased to cause human disease in countries where tuberculosis in cows has been eradicated and milk is pasteurized. It causes:
tuberculosis of cervical lymph nodes;
tuberculosis of the small intestine, intestinal and abdominal lymph nodes;
tuberculous peritonitis.

It can spread to other tissues and cause:
tuberculosis of bone.

Microscopy

Films of pus, sputum, pleural fluid, etc. are examined for acid-fast bacilli. The organism stains with Ziehl-Neelsen stain and resists decolourization by acids and alcohol, i.e. it is acid- and alcohol-fast.

Culture

Cultures are made on Löwenstein-Jensen medium, which contains eggs, potato, starch, mineral salts and malachite green (the last inhibits the growth of other organisms). Cultures can take up to 8 weeks to grow.

Animal inoculation

If necessary, suspect material is injected into a guinea pig to see if the animal develops tuberculosis. Post-mortem examination of the animal is made 6-8 weeks after inoculation.

Mycobacterium Leprae

Myco. leprae is a Gram-positive bacillus and causes:
leprosy.

It is probably spread from man to man by infected nasal secretion, and prolonged contact with a case is necessary for infection to take place. The organism produces chronic inflammatory changes in the skin, mucous membranes and peripheral nerves, with the production in them of severe degenerative changes.

Microscopy

Smears, scrapings and biopsies from lesions in the skin and nasal mucous membrane are taken and examined. The organism is acid-fast, but less so that *Myco. tuberculosis.*

Culture

It will not grow on any known culture medium.

Animal inoculation

A localized infection occurs when injected into the footpads of armadillos, rats, mice and hamsters.

Actinomyces

Actinomyces is a Gram-positive bacillus which grows in long branching filaments and lives as a parasite on man and animals, especially horses and cattle. It is normally present in the mouths and tonsils of 5 per cent of people. It causes:
actinomycosis.

Actinomycosis is a chonic infection occurring in the jaws and surrounding tissues, ileocaecal region and lungs. The pus which forms contains 'sulphur granules' — yellow, gritty and formed of tangles of filaments, sometimes with patches of calcification in them.

Microscopy

'Sulphur granules' from pus are crushed between microscope slides and stained. Filaments in tangled masses are seen.

Culture

Cultures are grown from 'Sulphur granules' on blood agar under anaerobic conditions and appear in about a fortnight.

Chapter 3   Bacteria, Part 2: Gram-Negative Bacilli, Cocco-Bacilli, Vibrios, Spirochetes, Rickettsiae, Fungi

GRAM-NEGATIVE BACILLI

Intestinal Bacilli (Coliforms)

Several types of Gram-negative bacilli (coliforms) can occur in the intestine, some of which are non-pathogenic there and some pathogenic. They include:

Non-pathogenic in intestine (lactose fermenting)	Pathogenic in intestine (non-lactose fermenting)
E. coli	Salmonella
Klebsiella	Shigella
	Proteus
	Pseudomonas

Microscopy

These bacilli are straight rods with a similar appearance.

Culture

Lactose fermentation. The non-pathogenic bacilli ferment lactose, the pathogenic ones do not. MacConkey's agar is used to distinguish them; it contains lactose and neutral red, and on it bacteria which ferment lactose have red colonies and those which do not have colourless or pink colonies.

Escherichia Coli

E. Coli (B. coli) is a normal inhabitant of the intestine. It causes disease when it gets out of its normal habitat. It can cause:
urinary infections, of which it is the most frequent cause (80 per cent);
gastroenteritis in infancy;
meningitis in infancy;   wound infection;
peritonitis;   cholecystitis;
bacteraemic shock, by a rush of organisms into the blood from the urethra after catheterization or cystoscopy, or from an area of sepsis in the abdomen or pelvis.

The number of *E. coli* in water is used as a measure of faecal contamination.

Microscopy

Most strains of the organism have a capsule and flagella.

Culture

Red cultures on MacConkey's agar show that it ferments lactose and is non-pathogenic in the intestine.

Biochemical tests

(a) Indole positive: a rose pink colour occurs when *E. coli* is grown on peptone water to which Ehrlich's rosindole reagent is added. This test distinguishes *E. coli* from *Salmonella*.

(b) Fermentation of carbohydrates: *E. coli* produces acid and gas from glucose, mannite and sucrose.

Klebsiella

Klebsiella are a genus of non-motile, lactose-fermenting bacilli found in the intestine and sometimes in the upper respiratory tract.
Kl. pneumoniae (Friedländer's bacillus) can cause:
Friedländer's pneumonia, a rare and severe kind of pneumonia;
urinary tract infections;
wound infections.

Salmonella

There are several kinds of salmonellae of which the most important are:
Salm. typhi
Salm. paratyphi A and *B*
Salm. typhi is the cause of:
typhoid fever.

Typhoid fever is water- or food-borne and spread by faecal contamination from a patient or carrier.

The organisms infect the lymph tissue of the intestinal tract, whence they pass into the mesenteric lymph nodes and the blood stream. They produce inflammatory changes in the organs they infect. Inflammation of Peyer's patches of lymph tissue in the small intestine can be followed by ulceration of them, and haemorrhage and perforation into the peritoneal cavity. The gall-bladder is likely to become infected and can become a reservoir of organisms. Patients can become temporary or chronic carriers.

Salm. paratyphi A and *B* are the causes of a similar but milder infection:
paratyphoid fever.

Salmonella food poisoning is a gastro-enteritis produced by various kinds of salmonella, especially *Salm. typhimurium*, *Salm. newport*, *Salm. thompson* and *Salm. paratyphi B*. Diagnosis of the cause is made by isolating the organism from the faeces. The spread is by faecally-contaminated water or food.

Microscopy

The organisms are motile and do not have a capsule.

Culture

Cultures are taken in the 1st week from blood (80 per cent positive); in the 2nd and 3rd week from faeces; from the 3rd week onwards from urine. The organism is isolated on a special medium which suppresses the growth of most bacteria, but not *salmonellae* and *shigellae*, and then subcultured onto MacConkey's agar where it forms colourless colonies because it does not ferment lactose.

Biochemical tests

(a) *Indole negative* (see p. 6).
(b) (i) *S. typhi* fails to produce gas from glucose.
(ii) *S. paratyphi* produces acid and gas from glucose.

Widal reaction

This is an agglutination test for antibodies to the organism, and is performed by adding the serum from a patient to a suspension of the organisms. The reaction is negative in the 1st week and likely to be positive in the 2nd. A positive reaction can appear after an injection of TAB vaccine.

Differentiation

The various types of salmonellae are differentiated by analysis of the antigens they possess.

Shigella

Shigella is a genus of Gram-negative bacillus which causes:
bacillary dysentery.
There are four species of the organism:
1. *Sh. sonnei:* causes a mild dysentery and is responsible for 95 per cent of cases in Britain;
2. *Sh. flexneri:* causes a moderately severe dysentery; occurs mainly in tropical and subtropical countries; is responsible for about 5 per cent of cases in Britain, most of them in psychiatric hospitals;
3. *Sh. boydii:* causes a moderately severe dysentery; occurs mainly in tropical and subtropical countries;
4. *Sh. shiga:* causes a severe dysentery; occurs in the Far East.

Infection is by the mouth. Dysentery is spread by faecal contamination of food and drink, lavatories, door-handles, linen, etc., and by flies. Epidemics occur where people live in overcrowded, insanitary conditions or where there is much incontinence. Dysentery is an acute inflammation of the colon with, in severe cases, ulceration, sloughing and later fibrosis of the mucous membrane of the colon. A carrier state can occur, but it does not usually last for more than a few weeks.

Faeces

Fresh specimens are necessary. Rectal swabs are unsatisfactory as they tend to produce negative cultures from definitely infected patients; if a rectal swab is taken, it must be from the rectum and not the anal canal. In the detection of carriers specimens should be tested on 3 successive days in each of 3 successive weeks.

Microscopy

The organism is non-motile – the only coliform which is not motile.

Culture

The organisms do not ferment lactose except *Sh. sonnei*, which ferments it slowly. On MacConkey's agar colonies turn pink after more than 18 hours.

Biochemical tests

(a) It does not produce gas from carbohydrates.
(b) It does not split urea (see p. 6).

Proteus

Proteus is a normal inhabitant of the bowel which can cause infections of the urinary tract, respiratory tract and wounds.

Microscopy

The organism has flagella.

Culture

It is non-lactose fermenting. On blood agar it swarms over the plate and has a fishy smell. It can be killed by ether if it is wished to isolate other organisms (e.g. staphylococci) from faeces.

Biochemical tests

(a) It is non-lactose fermenting.
(b) It splits urea (see p. 6).

Pseudomonas

Pseudomonas is frequently found living in the intestine where it does no harm. *Pseudomonas aeruginosa (pyocyanea)* is a species found as a pathogenic organism in:

wounds and burns: pus then has a blue-green colour and characteristic smell;
otitis externa;
urinary tract infections;
meningitis.

It is expected to become the great danger in hospitals in the future because of:
its ability to live in a wide range of temperature;
its resistance to antibiotics;
its resistance to weak disinfectants;
its ability to contaminate sterile solutions, corks of bottles, eye drops, ointments, humidifiers of mechanical ventilators, and babies' incubators.

Microscopy

It is a motile, non-sporing, non-encapsulated Gram-negative bacillus, indistinguishable microscopically from other species.

Culture

On MacConkey's agar it is non-lactose fermenting and has a characteristic smell of rotten apples. *Ps. aeruginosa* produces green discoloration of the medium.

Biochemical test

It produces acid from glucose.

Haemophilus Influenzae

H. influenzae is a cocco-bacillus which normally inhabits the upper respiratory tract of most people. It was once thought to be the cause of influenza, but it is now known to be a secondary invader. It can cause:
secondary infection in influenza and bronchiectasis;
upper respiratory tract infections;
otitis media;
acute epiglottitis and tracheitis in infants;
acute bronchitis;
meningitis in young children.

Microscopy

It is a Gram-negative cocco-bacillus, showing various shapes from long bacilli to cocci.

Culture

It is a 'blood-loving' organism which needs blood if it is to be isolated, and is grown on chocolate agar. Colonies often appear as satellites of colonies of *Staph. aureus* because *Staph. aureus* produces one of the factors necessary for its growth.

Bordetella Pertussis

Bord. pertussis resembles *H. influenzae* in appearance but is not present in the pharynx in health. It causes:
whooping cough.

Some viruses can cause a clinically indistinguishable disease.

Droplets

Cultures are made on a plate of an appropriate medium on to which the child has coughed. The colonies resemble drops or streaks of aluminium paint.

Brucella

Brucella are cocco-bacilli which cause brucellosis, an infection of animals transmissible to man. There are three types.
1. *Br. abortus:* an infection of cows; is responsible for most cases of human brucellosis in Britain, where it causes:
abortus fever (undulant fever).

2. *Br. melitensis:* an infection of goats in Mediterranean countries. It causes:
Malta fever.
3. *Br. suis:* an infection of pigs in Denmark and North and South America.

In all types infection is by milk or through abrasions in the skin of people handling infected animals. The organisms invade cells of the reticulo-endothelial system, producing inflammatory changes and an intermittently raised temperature.

Culture

Cultures are made from blood, bone marrow, lymph nodes and urine. Culture is made in an atmosphere of carbon dioxide 10 per cent as this is necessary for the growth of *Br. abortus*.

Agglutination tests

Agglutination tests are carried out on the patient's serum.

Microscopy

Organisms are found in fluid from buboes and in the sputum in pneumonic plague. They are short, oval and have a capsule. With methylene blue they stain more deeply at the ends than in the centre, and this gives them a distinctive appearance.

Culture

The organism grows best at about 27°C on ordinary media and on MacConkey's agar. Cultures can be made of the blood in septicaemic plague.

Pasteurella Pestis

P. pestis is a small Gram-negative bacillus and causes:
plague.

The organism is carried by rats and other rodents. Man is infected by the bites of fleas which have become infected by biting infected rats.

Plague is a severe disease with a high mortality. It occurs in sporadic and epidemic forms. Epidemics start in those parts of the world where rodents are most likely to be infected — India, other parts of Asia, parts of Africa and America. It occurs in three forms: *bubonic plague,* in which lymph nodes are enlarged and matted into masses called buboes; *pneumonic plague,* in which there is a severe and usually fatal haemorrhagic pneumonia; and *septicaemic plague,* in which there is a general blood-borne infection of the body.

VIBRIOS

Vibrios are comma-shaped organisms.

Vibrio Cholerae

V. cholerae and the closely-related *El Tor vibrio* cause:
cholera.

The organism is a curved, comma-shaped rod with a single long flagellum which enables it to move.

Cholera is an acute inflammation of the intestine, which produces severe diarrhoea, 'rice-water stools', dehydration, collapse and often death. It is spread by faecally contaminated water, food and flies. It is endemic in parts of India, Pakistan, Bangladesh and the Far East, and epidemics occur. It has spread to the Phillipines, the Middle East, Africa, USSR, Turkey and Spain.

The organism may be excreted in the faeces for a few days before and after an attack as well as being excreted in large numbers during it.

Chapter 3

> **Faeces**
>
> Films are made and the organism can be seen microscopically and then identified by cultural and biochemical reactions.

SPIROCHETES

Spirochetes are corkscrew-shaped organisms.

Treponema Pallidum

Tr. pallidum is a thin, spiral organism which moves slowly with corkscrew movements, often bending on itself or compressing or expanding its loops. It is unusual in that it probably reproduces by dividing by transverse fission instead of the usual longitudinal. It is rapidly destroyed by drying, heat and antiseptics. Washing with soap and water destroys all spirochetes which have contaminated the hands. It causes: syphilis.

Transmission is nearly always by sexual intercourse. It soon dies when not on the human body and is not often transmitted by contaminated articles. Congenital syphilis can be acquired *in utero* from a mother with syphilis in an active form.

Syphilis occurs in three stages.

Stage 1. After an incubation period of 10-90 days a primary chancre appears at the site of infection. The tissue reaction is a chronic inflammatory one, with invasion by plasma cells and inflammatory changes in the walls of the small blood-vessels. The chancre appears as a hard papule which goes on to ulceration, the fluid from the ulcer containing many spirochetes and being very infectious. Lymph nodes draining the part become inflamed. A general invasion of the body via the blood probably occurs shortly after infection.

Stage 2. This occurs a few weeks later or overlaps with the primary stage. It is an expression of the reaction of many tissues to the infection and is characterized by a rash, lesions of mucous membranes, enlarged lymph nodes, etc.

Stage 3. This occurs about 5-15 years after the primary infection. Among the conditions which can occur are: a *gumma,* a chronic inflammatory mass occurring in skin, bone, brain and cardio-vascular system; *meningo-vascular syphilis; general paralysis of the insane; tabes dorsalis; aneurysm of the aorta.*

> **Microscopy**
>
> *Dark-field microscopy* of fluid from a chancre is necessary because the organism is too thin to be visible with ordinary staining methods.
>
> **Serological reactions**
>
> Several tests are used to detect changes in the blood and CSF produced by infection. These tests depend upon antibody formation.
>
> (a) *Wassermann reaction (WR).* This reaction depends upon the similarity between a lipid present in *Tr. pallidum* and a lipid normally present in the tissues.
>
> WR is positive in the blood in:
> (i) primary syphilis 2-4 weeks after the appearance of the chancre;
> (ii) almost all cases of secondary syphilis;
> (iii) 80-90 per cent of cases of tertiary syphilis.
>
> WR is also positive in yaws, a tropical disease caused by a spirochete. Persistent false reactions can occur in systemic lupus erythematosus and other auto-immune diseases. Temporary false reactions can occur in the acute stages of some infections — infective hepatitis, malaria, glandular fever, leprosy, after smallpox vaccination and during pregnancy.

(b) *Kahn test:* a flocculation test positive in syphilis.
(c) *VDRL test* (Venereal Disease Research Laboratory test): is similar to the Kahn test.
(d) *TPI test* (Treponemal Immobilization test): uses the patient's serum and a suspension of the treponemes. If the patient has syphilis, an antibody in the serum causes the treponemes to become immobilized and then die.
(e) *FTA test* (Fluorescent Treponemal Antibody test): is a test similar to TPI and is sensitive in all stages of syphilis.

Borrelia Vincenti

Borr. vincenti is a large thick spirochete which is present with a bacillus called *Fusiformis fusiformis* in the gum margins of most people. Together they can cause:
Vincent's angina.

Vincent's angina is an acute ulcerative condition of the mouth and throat, which can go on to form gangrenous lesions of the skin and gangrene of the lung.

Swab from gums or throat

Microscopy: large numbers of both organisms can be seen on a slide stained with carbol fuchsin.

Leptospira Icterohaemorrhagiae

L. icterohaemorrhagiae is a spirochete with a tightly wound spiral. It is a parasite of rats and some dogs, from which it can be transmitted to man to cause:
Weil's disease.

This is an acute and severe disease with fever, haemorrhages, jaundice, etc. Infection takes place through the skin, mucous membranes of the mouth and nose, and the conjunctiva. The disease is an occupational hazard of sewer-workers, miners and farmers, and can be acquired by bathing in water contaminated by rats.

Dark-field microscopy

The organism can be recognized in the blood during the first week and in the urine during the second.

Serological tests

Tests for antibodies are performed with suspensions of the spirochete. Antibodies appear towards the end of the second week.

Culture

Cultures are made on special media.

Animal inoculation

Intraperitoneal inoculation of a guinea pig is performed with urine. The animal dies within 14 days and the organism is found in peritoneal fluid, blood, liver and spleen.

Rickettsiae

Rickettsiae are organisms biologically intermediate between bacteria and viruses. Like bacteria they contain both DNA and RNA, are visible with a light microscope, and reproduce by dividing down the middle. Like viruses they can live only within cells and cannot be grown on laboratory media. They have no cell wall.

Rickettsiae are the cause of:
epidemic typhus   scrub typhus
Rocky mountain spotted fever   Q fever.

Epidemic typhus is a purely human disease transmitted from person to person by the human body louse, a person becoming infected by a bite of by scratching a bite. It is a severe illness with fever, a rash and cerebral disturbance. Epidemics are liable to occur during wars and when people are living in overcrowded filthy conditions.

Rocky Mountain spotted fever is a severe infection spread by the bites of ticks, which transmit the infection from rats and other animals to man. A tick is a blood-sucking insect belonging to two families of the order of *Acarina*.

Q fever (the Q stands for 'Query?') is primarily a disease of sheep, cows and goats, being transmitted among them by ticks. Man is infected by inhaling infected dust or drinking infected milk. The organism produces an influenza-like illness with pneumonic consolidation.

Microscopy

The organisms are cocco-bacilli which stain poorly and are Gram-negative.

Culture

The organism is cultured on chorio-allantoic membrane or in the yolk sac of chick embryos.

Inoculation of animal

The isolation of rickettsiae from patients can be achieved by inoculating blood into the peritoneum of animals, but the procedure is dangerous to the operator and serological methods are used for diagnosis.

Serological methods

(a) *Weil-Felix test*. Certain strains of *Proteus* share carbohydrate antigens with *Rickettsiae*, and therefore the serum of a patient with typhus fever will agglutinate certain proteus suspensions in an antigen-antibody reaction. With the use of different proteus suspensions the method distinguishes between various rickettsiae infections, especially between epidemic typhus, Rocky Mountain Spotted Fever and scrub typhus.

(b) *Agglutination and complement fixation tests*. More precise diagnosis can be made using rickettsiae antigens obtained by growing the organism in the yolk sac of a chick embryo.

FUNGI

Fungi are members of a large group of organisms which includes the rusts, yeasts and moulds. They are usually larger than bacteria and can be multicellular or unicellular and have long filaments called hyphae. They reproduce asexually or sexually with the formation of spores. A few cause disease in man.

CANDIDA ALBICANS

This fungus is often present in the upper respiratory tract, vagina and intestine, and on the skin. It causes:
thrush   vaginitis
intertrigo in the skin folds of obese women
paronychia in people with hands in water a lot.

Antibiotic treatment for other diseases can cause a proliferation of *Candida* due to disturbance of the normal flora.

Swabs or skin scrapings

Microscopy

Large oval Gram-positive cells are seen.

> **Culture**
>
> Cultures can be grown on blood agar, with a visible growth overnight, or on Sabouraud's medium on which the growth of bacteria is inhibited and moist creamy colonies of *Candida* appear.

RINGWORM DERMATOPHYTES

These fungi by infecting the keratinized layer of the skin, hair and nails cause:
tinea pedis (athlete's foot);
ringworm of the scalp;
tinea cruris and other ringworm infections of the skin.

> **Scrapings, etc.**
>
> Scrapings are taken from the skin lesions with a blunt scalpel. Infected hairs are extracted from their hair follicles. Full thickness clippings are taken from infected nails.
>
> **Microscopy**
>
> Specimens are placed in a drop of potassium hydroxide on a slide. Hyphae are seen and sometimes spores.
>
> **Cultures**
>
> Cultures are made on Sabouraud's medium at room temperature. Colonies take 1-3 weeks to grow. Different species are identified by different appearances of cultures, rates of growth and microscopic appearances.

Chapter 4   Viruses

Viruses are small infective agents. The smallest of them consists of little more than nucleic acid contained within a coat of protein and can be converted into a crystalline state. Large viruses are more sophisticated. Viruses differ from bacteria in being:
  (a) much smaller
  (b) capable of division only within a living cell.
  Medically important viruses are usually cubical, helical or complex.
  The capsid or outer protein coat of a virus is probably used to attach the virus to the wall of the cell it is about to invade. Once the virus is attached, the nucleic acid inside it passes into the cell. Inside the cell the virus converts itself into sub-units, which can join together to form new viruses. Some cells are invaded at the same time by similar but different viruses, whose sub-units can combine to form a virus which has components of the two original viruses.
  The effects of the invasion are:
  (a) the host cell may be killed, the viruses in it being discharged to attack other cells
  (b) the host cells may be caused to fuse together to form giant cells or sheets of cells
  (c) some viruses have the ability to convert normal cells into malignant cells and so start a malignant growth
  (d) inclusion bodies may be formed: these are round, oval or irregular structures found in invaded cells; they may be clumps formed by particles of viruses or areas of degeneration
  (e) viruses may remain latent in cells for a long time, sometimes for years, and break out later into activity.

MUTATIONS

Viruses frequently develop mutations, i.e. they alter their biological properties a little and turn up in a slightly different form.

CLASSIFICATION OF VIRUSES

Viruses are difficult to classify. The main medical groups are:

1. *Poxviruses*	Smallpox virus, vaccinia virus, molluscum contagiosum virus
2. *Herpesviruses*	Chickenpox and herpes zoster virus, herpes simplex virus, cytomegalovirus
3. *Adenoviruses*	Viruses which cause respiratory tract infections and conjunctivitis
4. *Papovavirus*	Human wart virus
5. *Picornaviruses*	Poliovirus, Coxsackie viruses, ECHO viruses, rhinoviruses
6. *Reoviruses*	Viruses which cause respiratory tract infections
7. *Myxoviruses*	Mumps virus, influenza virus
8. *Arboviruses*	Yellow fever virus, several viruses which cause encephalitis
9. *Miscellaneous*	Measles virus, German measles (rubella) virus, hepatic viruses, rabies virus

CHEMICAL CLASSIFICATION

Viruses can be classified according to their chemical composition. They all contain protein and nucleic acid. In some viruses the nucleic acid is DNA (deoxyribonucleic acid) and in others it is RNA (ribonucleic acid). Medically important viruses are either DNA or RNA viruses.

DNA viruses	RNA viruses
poxviruses	picornaviruses
herpesviruses	reoviruses
adenoviruses	myxoviruses
papovaviruses	arboviruses
	rabies virus
	measles virus
	German measles (rubella) virus

POXVIRUSES

Smallpox Virus

The smallpox virus is a brick-shaped virus with rounded corners and is just large enough to be seen with a light microscope. It causes:
smallpox (variola major);
alastrim (variola minor), a mild form of smallpox.

Smallpox virus infects man only. It is spread mainly by droplet infection from the mouth and respiratory tract of a patient, but as the virus resists drying it can be spread by dust from infected clothing, bedclothing, floors, etc., also in later stages of the illness from desquamated skin. Patients do not become carriers.

VACCINIA VIRUS

Vaccinia virus is the one used to vaccinate people against smallpox. It is probably a hybrid of smallpox and cowpox.

Microscopy

Vesicular fluid (i.e. fluid from a vesicle on the skin): by electron microscopy a poxvirus can be seen to be present, but which one it is cannot be determined.

Culture

Material is inoculated into the chorio-allantoic membrane of a chick embryo. Spherical pocks appear, which distinguish smallpox from cowpox and vaccinia.

Gel diffusion test

The presence of pox antigen in material from skin lesions can be detected in 3 hours by a gel diffusion test (see p. 6), using known pox antiserum.

Molluscum Contagiosum Virus

This virus causes molluscum contagiosum, a disease of the skin characterized by multiple nodules in the epidermis.

HERPESVIRUSES

Chickenpox and Herpes Zoster Virus

The same herpesvirus causes:
chickenpox
herpes zoster

Chickenpox occurs in childhood as an acute infection. After an attack the virus can remain dormant in cells for many years without showing any signs of its presence. Herpes zoster is caused by a reactivation of the virus as the body's immunity to it becomes reduced. The virus attacks the sensory ganglia of the cranial nerves (most commonly that of the trigeminal nerve) or of the posterior roots of the spinal nerves, causing severe pain and a rash in the area of skin supplied by the nerve. Why it should attack cells in these ganglia is not known.

> **Electron microscopy**
>
> The virus looks like the virus of herpes simplex, but different from that of smallpox.
>
> **Culture**
>
> The virus does not grow in eggs, which distinguishes it from poxviruses. It grows in human tissue culture.

Herpes Simplex Virus

This is a common virus acquired by most people. It causes:
primary herpes
recurrent herpes

Primary herpes is an infection of the first few years of life, and causes vesicles in the mucous membrane of the mouth, the eye and the skin. Infection is usually spread by kissing. A generalized infection and encephalitis can occur. People who develop the illness remain carriers of the virus for life and are liable to have recurrent attacks of herpes on the face (cold sores), on the eyes and on the mucous membrane of the genitalia.

> **Microscopy**
>
> Vesicular fluid is examined with an electron microscope, but the virus cannot be distinguished in this way from that of chickenpox and herpes zoster.
>
> **Culture**
>
> The virus grows on the chorio-allantoic membrane of a fertile egg. This distinguishes it from the virus of chickenpox and herpes zoster, which will not grow on it.

Cytomegalovirus

Cytomegalovirus (CMV) produces in adults a mild primary infection, but — as with other viruses of the same group — the virus can remain latent in the tissues for years. About one per cent of pregnant women in Britain develop a primary infection during the pregnancy and many more have a reactivation of a latent infection. Pregnant women with the infection can excrete the virus in urine and secretions from the cervix uteri and later in the milk. A baby can be infected *in utero* if the mother develops a primary infection during the pregnancy, and about half the babies at risk are infected, especially if the infection occurs during the first six months of pregnancy. About 5-15 per cent of infected babies develop infection of the central nervous system. The disease can occur as a congenital cytomegalic inclusion disease, characterized by enlargement of the liver and spleen, jaundice, petechial haemorrhages and thrombocytopenia; or as a chronic condition in young children, producing microcephaly, mental retardation and intracerebral calcification.

> **Microscopy**
>
> The virus can be isolated from throat swabs, urine, cervical secretions.
>
> **Inclusion bodies**
>
> (See p. 7) can be seen in the nucleus in cells from a urinary deposit (hence cytomegalic *inclusion* disease).

ADENOVIRUSES

Adenoviruses get their name from being first identified in adenoids and tonsils removed surgically. They are a common infection of man: They cause:
acute inflammation of the upper respiratory tract;

conjunctivitis, kerato-conjunctivitis;
virus pneumonia;
an infection clinically indistinguishable from whooping cough;

Epidemics can occur, especially where children and adolescents are living closely together in schools, camps and training establishments. An adenovirus pneumonia can be fatal in an infant.

Isolation

The virus can be isolated from throat, conjunctiva, and faeces.

Culture

The virus grows in HeLa cells (see p. 7) and produces cytopathic effect (see p. 7).

PAPOVAVIRUSES

Papovaviruses get their name from their three main types: *pa*pilloma virus, *po*lyoma virus, *va*cuolating virus.

In man they cause:
warts.

Warts are infectious, benign tumours of epithelial tissue.

PICORNAVIRUSES

Picornaviruses get their name from: pico = small, and RNA.

Poliovirus

Poliovirus causes:
poliomyelitis.

The clinical features of poliovirus infection can be:

(a) no clinical features at all: probably the most common result of infection;
(b) a mild febrile illness;
(c) meningitis;
(d) a paralytic disease: the least common result, and due to destruction of the cells of motor nerves.

Isolation

The virus is found in faeces and throat swabs.

Culture

The virus is inoculated into tissue culture — monkey tissue and HeLa cells (see p. 7). A cytopathic effect is seen (see p. 7).

Serological test

Complement fixation test demonstrates the presence of antibodies (see p. 6).

Coxsackie Viruses

These viruses get their name from the town of Coxsackie, USA, where the first cases were identified. They are sometimes found in the throat and faeces of healthy people. They are divided into two groups, A and B. They cause:

Group A
herpangina, an acute pharyngitis with vesicles;
aseptic meningitis;   respiratory infections
a paralytic disease resembling poliomyelitis;
rashes with fever.

Group B
epidemic myalgia (Bornholm disease);
rashes with fever;   aseptic meningitis;
myocarditis;   pericarditis;
some cases of pancreatitis

Isolation

The virus can be isolated from faeces and throat swabs.

Culture

Group B virus grows in monkey kidney and HeLa cells (see p. 7) and produces a cytopathic effect (see p. 7). Group A virus: only one strain will grow in tissue culture.

Animal inoculation

In mice Group A causes a flaccid paralysis, Group B a spastic paralysis.

Serological tests

Neutralization tests (p. 6) demonstrate a rise in antibody titre in the patient's serum and so identify the virus.

Echoviruses

These viruses get their name from *e*nteric, *cy*topathogenic, *h*uman, *o*rphan, being called orphans because at first they could not be related to any known disease. They are now known to cause:
mild gastro-enteritis;
maculopapular rashes;
mild upper respiratory tract infections;
meningitis.

Isolation

The virus is isolated from faeces and the pharynx, and in meningitis from CSF.

Culture

The virus produces cytopathic effects (see p. 7) in monkey kidney.

Serological tests

Antibodies are detached by neutralization and complement fixation tests (p. 6, 7,).

Rhinovirus

Rhinovirus causes the common cold. Many types of it exist and antibodies against one do not confer immunity to another. Repeated infection therefore occurs.

Tissue culture

Rhinovirus grows and produces a cytopathic effect (see p. 7) in tissue culture.

REOVIRUSES

Reoviruses get their name from *r*espiratory, *e*nteric, *o*rphan. They cause:
upper respiratory tract infections;
febrile diarrhoea.

Culture

The virus grows on monkey kidney.

Serological test

Haemagglutination inhibition (see p. 7) is used to identify the strain of the virus.

MYXOVIRUSES

Influenza Virus

Influenza viruses are small spherical particles. They cause:

influenza;
influenzal pneumonia.

Epidemics occur, usually in the winter. Pandemics (affecting the whole world) have occurred. There are three types of the virus:
Type A: causes epidemics about every two years;
Type B: causes smaller epidemics about every three to six years;
Type C: a common infection; not known to cause epidemics.

New variants of established types arise and cause new epidemics against which people have little immunity.

The virus is spread by droplet infection from infected nasopharyngeal secretions.

Cultures

Cultures are made from throat swabs. Inoculation is made on to tissue culture or the amniotic sac of chick embryos. The virus causes haemadsorption (see p. 7) on monkey kidney.

Serological test

The virus can be identified by haemagglutination-inhibition and complement fixation tests (see p. 6, 7,).

Mumps Virus

Mumps virus resembles influenza virus. It causes:
mumps.

Mumps is primarily an infection of the salivary glands, especially the parotid glands. Orchitis, oophoritis, mastitis, meningitis and meningo-encephalitis can occur.

Tests

Swabs are taken from the openings of the parotid ducts into the mouth.

Isolation

Inoculation is made into the amniotic sac of fertile hens' eggs, and the amniotic fluid is tested for haemagglutination.

Culture

Cytopathic effect (see p. 7) is seen in HeLa cell culture and human amnion.

Serological tests

Haemagglutination inhibition and complement fixation tests are used (see p. 6, 7).

ARBOVIRUSES

Arboviruses get their name from *ar*thropod-*borne*, i.e. spread by arthropods (mosquitoes, ticks, sandflies). They cause:
yellow fever;
several kinds of encephalitis.

Yellow fever occurs in the tropics and gets its name from the jaundice that is one of the signs of it. The virus is a parasite of monkeys and is transferred to man by the bite of mosquitoes.

Tests

Samples of blood are taken in the early stages of the disease.

Culture

Many arboviruses grow on tissue culture and in chick embryos.

Serological tests

Haemagglutination-inhibition, complement fixation and neutralization tests (see p. 6, 7,) are performed.

Inoculation

Encephalitis is produced by inoculation into suckling mice and is prevented by specific yellow fever antiserum.

MISCELLANEOUS VIRUSES

Measles Virus

Measles virus causes:
measles;
subacute sclerosing encephalitis.

Measles is very infectious and affects almost all children. It is spread by droplet infection. Subacute sclerosing encephalitis is an uncommon disease which occurs several years after an attack of measles, producing degenerative changes in the brain. The virus can be isolated from brain tissue which it is thought to have entered during the original attack of measles. A connection has been suggested between the measles virus and multiple (disseminated) sclerosis, a chronic degenerative disease of the brain and spinal cord.

Isolation

The virus is isolated from blood and secretions of the upper respiratory tract.

Culture

On inoculation into monkey kidney, HeLa cells and human amnion, giant cells, syncitia and inclusion bodies are seen.

Serological tests

Haemagglutination-inhibition and complement fixation tests are carried out (see p. 6, 7,).

German Measles (Rubella) Virus

German measles virus causes:
German measles (rubella);
abortion or congenital deformities in about 10 per cent of the children of mothers who develop German measles during the early months of pregnancy.

The disease is spread by droplet infection and the patient is infectious from about nine days before the appearance of the rash. The virus can be isolated from the tissues of an aborted fetus, from a child with congenital abnormalities produced by it, and from an apparently healthy child whose mother has had German measles late in pregnancy.

Isolation

The virus can be isolated from the throat.

Tissue culture

The virus can be detected by adding it to Echovirus in tissue culture for it interferes with the cytopathic effect produced by the Echovirus. The virus can be identified by the inhibition of this interfering effect by specific antiserum.

Serological tests

Antibodies to rubella can be detected by haemagglutination inhibition and complement fixation tests (see p. 6, 7). By testing antibody titres at appropriate times, past infection can be distinguished from an active or recent infection, an important distinction in early pregnancy.

Rabies Virus

Rabies virus infects dogs, monkeys, foxes, wolves and other warm-blooded animals. The main cause of infection in man is a bite from a dog. Dogs are not infectious unless they have the clinical disease as the virus must be present in sufficient numbers in the saliva. From a bite the virus passes to the central nervous system mainly along sensory nerves. The incubation period is 3-12 weeks. Clinical features are pain at the site of the bite, restlessness, pharyngeal spasms which cause difficulty in swallowing, and fits. The disease is usually fatal. It has been eradicated from the British Isles and is kept out by strict quarantine of imported animals, but it is spreading across France towards the Channel, being spread mainly by foxes.

Diagnosis

1. In life the virus can be isolated from the saliva of infected animals.
2. After death Negri bodies, which are characteristic inclusion bodies, are found in nerve cells in the brain.

Hepatic Viruses

The hepatic viruses have not yet been completely identified and theories about them are speculative. They are thought to cause:
infective hepatitis;
serum hepatitis.

In both these conditions the patients have the same symptoms: loss of appetite, nausea, vomiting, fever; some become jaundiced. Pathological changes in the liver are identical in them. The liver cells show degenerative changes, with an increase in the number of cells surrounding the small portal vessels. Liver function tests show evidence of liver damage.

There appear to be two different viruses, virus A and virus B.

Virus A is thought to cause:
infective hepatitis.

Infective hepatitis is an acute infection, endemic in most countries. Small epidemics can occur. Infection is usually by faecal contamination of food or water. The incubation period is 15-40 days. During an attack the virus is present in blood and faeces; some patients may be carriers of it for months.

Virus B is thought to cause:
serum hepatitis;
polyarteritis nodosa (possibly).

Serum hepatitis is spread mostly by transfusion or injection of human blood, plasma, serum or blood-products such as anti-haemophilic globulin, and to a lesser degree by faecal contamination of food or water. The commonest source is a needle or syringe in which there is a trace of contaminated blood, and much infection can be prevented by the use and subsequent destruction of disposable syringes and needles. Drug-addicts who swap syringes and needles frequently infect themselves. Infection can be spread by blood transfusion, especially when blood-donors are not tested. In some cases sexual or domestic contact appears to be the cause of infection.

The incubation period is longer than that of infective hepatitis, being 40-150 days. 5-10 per cent of infected persons become carriers.

Virus hepatitis is a grave risk to staff and patients in a haemodialysis unit (artificial kidney unit).

AUSTRALIA ANTIGEN

Australia antigen or hepatitis B surface antigen (Hbs Ag) is an antigen present in the blood of people who have had serum hepatitis and indicates that they are potential carriers of virus B. It gets its name because it was first identified in Australia. The antigen is identified by immunological tests. It is commonly found in association with liver disease and is a possible cause of hepatitis, acute and chronic. There is a high incidence of it in mongolism and professional blood-donors. The incidence of symptomless carriers is higher in many tropical countries than in northern Europe, North America and the Antipodes.

The carrier of HB Ag is not thought to be much of a risk in ordinary life, but he becomes dangerous if his skin is pricked and his blood shed. This is most likely to happen in medical and surgical procedures, but it can occur in ear-piercing, tattooing, acupuncture and self-injection.

People who are HB Ag carriers should be identified and special precautions should be taken when they are in hospital. People to be regarded with suspicion are:

(a) patients with acute or chronic liver disease, mongolism (Down's syndrome) and polyarteritis nodosa;

(b) patients from a high-risk country;

(c) patients who have had a blood transfusion within the preceding six months because they might have had an untested transfusion;

(d) people repeatedly offering blood;

(e) pregnant women because of the loss of blood at childbirth and the danger of infecting baby and staff;

(f) drug addicts, tattooed persons, male homosexuals, sexually promiscuous people.

Precautions with HB Ag patient

1. Blood, urine and faeces are regarded as highly infectious.

2. Laboratory tests are reduced to a minimum and blood taken only when absolutely necessary.

3. In taking blood staff should wear protective clothing and gloves. A plastic sheet is placed under the patient's arm.

4. Blood is transferred gently into the container. Care is taken to avoid droplet and aerosol formation and not to contaminate the rim and the outside of the container.

5. The container must be perfect and have a screw-cap. It is placed in an individual plastic bag. The bag is heat-sealed and marked with a self-adhesive label, which is not licked. The bag is not stapled. The laboratory request form is not put in the bag.

6. The label of a known case is marked: HIGH RISK SPECIMEN. AUSTRALIA ANTIGEN POSITIVE.

7. Any spilt blood is diluted at once with strong hydrochlorite solution and then wiped up.

8. Needles and syringes are placed in a rigid container and sent for destruction.

9. Porters and drivers are warned to take special care of the specimen.

Chapter 5 Parasites

Fleas

Fleas are small wingless insects, flattened from side to side, with long legs for leaping and mouths adapted for piercing the skin and sucking blood. Different kinds of flea prefer to live on particular kinds of animal, but in some circumstances will migrate to another type, e.g. from rat to man. They live by sucking blood, but can survive for months without feeding. They drop their eggs anywhere. The eggs hatch in larvae in 3-4 days. Larvae can, like the adult flea, lie dormant for long periods.

The medically important fleas are:

(a) *Pulex irritans.* This is the common human flea. It will also live on rodents, dogs and cats. The bites appear as small, irritating spots.

(b) *Xenopsylla cheopsis.* This flea lives on rats. It is the transmitter of *Pasteurella pestis,* the plague bacillus. When an infected flea transfers from rat to man it infects man by biting and causes him to develop bubonic plague.

(c) *Tungida penetrans.* This is the jigger flea, an inhabitant of tropical countries. It produces chigos by the burrowing of the female into the skin and secondary infection of the burrows.

Lice

Lice are small flat wingless insects with legs adapted for grasping hairs. They live on the body for 4-6 weeks, taking two meals of blood a day. Their bite causes a small haemorrhagic irritating spot. The female lays up to 6 eggs a day. The eggs are called nits and are adherent to hairs. There are 3 types which infest human beings.

Pediculus humanus corporis (body louse) lives in the hair of the body, avoids light and will transfer itself to clothing where it will survive, in cold conditions, up to a week. By its bite it is the transmitter of:
louse-borne typhus fever;
louse-borne relapsing fever, caused by *Borrelia recurrentis,* a spirochete.

Pediculus humanus capitis (head louse) is smaller, lives on the hair of the scalp, and avoids light. It does not usually transmit any disease.

Phthirus pubis (crab louse) is broader and flatter than the other lice, lives in the hair of the public region, and can spread from person to person at sexual intercourse. It does not usually transmit any disease.

Scabies Mite

Sarcoptes scabei (scabies mite) lives on the skin. The male and female come together at the orifice of a hair follicle. The male dies after impregnating the female. The female is oval and about 0.4 mm long, just large enough to be seen with the naked eye. She has two pairs of legs with suckers in front and two pairs of legs with trailing bristles behind. When she has become pregnant, she burrows into the horny layer of the skin, lays up to 30 eggs in her burrow, and then dies. The burrow is visible as a thin, slightly raised, slightly wavy line, with the mite visible at the end as a dark spot. The eggs hatch into larvae and the larvae become adult mites. The complete life cycle lasts about 10 days. The burrows itch intensely and affected parts are likely to be scratched and may become secondarily infected.

The common sites for burrows are:
inner aspect of wrists
clefts between fingers
inner aspect of hands
soles of feet
male external genitalia.

Trichomonas Vaginalis

Trichomonas vaginalis is an oval or pear-shaped organism, which varies in size from that of a leucocyte to about two and a half times that size. It has a nucleus near its anterior end. The axostyle is a long tapering structure which arises in the nucleus, passes through the organism, and sticks out from the posterior end. Four thin, long flagellae project out of the anterior end and by their movements give the organism a typical jerky movement. An undulating membrane attached to one side is in a state of constant undulating movement.

Trichomoniasis is a sexually-transmitted infection with an incubation period of 1-3 weeks. Other possible methods of spread are by imperfectly sterilized gynaecological instruments, rubber gloves or douche nozzles, by wearing borrowed unwashed clothing, and from recent secretions on lavatory seats and by splashing from recently infested lavatories.

Trichomoniasis in women occurs as:

(a) *Vaginitis:* the vagina is inflamed and reddened; and a thin, yellow offensive discharge is present and may inflame the upper thighs. There is sometimes no discharge.

(b) *Skenitis and bartholinitis:* an inflammation, which may go on to abscess formation, of Skene's glands (on either side of the urethra) and of Bartholin's glands (in the labia majora).

(c) *Urethritis:* the urethra is inflamed in about half the cases.

(d) *Cervicitis:* the surface of the cervix may be inflamed, but the infection does not spread into the body of the uterus or into the uterine (Fallopian) tubes.

Associated condition: about half the women with gonorrhoea have also got trichomoniasis.

Trichomoniasis in the male

Urethritis: the urethra has a low grade infection with a mucous or mucopurulent discharge. Some infected men show no signs of it.

Microscopy

The organism is recognized by its appearance and jerky movements in a fresh drop of discharge from the vagina or urethra.

Culture

The organism can be cultured on a special medium.

Threadworms

Threadworms (pin worms, *Enterobius vermicularis*) are the commonest worms to be found in the intestine. The worm is a parasite of human beings only. It looks like a thin white thread, and inhabits the small and large intestine. The male is about 0.5 cm long and lives and dies in the intestine. The female is about 1.0 cm long and escapes through the anus to die on the adjacent skin, disintegrating and discharging large numbers of eggs which stick to skin and clothing. Infection and reinfection are due to swallowing the eggs, which in the intestine become the larvae from which male and female worms develop.

Worms and eggs

The female worms can be seen in the faeces or emerging through the anus. The eggs can be picked up on sticky tape pressed over the perineal region.

Roundworms

Ascaris lumbricoides is a roundworm which can inhabit the intestine. Its incidence is worldwide. It is similar to the earthworm but white and longer. Female worms are longer than males and can measure up to 25 cm. The worms live in the intestine off the intestinal contents. Hundreds of worms can be present at the same time. The eggs escape in the faeces; they are resistant to heat, drying and antiseptics.

Infection is due to swallowing the eggs. The larvae hatch out in the small intestine, penetrate its wall and are carried in the blood to the lungs. There they pass through the alveolar wall into the alveoli and pass up the respiratory passages into the pharynx. They are then swallowed and arriving again in the small intestine are now converted into adult worms.

Complications

Obstruction to the bile or pancreatic duct by a worm trying to pass up it.
Intestinal obstruction, volvulus, intestinal perforation, in heavily infected children.
Pneumonitis: due to presence of larvae in the lungs.
Allergic reactions: eosinophilia, enlarged lymph nodes.

Faeces

Worms and eggs are visible.

Blood

Eosinophils may be increased. Normal: 40-440 per mm^3.

Sputum

Sputum may be blood-stained and contain larvae.

Tapeworms

Tapeworms are long white ribbonlike worms which inhabit the intestine. They occur in all parts of the world, especially in the tropics and subtropical regions. Infection by the larger tapeworms (the beef tapeworm and the pork tapeworm) is usually by a single worm, but there are some dwarf tapeworms with which infestation is usually multiple.

The tapeworm attaches itself by its small head to the mucous membrane of the intestine. From the head end segments are produced which push away the segments previously formed. The worm has no mouth or alimentary tract and absorbs its nourishment through its surface from the contents of the intestine. Segments laden with eggs are discharged through the anus or in the faeces, and the eggs are then discharged from it. If the eggs are eaten by an appropriate animal, larvae develop and migrating into the tissues form cysts there. The cyst contains the head of what could become an adult worm.

Taenia saginata (beef tapeworm) can grow up to 6 or more metres long and have a thousand or more segments, which can be up to 1.5 cm wide. If the eggs are eaten by cattle, cysts develop in their muscles, causing what is called 'measly' beef. The infection is transmitted to man if he eats infected meat raw or imperfectly cooked.

Taenia solium (pork tapeworm) is a smaller tapeworm transmitted in pork.

Cysticercosis is a condition in which cysts containing the larvae of the *T. solium* develop in man as a result of the eggs from infected meat being in the stomach. The larvae develop from the eggs and penetrate the mucous membrane of the small intestine and are then distributed through the body in the blood stream. Cysts are formed (especially in the brain, connective tissue and muscle) and can become calcified.

> **Faeces**
>
> Segments of tapeworm may be found in the faeces or discharged through the anus.
>
> **Biopsy**
>
> Specimens of muscle or connective tissue are removed by biopsy and examined for cysts.

Hydatid Infection

Hydatid infection is an infection of man in which cysts are formed by *Echinococcus granulosus* or *Echinococcus multilocularis,* tapeworms found in many parts of the world and especially in Australia, South Africa, Argentina, Middle and Eastern Europe.

Cattle and sheep are intermediate hosts which become infected with the larvae of the worm. If their viscera are eaten by other animals (dogs, cats, foxes, wolves), the adult worm develops in the small intestine of these animals and produces eggs which are discharged in the faeces. Infection of man follows ingestion of the eggs, and the dog is the commonest source of them.

In the alimentary tract of man the eggs develop into larvae. The larvae pass into the wall of the small intestine and are spread round the body in the blood. The liver and lung are particularly liable to be infected. In the tissues the larvae stimulate a cellular reaction round them – of lymphocytes, eosinophils and plasma cells; fibrous tissue develops and forms the wall of the cyst, in which the larvae can live for years. A cyst can be up to 25 cm diameter. The walls of the cyst can eventually become calcified.

E. granulosus forms a unilocular cyst and *E. multilocularis* a multilocular one. Within the cyst 'brood capsules' or daughter cysts form containing the head of a worm, and if the cyst wall ruptures, these brood capsules are discharged and infect other tissues.

Complications

Rupture of a cyst.
Acute anaphylactic reaction to leakage of cyst fluid or rupture of cyst wall.
Abscess formation in cyst.

> **Blood**
>
> *White cells:* increase in number of eosinophils during an anaphylactic reaction. Normal number: 40-440 per mm^3.
>
> **Skin test**
>
> In the Casoni skin test 0.1 ml of an antigen prepared from hydatid cyst fluid is injected intradermally. A positive reaction is one in which a large wheal surrounded by a zone of erythema develops in 15-20 minutes.
>
> **Complement fixation test**
>
> A complement fixation test is used employing the same fluid as that used in the Casoni skin test.

Toxocara Infection

Toxocara is a common intestinal worm of dogs and cats, especially puppies and kittens. Children and adults can be infected by handling the animals and getting eggs of the worm on their hands. The eggs are ingested and in the intestine develop into larvae. The larvae pass through the mucous membrane and invade the venules and lymphatics of the intestine, and so are distributed throughout the body. They produce granulomatous reactions in many organs, especially:

eye   brain   liver
lungs   heart   kidneys.

The granulomatous lesions can become necrotic, enclosed within fibrous tissue, and calcified.

> **Blood**
>
> *White cells:* there is usually an increase in the number of eosinophils. Normal: 40-440 per mm^3.

Trichiniasis (Trichinosis)

Trichiniasis is the disease produced by *Trichinella spiralis,* a nematode worm.

Trichinella spiralis infects many animals, especially pigs, and eating raw or undercooked pork is the usual cause of infection in man.

Infected meat contains small cysts in which live the larvae of the worm. When infected meat is eaten, the cyst wall is digested by gastric juice and the larvae escape and attach themselves to the mucous membrane of the small intestine. The larvae develop into adult worms, of which the male is 1.5 mm and the female 3-4 mm long. The male dies after impregnating the female. The pregnant female burrows into the mucous membrane of the small intestine, deposits there several hundred larvae and then dies. The larvae pass into the blood stream and are disseminated throughout the body. Their tissue of choice is striated muscle (especially the diaphragm, pectoral, deltoid, intercostal, gluteal and gastrocnemius muscles). The tissue reacts to the presence of larvae by forming small cysts in which they are enclosed. In 6-18 months calcification appear in the wall of the cyst, and the larvae can live within it for many years.

> **Muscle**
>
> *Biopsy specimens* are examined for the presence of cysts.

> **Blood**
>
> *White cells:* there is an increase in the number of eosinophil cells, which in acute infections may be raised to 20,000 per mm^3. Normal: 40-440 per mm^3.
>
> **Immunological tests**
>
> Precipitin and complement fixing antibodies may be found in the serum. Precipitins are antibodies which can be detected by precipitation (i.e. an antigen-antibody complex comes out of solution).

Hookworm Infection

Ancylostoma duodenale and *Necator americanus* are the two hookworms which infect man.

A. duodenale occurs mainly in temperate climates and *N. americanus* mainly in tropical and subtropical countries. In some parts of the world both worms are present.

Both kinds have a hooked appearance. *A. duodenale* is up to 1 cm long. *N. americanus* is shorter and thinner.

Infection is by the penetration of the skin by the larvae. Eggs of the worms passed in faeces will in moist conditions hatch into larvae. The usual method of infection is walking barefoot on contaminated soil. The larvae penetrate the skin of the feet (or any other part of the skin they come into contact with) and eventually reach the lungs. There they pass through the alveolar wall and up the respiratory passages to reach the pharynx. They are then swallowed. In the gastro-intestinal tract the larvae become worms, which attach themselves to the mucous membrane of the small intestine. The eggs are excreted in the faeces.

Each adult worm attached to the mucous membrane of the small intestine causes a daily loss of 0.03-0.1 ml of blood, and in heavy infections the loss can be serious.

Complications

Hypochromic anaemia: due to loss of blood. This anaemia may occur only in people who have deficient iron reserves or are suffering from protein deficiency.
Ascites.
Oedema.

Faeces

Specimens of faeces are examined for the presence of eggs.

Blood

Red cells: may be reduced. Normal $4.5\text{-}6.5 \times 10^{12}/l$. in male adults; $3.9\text{-}5.6 \times 10^{12}/l$. in female adults
Haemoglobin (Hb): may be reduced. Normal: 13.5-18.0 g/dl in male adults; 11.5-16.5 g/dl in female adults.

Filariasis

Filariasis is infection by filarial worms, of which there are several kinds which produce various lesions. It occurs in tropical and subtropical countries.

Bancroftian filariasis occurs in many parts of the world. *Malayan filariasis* occurs in Malaya and adjacent regions. Infection of man is produced by the bite of infected mosquitos. Larvae are transmitted in the bite and develop in about 6 months into worms, which are thin and threadlike, grow up to about 10 cm long, and lie coiled up in lymph vessels and nodes, especially of the pelvis and external genitalia.

Lymphangitis and lymphadenitis develop. Blocking of the lymph vessels produces elephantiasis – a thickening of the skin and subcutaneous tissue and oedema, often to a very severe degree.

Blood

Microfilariae (a small form of the worm) may be found in the blood if a specimen is taken at the time of day (20-0.2 hours) when they appear there in the greatest number.

Onchocerciasis (River blindness) is caused by *Onchocerca volvulus*, a filarial worm transmitted by the bite of a genus of bloodsucking blackflies, which breed in fast flowing rivers of tropical Africa and America. Over 20 million people are affected. The blindness is due to invasion of the eye by the larvae, and in some communities is present in 20 per cent of adults. The skin is invaded by millions of larvae, causing chronic inflammatory changes (which may be mistaken for leprosy) and a prematurely aged appearance.

Schistosomiasis

Schistosomiasis (bilharziasis) is due to infection by *Schistoma*, a blood fluke, of which there are 3 major species present in tropical and subtropical countries.
S. japonicum: causes Asian schistosomiasis. Other animals can be affected. Occurs in Japan and Pacific islands.
S. haematobium: causes genito-urinary schistosomiasis. Occurs in Africa and Arabia.
S. mansoni: causes intestinal schistosomiasis. Other animals can be affected. Occurs in Africa and South America.

The life-cycle of each species is essentially the same. The larvae hatch out of eggs in contaminated water and swim about and enter a susceptible water snail (the species of snail varies with the species of *Schistoma*), develop further in it, and are discharged again into water. Man is infected through the skin by wading or swimming in contaminated water or through the alimentary tract by drinking the water. The larvae enter the blood and are distributed around the body. They become adult male or female worms 1-2 cm long, which live mainly in the venules of the intestine and pelvis. The female produces eggs which escape from the venules and invade various organs, especially the intestine and bladder. Some eggs are discharged in faeces or urine, and complete the life-cyle by entering water. Transmission from man to man is impossible.

Pathological changes produced are:
(a) A granulomatous reaction around the eggs and worms. The organs particularly liable to be affected are:
liver   intestine   lung
kidneys   ureters   bladder.
The granulomatous reaction is severe and followed by fibrosis.
(b) Schistosomiasis of the bladder produces severe fibrosis, contraction of the bladder, and calcification. Similar changes can occur in the rest of the urinary tract. Carcinoma of the bladder is a complication, but it has not been definitely proved to be due to schistosomiasis.
(c) Schistosomiasis of the intestine produces ulceration, granulomatous and fibrous changes, and polyposis.
(d) Immunity reactions and allergic manifestations.

Faeces, urine

Eggs are identified by their size and shape, which are slightly different in the 3 species.

Rectal biopsy

A specimen of rectal mucous membrane is removed and examined for eggs.

Blood

Hospitals for tropical diseases have laboratories with facilities for carrying out immunodiagnostic tests for schistosomiasis. Antibodies appear in the blood about 4 weeks after infection.

Amoebiasis

Amoebiasis is due to infection by *Entamoeba histolytica,* an amoeba. It occurs in all parts of the world and especially in the tropics.

Infection is by swallowing faecally contaminated food or water containing cysts of the organism. The cyst wall is dissolved in the small intestine and the amoeba released. The amoebae can live for years in the small and large intestine and not do any harm. Influenced by some unknown factor they can, however, penetrate the mucous membrane and cause a little inflammation and some superficial ulceration. Serious complications can develop if the amoebae penetrate the portal venous system and are carried to the liver.

Complications

Amoebic hepatitis.
Amoebic abscess: can be large, contain necrotic liver tissue, and rupture into the peritoneal cavity or through the diaphragm.
Infection of lungs and brain: can follow rupture of an abscess.

Faeces

Faeces are examined for amoebae and cysts. Amoebae have to be distinguished from *E. coli,* a normal and harmless inhabitant of the colon.

Biopsy

Scrapings from the mucous membrane of the colon are examined for amoebae and cysts.

Pus from hepatic abscess

Pus can be aspirated and examined for amoebae.

Toxoplasmosis

Toxoplasmosis is due to infection by *Toxoplasma gondi*, a protozoon found in many species of birds and animals and some reptiles, and with a world-wide distribution.

The parasite is a slender, crescent-shaped organism, with one end blunt and the other pointed. It is about 4-6μ long and about 2μ at its broadest. It lives in cells of the reticulo-endothelial system and in tissue fluid. In the cell it divides by longitudinal fission, after which the cell ruptures and the new parasites are liberated and enter other cells.

Human infection can be:
(a) *Acquired:* from animals, probably cattle, sheep, pigs, cats, dogs and rodents. The method of transmission from animal to man is probably (i) by ingestion, (ii) by inhaling infected droplets, (iii) in laboratory workers by direct contact with infected tissues.
(b) *Congenital:* transmitted from an infected mother through the placenta to her child. If the mother becomes infected early in pregnancy the child may be aborted or still-born. If the mother is infected late in pregnancy, the child is likely to be born alive but may develop signs of infection some weeks or months later. Transmission through the milk of a lactating mother is a possibility.

The organism is thought to be distributed throughout the body in the blood-stream. Tissues particularly likely to be affected are:

brain	lung	liver
spleen	kidney	lymph nodes
muscle	bone marrow	adrenal glands.

Small areas of necrosis occur, each surrounded by a zone of inflammation. Large cells distended by parasites are often present. In congenital infections small granulomata can occur in the brain and go on to calcification.

In many cases there are no signs or symptoms of infection, which can then be diagnosed only by special tests.

In *congenital infections* the following can occur:
encephalitis;
patches of calcification in the brain;
hydrocephalus;
choroido-retinitis of the eye.

In *acquired infections* the following can occur:
fever; pneumonitis;
myocarditis; enlarged lymph nodes;
acute meningo-encephalitis.

Bone marrow, splenic tissue, exudates, CSF

In acute infections fresh and stained specimens are examined for the parasite.

Animal inoculation

Mice, hamsters and guinea pigs are inoculated with infected material and examined later for the parasite.

Toxoplasmin skin test

A toxoplasmin is prepared from a strain of *Toxoplasma* and injected intradermally. A control injection of a fluid not containing the toxoplasmin is injected at the same time. A positive reaction is an area of erythema and induration exceeding 10 mm diameter occurring in 48-72 hours with an absence of reaction in the control site. About 10-20 per cent of apparently uninfected people give a positive reaction.

Complement fixation test

This test uses an antigen obtained from a chick embryo. Antibodies develop 3-4 weeks after infection and can either disappear within 6 months or persist for years. About 10 per cent of apparently uninfected people give a positive reaction.

Blood

Red cells and haemoglobin usually reduced.
Lymphocytes and monocytes usually increased; eosinophils sometimes increased.

CSF

In meningo-encephalitis CSF may be yellow with protein increased; white cells up to 50-1500 per mm^3. and sometimes red cells are present.

Giardiasis

Giardiasis is infection by *Giardia lamblia,* a pear-shaped organism, 10-18μ long and possessing a flagellum and sucker. It occurs in all parts of the world. Man is the only host.

Infection is due to swallowing cysts of the organism in faecally contaminated food or water. The organism takes on its active form and attaches itself by its sucker to the surface of the mucous membrane of the upper part of the small intestine. Slight infection produces no symptoms. Severe infection produces diarrhoea and abdominal pain.

Complication

Steatorrhoea occurs if the infection is so severe as to interfere with intestinal function and cause malabsorption.

Faeces

Specimens of faeces are examined for the parasites, which can by present in large numbers.

Malaria

Malaria is due to infection by a parasite of which there are 4 kinds:
Plasmodium vivax: causes a benign tertian malaria.
Plasmodium ovale: causes a benign tertian malaria.
Plasmodium malariae: causes a quartan malaria.
Plasmodium falciparum: causes malignant tertian malaria, a severe, progressive and often fatal disease.

The terms 'tertian' and 'quartan' refer to peaks of temperature arising on the 3rd and 4th days of the illness.

The disease occurs mainly in tropical and sub-tropical countries, and can occur in temperate countries where conditions are suitable for the *Anopheles* mosquito.

The life cycle of the parasite is mainly the same for all four kinds.

The parasite spends half its life in man and half in the *Anopheles* mosquito, and passes through various stages of development.

Man is infected by the bite of an infected female *Anopheles* mosquito. At the time of biting the mosquito injects into the skin some saliva from its salivary glands. If the *sporozoites* of the plasmodium are present in the saliva, the man becomes infected. The sporozoites enter the blood and are transmitted to the liver and there develop into merozoites. The *merozoites* are discharged into the blood where they invade red blood cells. In the red blood cells they pass through various stages and again become merozoites. The merozoites are discharged in large numbers at regular intervals producing the rise of temperature that is the typical feature of the disease. With *P. falciparum* the parasites in the liver die after the first discharge into the blood, but with the other kinds some parasites continue to live and reinfect the blood. Some of the merozoites develop into *gametocytes,* the male and female sexual forms of the plasmodium.

In the *mosquito:* the mosquito becomes

infected by biting an infected man and sucking up some of his blood at the time the gametocytes are present in it. The gametocytes eventually become sporozoites, and the life cycle of the plasmodium is completed by the mosquito biting a man.

A partial immunity can develop after long continued infections or repeated infections, and so attacks become less frequent and milder in people living in malarious areas.

Complications

Anaemia: as a result of the destruction of red cells by the parasite.
Cerebral malaria: the brain is congested and has small haemorrhages and patches of necrosis due to the blocking of small blood vessels by parasite-laden red cells.
Blackwater fever: jaundice due to a failure of the liver to deal with large amounts of bilirubin presented to it by the destruction of many red cells.
Malaria nephrosis: can occur in children with *P. malariae* infection and thought to be due to a deposit of antigen-antibody complex on the basement membrane of the glomeruli of the kidneys.

Blood

Films are stained and examined for the presence of the parasite in various forms within the red cells.
White cells: often reduced in number (leucopenia), especially the granulocytes.
Erythrocyte sedimentation rate (ESR): raised.

Leishmaniasis

Leishmaniasis is due to infection by a protozoon of the genus *Leishmania* transmitted by the bite of a sandfly. Two kinds occur.

1. *Visceral leishmaniasis* (Kala-azar) is due to infection by the *L. donovani*. It occurs mainly in the Near and Middle East, Africa and Central and South America. The organism is 2-5μ long. It invades cells of the reticuloendothelial system and causes enlargement of the liver, spleen and lymph-nodes.

Smears

Smears obtained from bone marrow, blood, liver and spleen are examined for the organism.

Culture

The organism is cultured on rabbit-blood agar.

---

2. *Cutaneous leishmaniasis* (Oriental sore) is due to infection by *L. tropica*, a round or oval organism 2μ long. It occurs mainly in the Near and Middle East, West Africa and Central and South America. It invades cells of the reticuloendothelial system and produces granulomatous lesions in the skin which break down into ulcers.

Smears

Smears of tissue obtained from the margin of an ulcer are examined for the organism.

Culture

The organism is cultured on rabbit-blood agar.

Trypanosomiasis

Trypanosomiasis is due to infection by a *Trypanosoma,* a protozoal organism about 15μ long, 3μ wide, and with a flagellum. It occurs in African and South American forms.

1. *African trypanosomiasis* (sleeping sickness) occurs in Central and West Africa. It is spread by the bite of the tsetse fly, which likes moderate heat, bites in daylight, and breeds in moist shady places. The organism spreads through the lymph vessels and nerves into the blood stream. The central nervous system is invaded with the production of meningo-encephalitis, oedema of the brain, small haemorrhages and congestion of the choroid plexuses.

2. *South American trypanosomiasis* (Chagas' disease) is produced by a trypanosome similar to the African one. It is spread by the bite of certain bugs. Having spread through the lymph vessels and nodes into the blood stream, the organism invades liver, spleen, thyroid gland, myocardium, brain and meninges, producing an inflammatory reaction which is followed by fibrosis. The oesophagus and colon dilate enormously if their nerve-plexuses become invaded and paralysed.

Blood etc.

The blood, CSF and lymph node juice are examined for both forms of parasite.

Chapter 6 Inflammation

Inflammation is the reaction of a tissue to any damage not severe enough to kill it. Tissues can be damaged by:
infection by micro-organisms;
injury;
chemical and physical poisons.
Acute inflammation is an immediate response to a harmful stimulus.
Chronic inflammation is the response to a less intense but more persistent stimulus.

Acute Inflammation

When a tissue is acutely inflamed, it is:
red   swollen
hot   painful
and suffers impairment of function. These changes are due to the following reactions.

1. RESPONSE OF THE BLOOD-VESSELS

Histamine (a chemical substance stored in cells in the tissues) or a histamine-like substance causes the arterioles at first to contract and then to dilate. The capillaries and venules dilate. The redness and heat of inflamed tissue is due to this dilatation. The swelling is due partly to this dilatation, partly to the fluid that passes out of the blood-vessels into the tissues. The pain is due to the action of histamine on sensory nerve endings. The impairment of function is due to the abnormal chemical and physical state of inflamed cells.

2. FORMATION OF AN EXUDATE

An exudate is the fluid that passes out of the blood into the tissues. In the fluid are some cells.

(a) *Fluid*.

The amount of fluid in inflamed tissues is increased because:
(i) The capillary wall becomes more permeable.
(ii) The dilatation of the arterioles causes a rise of pressure within the capillaries, forcing more fluid out of them.

The effects of this increase of fluid in the tissues are:
(i) The 'toxin' which caused the inflammatory responses becomes diluted and therefore less toxic.
(ii) Certain anti-toxic agents in the fluid neutralize the toxin.
(iii) Fibrinogen in the fluid clots and forms fibrin, a dense substance which walls off the inflamed area (or at least attempts to do so) and prevents it from getting any larger.

(b) *Cells*.

Cells from the blood pass out of the blood-vessels.
(i) *Polymorphs* (polymorphonuculear leucoytes), which normally keep to the centre of the blood stream in any blood-vessel, move to the edge and then pass, with amoebic movements, through the capillary walls. They are thought to do this under the influence of some chemical stimulation. At the same time the bone marrow is stimulated to produce more polymorphs. The polymorphs are phagocytic, i.e. they destroy and absorb bacteria and dead cells. They themselves die in the process and become liquified.

Pus is a creamy, green or greenish-yellow fluid formed of dead and living polymorphs, cell debris and bacteria. An *abscess* is a collection of pus.

(ii) *Monocytes* tend to behave like polymorphs, but their number is not greatly increased.
(iii) *Lymphocytes* usually remain in the blood.
(iv) *Red cells* leak through the capillary wall, sometimes in numbers big enough to make the exudate appear blood-stained or, with a big leak, 'haemorrhagic'.

THE SPREAD OF BACTERIAL INFLAMMATION

An acute inflammatory reaction to harmful micro-organisms may be limited to a small area of the body (e.g. a boil) or may extend to other parts of the body or to the whole body. It can spread:
(a) *Directly through a tissue.* Healthy tissue offers resistance to the spread or the spread may be halted by a barrier of fibrin. Some micro-organisms (e.g. *Str. pyogenes*) contain an enzyme that dissolves fibrin and so breaks down this barrier. Other organisms may overcome local resistance and spread extensively.
(b) *Along the lymph system.* Infection commonly spreads along lymph vessels into lymph nodes. *Acute lymphangitis* is an inflammation of the walls of a lymph-vessel, which in the skin becomes visible as a thin red line. *Acute lymphadenitis* is an inflammation of lymph nodes; like other inflamed tissues they become red, hot, swollen and painful.
(c) *Into the blood stream.* The spread may be directly into a blood-vessel involved in the inflamed area or indirectly through the thoracic duct (the main lymph vessel through which lymph passes out of the lymph system into the blood at the junction of the left internal jugular and left subclavian veins).
Bacteraemia is the presence of micro-organisms in the blood.
Septicaemia is the disease-state due to the multiplication of micro-organisms in the blood.
Pyaemia is the carriage of pyogenic micro-organisms in the blood, with the production of abscesses in the tissues.
(d) *Along a serous membrane,* i.e. the pericardium, the pleura, the peritoneum, producing a pericarditis, a pleurisy or a peritonitis.

(e) *Along a nerve.* Some micro-organisms, e.g.:
polio virus   herpes viruses
virus of rabies
can pass along a nerve-fibre.

Chronic Inflammation

Chronic inflammation is the response of tissues to harmful stimuli less severe than those that cause acute inflammation but more persistent. In many chronic inflammations, some degree of acute inflammation is going on at the same time.

A *granulomatous inflammation* is a chronic inflammation in which there are clumps of histiocytes (phagocytic cells found in connective tissue) and multi-nucleated giant cells.

In chronic inflammation the response of the blood-vessels is less marked and the amount of exudate is much less. Lymphocytes and plasma cells are the commonest kinds of cells in the exudate. Polymorphs are present if there is any acute inflammation in the tissues. Repair of the tissue by fibroblasts is likely to be going on at the same time as the inflammation in some areas.

Healing Processes

Healing of damaged tissues is either by first intention or by second intention.

HEALING BY FIRST INTENTION

Healing by first intention is the term used to describe the kind of healing that takes place in 'clean' incisions where there has been no extensive loss or damage of tissues and no infection of the wound. It is the sort of healing that is expected of a surgical incision.

The following stages take place:
(a) Blood from cut vessels clots and sticks together the edges of the wound.
(b) Phagocytic cells move into the clot to

absorb any dead or dying cells and bacteria.
(c) New capillaries grow out of adjacent ones into the clot, at first as solid rods of cells, which later become canalized and let in the blood.
(d) Fibroblasts move in and lay down fibrous tissue at right angles to the original wound.
(e) The fibrous tissue contracts; capillaries in excess of what is now required are absorbed, and the phagocytic cells disappear.

HEALING BY SECOND INTENTION

Healing by second intention is the kind of healing that occurs where there has been extensive tissue loss or damage or the wound has become infected. Healing is a much slower process than by first intention.
(a) Attempts are made to localize infection by walling it off with fibrous tissue. This is likely to produce an abscess. An abscess is not likely to clear up unless it is drained surgically or bursts spontaneously on to the skin or into a hollow organ such as the intestine.
(b) Granulation tissue appears at the bottom of the wound. Granulation tissue is formed of phagocytic cells, fibroblasts and capillaries and grows upwards as rough, brown, weeping tissue, which eventually plugs the hole with fibrous tissue. A permanent scar is formed. The scar either contracts or, if it is subject to tension, stretches.

Regrowth of Specialized Tissues

Specialized cells are divided into 3 classes according to their ability to regenerate after injury.

1. *Labile cells.*

These are cells which are normally dividing and regrowing continually throughout life, and which when damaged can be quickly and fully replaced. These cells form:
the skin; the lymph nodes;
the bone marrow;
the mucous membrane of the stomach and intestine.

2. *Stable cells.*

These are cells which normally do not multiply after full growth has been reached but will regenerate if the organ is damaged. They include the cells of:
the liver; the pancreas;
the thyroid gland; the adrenal glands.

3. *Permanent cells.* These are cells whose number is fixed before birth and which if they are damaged are not replaced:
cells of nervous system;
cells of voluntary muscle.

Chapter 7 Immunity, Hypersensitivity, Autoimmunity, Collagen Diseases

In addition to the local reactions which they produce when they invade the body, micro-organisms produce general reactions in certain tissues and so affect the body as a whole. Micro-organisms contain antigens. An *antigen* is usually a protein (it can be a polysaccharide) which stimulates the lymph tissue of the body to produce antibodies. An *antibody* is an immunoglobulin and anti-infective factor. There are 5 principal types of antibody:
IgG: present in blood and tissue fluids;
IgA: present in secretions;
IgM: present in blood early in infections;
IgD: functions unknown;
IgE: responsible for certain allergic phenomena.

Immunoglobulins are produced in lymphoid tissue, probably by plasma cells, mainly in the spleen and lymph nodes.

When a particular micro-organism invades the body, its antigen stimulates the production of an antibody. The antibody is a specific one — one produced only against one particular type of organism or against one particular strain of that organism. The presence in the blood, tissue fluid and secretions of an adequate amount of an antibody will modify or prevent the invasion of the body by the particular micro-organism whose antigen has stimulated the production of that particular antibody.

Immunity

Immunity in a clinical sense is the ability to withstand the harmful effects of pathogenic organisms. In a more specific sense it means an altered reaction to any antigen, by a process of sensitization, the result of which may be beneficial or harmful. The factors upon which it depends are:

(a) Inheritance

If one's ancestors have been repeatedly subjected to attacks by a particular micro-organism, one has some degree of resistance to that organism so that its effects are weakened. People whose ancestors have not had this experience can suffer severely if attacked by the organisms, and a usually mild infection can for them be a killer.

(b) A previous attack by a micro-organism

The antibodies produced in response to the antigens of a micro-organism persist for a variable time in the blood and tissues. If, for example, a person has mumps, the production of antibodies is so great and they persist so long that he is not likely to have another attack however long he lives. Some infections do not stimulate much antibody reaction, e.g. the common cold, of which a person may have many attacks. Some organisms, e.g. influenza virus, have the ability to turn up with a slightly modified chemical constitution, and the antibodies produced by one attack may not be quite the right ones to cope with a later attack. Antibodies may disappear after years and render a person liable to another attack. Herpes zoster, an infection of nervous tissue, is thought to be a response to the reactivation of chicken pox virus which has lain dormant in the tissues since the original attack and is reawakened into activity when the amount of antibody falls below the level necessary to keep the virus inactive.

Chapter 7

(c) Vaccination

Vaccination is the inoculation of the body with micro-organisms in order to stimulate in it the production of antibodies. The micro-organisms used are specially grown for the purpose in a laboratory and are either killed before use or have their toxic effects diminished by having been grown on media known to weaken them. Diseases against which vaccination can be used include:

smallpox	typhoid fever
measles	German measles
poliomyelitis	tetanus
diphtheria	influenza
tuberculosis	whooping cough
cholera	yellow fever
rabies	

Vaccination has to be repeated at intervals to maintain the amount of antibody at a sufficiently high level; these secondary doses are known as booster doses. The degree of protection produced by any form of vaccination is usually not as great as that produced by a natural infection.

For the first few months of life a baby is protected by those maternal antibodies which have passed into it in fetal life through the placenta; and immunization against a particular infection is not carried out in infants until the time when their antibody protection is likely to have fallen to a level at which infection becomes possible.

Toxoids

The harmful effects of some organisms are due to toxins they produce; immunity is conferred by inoculating with a harmless toxoid (developed from the toxin) which stimulates the production of antitoxin. Toxoids are given against:

diphtheria	tetanus.

HYPERSENSITIVITY

Hypersensitivity (allergy) is a state in which a person has become sensitized to a particular antigen; stimulation of that antigen causes an abnormal reaction.

There are two types of hypersensitivity.

I. Immediate type hypersensitivity

This type is a result of a production of gamma globulin antibodies.

II. Delayed type hypersensitivity

This type is caused by cells. The response is due to invasion of the tissues by inflammatory cells, mostly lymphocytes, which have antibody bound to their cytoplasm. The reaction occurs 24 hours or more after stimulation by the antigen.

I. Immediate type hypersensitivity

1. ANAPHYLACTIC SHOCK

This is an immediate reaction due to the liberation of large amounts of histamine, liberated by the rupture of mast cells on whose surface an antigen-antibody reaction has occurred. The antigen can be in serum or a drug (especially penicillin) or vaccine, rarely a bee sting. The antibody is a reagin (IgE). Some antibodies are called *reagins* or non-precipitating antibodies because they cannot be detected by tests of precipitation and agglutination.

Anaphylactic shock is an acute and sometimes fatal condition characterized by:

spasm of bronchial muscle;	fall of BP;
rapid pulse;	shock;

and sometimes by:

oedema of larynx;	diarrhoea;
angioneurotic oedema of skin;	vomiting;
conjunctivitis.	

It is likely to occur if a protein-containing substance is injected into the body 10 days after an injection of the same substance.

2. HAY FEVER AND ASTHMA

These allergies are associated with the same antibody (IgE) which is involved in the anaphylactic reaction. People who produce the IgE antibody are likely to suffer general anaphylactic reactions and local reactions such as hay fever and asthma. IgE antibody becomes attached to tissue mast cells; and when antigen combines with it histamine and other substances are released, causing the symptoms.

Hay fever

Hay fever is a local reaction. When the antigen (usually a pollen) comes into contact with the mucous membrane of the nose and conjunctiva, excessive secretion is produced.

Asthma

The allergens are usually pollens (especially timothy grass in Britain and ragweed in USA), mites of house dust, spores and moulds. The antigen is inhaled and reaches the bronchial mucous membrane via the upper respiratory tract, or it may arrive via the blood stream from the alimentary tract. It combines with antibody attached to the cells of the bronchial mucous membrane; this antigen-antibody reaction damages the cells, and histamine is produced and causes bronchospasm.

Hay fever and asthma are partly due to hereditary predisposition.

3. HAEMOLYTIC DISEASE OF THE NEWBORN

This disease is due to antibodies to Rhesus positive blood passing through the placenta from a Rhesus negative mother to a Rhesus positive fetus. The antibody reacts with a naturally occurring antigen present on the surface membrane of fetal Rhesus positive red blood cells, causing haemolysis.

The mother can become sensitized, i.e. develop antibodies:
1. At the birth of a previous Rhesus positive baby, a few red cells having entered her circulation when the placenta became detached.
2. Because of a previous Rhesus positive blood transfusion.

4. SERUM SICKNESS

A reaction may occur in response to a first administration of serum, especially to horse serum. In this reaction antibodies (IgG) to the serum develop within 8-12 days and react with the foreign serum still remaining in the body, and this antigen-antibody complex damages the vascular endothelium, causing:
swelling of the face;   urticarial rashes;
proteinuria;   effusions into joints;
enlarged lymph nodes; fever.

Accelerated serum sickness is a reaction occurring within a few hours when the patient is already sensitized to the foreign serum.

Rarely an anaphylactic reaction, with hypotension and cyanosis, occurs, the antibody being in these cases IgE.

5. FARMER'S LUNG

This is a result of exposure to actinomycetes (members of an order of Gram-positive bacteria with cells arranged in filaments) found in damp hay. In this type of hypersensitivity the inter-reaction between antigen and antibody causes an immune-complex to be deposited in the walls of the blood vessels, causing damage to the vessels and degeneration of the tissues supplied by them. In farmer's lung, vascular damage is followed by a pneumonia-like illness and eventually fibrosis of the lung.

II. Delayed type hypersensitivity

1. MANTOUX REACTION

The Mantoux reaction used to detect tuberculosis is a delayed-type hypersensitivity involving lymphocytes and other cells. A positive reaction is one in which an area of induration (due to a cellular response) occurs 24-72 hours after the injection of tuberculin (a preparation derived from fluid in which *Myco. tuberculosis* has been grown, but not containing any organisms) into the skin of a person, and is an indication that he has or has had tuberculosis. A patch of erythema at the site of injection is not a positive reaction.

2. CONTACT DERMATITIS

In this condition the allergen causes sensitisation by contact with the skin. Many substances can act as allergens, e.g. nickel, chemicals, cosmetics, deodorants, hair lotions, rubber, and plants, especially primulas and chrysanthemums.

3. GRAFT REJECTION

Rejection of a homograft (i.e. a graft from an animal of the same species) is probably a delayed hypersensitivity reaction. The graft is recognized as foreign, is infiltrated by lymphocytes and destroyed.

Autoimmune Diseases

An *autoimmune disease* is one in which certain antibodies called autoantibodies have a harmful effect upon healthy tissues. These autoantibodies are antibodies to the patient's own tissues. Lymphocytes also play a part in the production of autoimmune diseases.

Normally in fetal life a tolerance develops to the body's own antigens, which are recognized as 'self'. This is possibly because the body's own antigen is present in such great amounts that the cells which would have manufactured antibody to it are eradicated. These cells are known as 'forbidden clones', i.e. groups of cells which are dangerous to the body.

POSSIBLE CAUSES OF AUTOIMMUNE DISEASES

Autoimmune diseases may be due to:
I. Disorder of the immune mechanism;
II. Failure of recognition of 'self' antigens;
III. A similarity between 'self' and foreign antigens.

I. Disorder of the immune mechanism

1. There is a loss of tolerance to 'self' antigens. There may be a malfunctioning of antibody-producing cells so that abnormal antibody is produced, or there may be a failure of suppression of 'forbidden clones'.
2. Lymphocytes may undergo mutation and produce antibodies to 'self' cells, e.g. (i) to red blood cells in autoimmune haemolytic anaemia; (ii) to platelets in autoimmune thrombocytopenia.

II. Failure of recognition of 'self' antigens

1. ALTERATION OF ANTIGEN

Substances normally present have their surface chemical arrangement altered, e.g. by irradiation, infections, drugs, burns, and are not recognized as 'self'.

In disease new antigens may be formed.

2. EXPOSURE OF PROTECTED CELLS TO THE IMMUNE SYSTEM

Some tissues are anatomically segregated from the immune system, e.g. the lens of the eye, the brain, spermatozoa. Damage to them can result in the tissue antigen coming into contact for the first time with the immune system, which cannot recognize the tissue antigen as 'self'. This mechanism is thought to be the cause of sympathetic ophthalmia.

3. LATE MATURATION OF ANTIGEN

When new antigens are formed after the immune system has become fully matured (e.g. spermatozoa), they may not be recognized as 'self'. Some cases of male sterility are thought to be due to auto-antibodies against spermatozoa. But this occurs only if spermatozoa come

III. Similarity between 'self' and foreign antigens

A foreign substance may share antigens with a host tissue; therefore antibodies formed to combat the invader may also act against self-tissue. This is thought to be the mechanism operating in rheumatic fever. The group A beta haemolytic streptococcus has an antigen very similar to one present in heart muscle. Streptococci are not found in Aschoff nodes (inflammatory lesions in the myocardium); but antibodies in the serum of patients recovering from group A streptococcal infections react against heart muscle and against the similar antigen present in the streptococci.

THE THYMUS GLAND

The thymus gland is essential for the development and maintenance of some immunological mechanisms.

In fetal life it produces lymphocytes from primitive cells which have moved into it from the liver and yolk sac.

After birth it maintains a pool of circulating, immunologically competent lymphocytes, which are responsible for cell-mediated immunity (see T lymphocytes below). It does this probably by producing a factor which causes cells passing through it to become sensitive to antigen.

It may also be responsible for suppressing 'forbidden clones' or for failing to suppress them.

T AND B LYMPHOCYTES

T lymphocytes (thymus dependent lymphocytes) travel in the blood from the bone marrow as primitive lymphoid cells, and pass through the thymus, where they are 'processed': they become lymphocytes sensitive to antigens and circulate in the bloodstream, mediating cellular immune responses anywhere in the body, e.g. rejection of grafts and delayed hypersensitivity reactions.

B lymphocytes are not dependent on the thymus for 'processing'. They also originate in the bone marrow and are the precursors of plasma cells, which produce and release antibodies into the plasma.

INTERACTION BETWEEN T AND B LYMPHOCYTES

The ability of B lymphocytes to form antibodies against certain antigens depends on 'help' or stimulation from T lymphocytes.

PROBABLE AUTOIMMUNE DISEASES
myasthenia gravis; rheumatoid arthritis; haemolytic anaemia; pernicious anaemia; Sjögren's disease; ulcerative colitis; Hashimoto's disease. sympathetic ophthalmia;

DISEASES WITH A POSSIBLE AUTOIMMUNE FACTOR

Diabetes mellitus; multiple (disseminated) pemphigus; sclerosis; acute peripheral neuritis.

The evidence for the existence of autoimmune disease includes:
(a) patients with an autoimmune disease show an increase in the amount of serum gamma-globulin;
(b) autoantibodies can be identified in the serum;
(c) the diseases show a common pathological pattern of invasion of tissues by lymphocytes, plasma cells and histiocytes;
(d) the thymus gland may be enlarged or persist into adult life, or there may be a tumour of it;
(e) there may be a family history of the various autoimmune diseases;
(f) improvement may be produced by corticosteroid and cytotoxic drugs.

Collagen Diseases

The *collagen diseases* are diseases of connective tissue and considered as autoimmune diseases. They present a varied clinical picture, but have some pathological and clinical features in common.

The collagen diseases include:
systemic lupus erythematosus;
dermatomyositis;
rheumatoid arthritis;
polyarteritis nodosa;
systemic sclerosis;
rheumatic fever.

The essential pathological feature which occurs in these diseases is the appearance in connective tissue in various parts of the body of a kind of degeneration called 'fibrinoid degeneration' because its staining reactions resemble those of fibrin. Common clinical features are pyrexia, joint pain and swelling, a poor prognosis (except in rheumatic fever), and usually some response to treatment by cortisone.

Blood

Erythrocyte sedimentation rate (ESR): raised
White cell count: normal or low

SYSTEMIC LUPUS ERYTHEMATOSUS (SLE)

This condition appears most commonly in middle-aged women. Chronic degenerative changes appear in many organs, especially:
(a) joints: swollen and painful;
(b) skin: areas exposed to light become erythematous and thickened; on the cheeks and nose this forms a 'butterfly rash';
(c) kidney: glomerulonephritis occurs; the basement membrane of the glomerular capillaries becomes thickened by the deposit of immunoglobulins in it; renal arteries show fibrinoid degeneration;
(d) heart: fibrinoid degeneration of the pericardium; small vegetations on the cusps of the valves;
(e) spleen: fibrinoid degeneration of its arteries;
(f) liver: acute or chronic hepatitis.

Blood

LE cells can be seen. An LE cell is a polymorph which has absorbed a large nucleus. This nucleus fills most of the cell, stains differently from the polymorph nucleus, and squashes the polymorph nucleus against the cell membrane.

POLYARTERITIS NODOSA

This condition can occur without obvious reason or as a hypersensitivity reaction to a drug. Collagen degenerative changes appear in the arteries of skeletal muscle, heart, kidneys, liver, gastro-intestinal tract, nervous system, etc. Joints can become painful and swollen. Patients are likely to die within a few years because of the damage to heart, brain or kidneys.

Blood

Erythrocyte sedimentation rate (ESR): raised.
White cells: usually normal or low count, but there is sometimes an increase in the number of eosinophils – normal: 40-440 mm^3

DERMATOMYOSITIS

This collagen disease is characterized by rashes of various kinds, muscular degeneration, and myocarditis. In about 20 per cent of patients it occurs as a complication of a malignant neoplasm somewhere in the body.

SYSTEMIC SCLEROSIS (SCLERODERMA)

This collagen disease is characterized by thickening and hardening of the skin and by collagen degeneration in blood vessels, heart, kidney and gastro-intestinal tract.

RHEUMATOID ARTHRITIS

See p. 187

RHEUMATIC FEVER

This condition follows infection with a haemolytic streptococcus, the first attack being preceded by a sore throat or tonsillitis about 3 weeks previously. It is an acute condition with fever, arthritis, anaemia, nodules in the skin, and degeneration of the heart. The basic lesion in the heart is an Aschoff node – a small area of fibrinoid degeneration surrounded by lymphocytes, giant and other cells. Multiple nodes are present in all the tissues of the heart, producing endocarditis, myocarditis and pericarditis. The streptococci cannot be found in the lesions. The heart valves are likely to be swollen and inflamed; they may recover completely, but in severe infections they become fibrosed and stiff.

Chapter 8 Disorders of Fluid and Electrolyte Balance

Many of the body's activities are directed at keeping within narrow limits the volume and composition of the body fluids. A number of chemical and physical adjustments are continually being made in order to maintain an essential balance of fluid and electrolyte. If these mechanisms are overloaded or break down serious illness can result.

Water Balance

Water forms about 50-60 per cent of the body of an adult, i.e. about 45 litres in an average man weighing 70 kg. Of this:
intracellular fluid (ICF) forms 25-30 litres;
extracellular fluid (ECF) forms 13-16 litres.
 Of the ECF:
plasma forms 3-3.5 litres;
lymph forms 1.5 litres;
secretions, CSF, etc. form 1.5 litres.

Solids form 40-50 per cent of the body. Of this, about one-third is fat, which contains little water and is not much involved in water-exchange.

In a healthy person in normal conditions water intake = water output.

Short term variations are adjusted by alterations in the volume of ICF.

Water Depletion

Causes:
1. *Failure of intake*
no water available
inability to swallow – weakness, coma, oesophageal stricture

2. *Excessive loss of water with low sodium concentration*
diabetes insipidus

Even when there is a failure of intake, a physiological loss of water, up to 1 litre a day, occurs in urine, respiration and perspiration.

The loss of water without loss of salts produces a rise in the osmotic pressure of the extra-cellular fluid. At the beginning of water deprivation, the osmotic pressure of the intra-cellular fluid is lower than that of the extra-cellular fluid, and water therefore passes from the intra-cellular fluid into the extra-cellular fluid and maintains the plasma volume. With the loss of water from the intra-cellular fluid, its osmotic pressure rises until it equals that of the extra-cellular fluid, and therefore no more water passes into the extra-cellular fluid. If the water is still not replaced, the plasma volume falls, leading to haemoconcentration and a failure of peripheral circulation.

The patient is likely to show thirst, weakness, apathy, oliguria, loss of body weight, and coma, as the depletion progresses. Symptoms start to appear when about 2 litres of fluid have been lost. Death occurs when about 15 per cent of body weight has been lost; this occurs in infants without water in less than a week and in an adult in about 10 days.

Blood

Haemoconcentration: haematocrit raised because the plasma volume is reduced. Haematocrit is the percentage of red cells in a volume of blood. Normal: 40-47 per cent.
Plasma proteins: raised.

> **Urine**
>
> *Volume:* less than 500-750 ml in 24 hours.
> *S.G.:* high, 1 040.

Sodium Depletion

1. LOSS OF SODIUM-CONTAINING FLUID

(a) *In gastrointestinal secretions*
Diarrhoea; vomiting; fistulae; obstruction of small intestine.
(b) *Urinary loss*
Diuretics;
Addison's disease and after adrenalectomy, because lack of adreno-cortical hormone results in a failure of the renal tubules to reabsorb sodium.
(c) *Through the skin*
severe sweating; burns.
(d) *Into oedema or ascites*

2. LACK OF INTAKE OF SODIUM

Starvation; anorexia.

Sodium depletion occurs when fluids containing sodium are replaced by water only. It is more serious than loss of water only as the plasma volume falls quickly and therefore complications occur more quickly.

The extra-cellular fluid is hypotonic, having a lower osmotic pressure than fluids of the intra-cellular compartments. The body tries to restore the osmotic pressure: water passes from the extra-cellular fluid to the intra-cellular fluid. Therefore the volume of extra-cellular fluid is lowered and the plasma volume falls quickly. The result is haemoconcentration, circulatory failure, and secondary renal damage.

CLINICAL PRESENTATION

Symptoms of loss occur when the patient has lost the amount of sodium present in 4 litres of isotonic (physiological) saline. A common symptom is painful muscular cramp, which occurs in men working very hard in hot atmospheres and is due to heavy sweating. When depletion is severe, the skin is flabby due to loss of water. The patient may not be thirsty, which contrasts with the thirst of water depletion. There may be nausea and vomiting. There is a low blood pressure, which may cause fainting, and a rapid pulse. Death can occur from circulatory failure.

> **Blood**
>
> *Plasma sodium and chloride:* normal at first; fall as loss becomes more severe.
> *Haemoconcentration:* haematocrit raised. Normal 40-47 per cent.
> *Plasma proteins:* raised.
> *Urea:* raised.
>
> **Urine**
>
> *Volume:* at first normal; falls as depletion becomes worse.
> *Sodium:* reduced.

DEPLETION OF BOTH SALT AND WATER

A combined loss is more common than a depletion of salt or water separately. It occurs:
1. when salt-containing fluids are lost from the body and not replaced;
2. when fluid is lost into parts of the body and is not taking part normally in ionic exchanges – in ascites, oedema, paralytic ileus;
3. after surgical procedures, when fluids have been restricted and sodium has been lost in sweating.

When sodium and water are both lost, the volume of extra-cellular fluid is lowered but the composition remains the same. The extra-cellular fluid is therefore isotonic (i.e. at the same osmotic pressure as the intra-cellular fluid) and there can be no movement of fluid from the intra-cellular fluid to the extra-cellular fluid. The plasma volume falls quickly, leading to haemoconcentration. The loss of sodium-containing fluid is therefore more serious than the loss of an equal amount of water, as a fall in plasma volume and complications occur more quickly.

CLINICAL PRESENTATION

The patient has thirst and oliguria due to water deprivation and the circulatory symptoms of sodium deprivation.

> **Blood**
>
> *Electrolytes:* probably low.
> *Haemoconcentration:* haematocrit raised.

Water Excess

An overload of water can occur when there is oliguria for any reason:
in chronic renal failure;
when there is excessive secretion of anti-diuretic hormone (this may happen post-operatively);
with excessive amounts of intravenous glucose.

CLINICAL PRESENTATION

The patient suffers lethargy and loss of appetite. Headache occurs due to raised intracranial pressure as a result of an excessive volume of body fluids. With a deterioration of his condition he suffers delirium and fits.

Sodium Excess

Causes:
1. *Failure of excretion of sodium*
renal failure;
excessive secretion of adreno-cortical hormones (aldosterone and cortisol) in disease or post-operatively.

2. *Excessive intake of sodium*
Over-transfusion with saline.

The normal kidney has a limit beyond which it cannot excrete more sodium. When sodium is retained, water is also retained. Fluid passes from the intra-cellular fluid into the extra-cellular fluid. This rise in extra-cellular fluid volume causes peripheral oedema, raised venous pressure, and pulmonary oedema leading to respiratory failure. The rise in blood volume leads to an increase in cardiac output and hypertension, and a rapid increase in blood volume causes cardiac failure. If sodium retention is prolonged, death occurs due to dehydration of cells.

> **Blood**
>
> *Serum sodium:* may not be raised owing to the retention of fluid.

Oedema

Oedema is an excess of fluid in the tissues. Normally fluid is forced into tissue spaces by the force of the blood pressure at the arterial end of capillaries. At the venous end of the capillary the blood pressure has dropped and the plasma proteins exert an osmotic pressure which draws the fluid back. The lymphatics drain any excess fluid.

CAUSES OF OEDEMA

1. *Increased blood pressure in capillaries*
An increase of pressure at the venous end of the capillary can overcome the osmotic pressure of the plasma proteins, so that fluid is not reabsorbed. Venous pressure increases in cardiac failure and obstruction to venous drainage for any reason, e.g. venous thrombosis, varicose veins, pressure of pregnant uterus on the pelvic veins.

2. Reduced osmotic pressure of blood

When the osmotic pressure is lower than the blood pressure at the venous end of the capillary, the tissue fluid is not reabsorbed. Osmotic pressure can be reduced because of lack of plasma proteins or because of capillary damage.

(a) *Plasma protein deficiency* can be due to a failure of intake or of absorption, or to excessive loss as in albuminuria of the nephrotic syndrome.

(b) *Increased capillary permeability* can be due to damage by burns, chemicals, infections and insect bites. Proteins pass through the capillary into the tissue fluid; the osmotic pressure of the blood is lowered and fluid is not withdrawn from the extra-cellular fluid into the blood.

3. Retention of sodium

Retention of sodium causes increased osmotic pressure in the extra-cellular fluid and therefore water is retained.

4. Obstruction of lymphatics

When lymphatics are removed surgically or blocked (e.g. by neoplasms, infections) fluid cannot drain into them from the tissues.

Potassium

Potassium is present in nearly all food, so a dietary deficiency is unlikely except in starvation. Most of the body potassium is in the cells, but the maintenance of a normal level in the plasma is vital (normal: 3.5-5.0 mmol/l.).

Potassium is important in normal neuromuscular conduction in skeletal, cardiac and intestinal muscle. Plasma levels which are too high or too low interfere with normal functioning.

The level of potassium in the plasma is not always an indication of overall potassium level.

POTASSIUM EXCESS

If potassium is retained in excess in the body, hyperkalaemia (excess of potassium in the blood) occurs. Excess in the cells does not occur. Retention of potassium is due to failure of the kidney to excrete excess potassium ions. This may happen:
1. in chronic renal failure;
2. when there is deficiency of adreno-cortical hormone (e.g. in an Addisonian crisis), because the function of renal tubules is impaired and potassium is not excreted;
3. when a patient who has impaired renal function is given too much potassium for the treatment of hypokalaemia.

There may be a temporary raised plasma potassium level when potassium moves from the cells into the extra-cellular fluid. A normal kidney excretes the excess and the shift may result in an overall deficiency of potassium.

POTASSIUM DEFICIENCY

Potassium deficiency in the cells and hypokalaemia (potassium deficiency in the blood) are due to excessive loss of potassium in gastrointestinal secretions and in urine.

1. Gastrointestinal loss

Potassium deficiency can be due to prolonged loss of gastrointestinal secretions, e.g. by diarrhoea or vomiting.

2. Urinary loss

(a) Prolonged use of diuretics without potassium supplements.
(b) In disorders of the renal tubules.
(c) An excess of adreno-cortical hormone (aldosterone) alters renal tubular function and causes too much potassium to be excreted.

A shift of potassium from cells into the extra-cellular fluid may cause a temporary raised plasma potassium, but excretion in the urine may lead to an overall potassium deficiency. A shift of potassium from the plasma into the cells can cause hypokalaemia.

POTASSIUM SHIFT FROM EXTRA-CELLULAR FLUID INTO CELLS

This happens:
1. with prolonged intravenous infusion of glucose-saline without potassium supplement
2. by the action of insulin given for the treatment of ketosis
3. in alkalosis potassium moves into cells to replace deficient hydrogen ions.

POTASSIUM SHIFT FROM CELLS INTO EXTRA-CELLULAR FLUID

Potassium can be lost in the urine when there is a movement of potassium from cells into the extra-cellular fluid. There may be a temporary raised potassium level, but with normal excretion the body loses potassium. This can happen:
1. in ketosis of diabetes and other acidoses, hydrogen ions displace potassium ions from the cells; potassium passes into the extra-cellular fluid and is excreted;
2. during haemolysis, because a lot of potassium is released from red blood cells;
3. during necrosis of cells, e.g. burns, crush injuries, after operations.

CLINICAL EFFECTS OF POTASSIUM ABNORMALITIES

Potassium deficiency

This causes abnormalities of neuromuscular activity:
1. muscular weakness and paralysis, including the respiratory muscles;
2. cardiac arrhythmias, weakness of heart muscle, fall of blood pressure;
3. ileus – a dilatation of the bowel due to weakness of muscle.

Hyperkalaemia

This causes abnormal neuromuscular functioning, particularly affecting the conducting tissue of the heart. ECG changes occur, the heart rate is slowed, and cardiac arrest can occur.

Acid-Base Balance

The acidity or alkalinity of a solution depends on the hydrogen ion concentration. The pH scale has been derived mathematically to give a simple numerical scale of hydrogen ion activity. (pH is actually the negative logarithm of hydrogen ion concentration.) 6.8 represents the neutral point at 37°C. The pH of the blood is normally between 7.36 and 7.42, i.e. blood is slightly alkaline. In a healthy person it varies only a little within this range. Arterial blood is slightly more alkaline than venous blood because it contains less carbon dioxide in solution (see below). A pH below 7.0 or above 7.8 is not compatible with life.

Normally the pH is kept within the narrow range necessary for health by temporary and then by permanent biochemical adjustments.

Buffers are biochemical systems which make the temporary adjustments by mopping up extra hydrogen (acid) or hydroxyl (base) ions. The extra acid or base is temporarily neutralized and the pH is kept constant or changed only slightly.

Permanent adjustments are made by the lungs and kidneys.

One of the important buffer systems in the blood is the bicarbonate/carbonic acid system in the plasma. It should be noted that all the carbon dioxide in solution is referred to as carbonic acid although most of it is not actually carbonic acid. The pH of the blood remains constant if the ratio between bicarbonate and carbon dioxide remains constant at 20:1.

Other important buffering in the blood is carried out by haemoglobin in the red blood cells and by plasma proteins.

The respiratory centre in the brain responds to changes in pH by increasing or decreasing carbon dioxide excretion.

RESPIRATION

Metabolism in the body produces carbon dioxide as an end product. In solution some of this becomes carbonic acid. Extra hydrogen ions are neutralized by combining the bicarbonate to form carbonic acid.

When there is a lowering of pH the lungs excrete more carbon dioxide and the level of carbonic acid in the plasma falls.

When the pH rises respiration is reduced in rate and depth, carbon dioxide is retained and plasma carbonic acid rises.

The normal response of the respiratory centre is important in maintaining the correct ratio of bicarbonate to carbonic acid, and therefore in maintaining the pH.

For as long as the ratio is maintained between carbonate and carbon dioxide, the acidosis or alkalosis is compensated. In the early stages of acidosis the bicarbonate will rise and in the early stages of alkalosis fall. When the disturbances becomes more severe, the bicarbonate will not remain in the constant ratio to carbon dioxide and the disturbance will be uncompensated.

RENAL MECHANISM

Final adjustment is made by the kidney which can secrete an acid or alkaline urine with a wide pH range of 4.5-8.5. In order to reduce the acidity of the extra-cellular fluid the kidney excretes phosphoric acid and sulphuric acid (derived from ingested protein) as acid phosphate and sulphate. Hydrogen ions combine with ammonia to be excreted as ammonium salts. Bicarbonate is reabsorbed.

If there is alkalosis, the kidney excretes an alkaline phosphate instead of the acid form, and also excretes bicarbonate.

If the normal mechanisms fail and the pH falls to 7.3 or rises above 7.5, an acidaemia or alkalaemia exists. The cause of this acid-base disturbance may be respiratory or metabolic.

Tests for acidaemia and alkalaemia

pH of blood (plasma): is measured by specially designed instruments. Particular precautions must be taken: blood must be arterial or treated to be identical with arterial blood; it must be collected anaerobically and kept at 0°C.

Pco_2. The partial pressure of carbon dioxide in the blood (partial pressure is proportional to volume) is: 1. directly measured by special instruments, 2. indirectly measured by measuring the carbon dioxide in alveolar air or in expired air.

The Pco_2 represents the plasma carbonic acid level and is useful when the acid-base abnormality is due to respiratory causes.

Plasma bicarbonate: measured indirectly from total plasma carbon dioxide.

Standard bicarbonate: this is the concentration of bicarbonate in plasma after the sample of whole blood has been standardized, i.e. brought to standard conditions of Pco_2 40 mmHg at 37°C. Bicarbonate levels are particularly useful when the acid-base disturbance is metabolic.

Plasma potassium: should be measured in all cases of alkalaemia.

Respiratory Disturbances

1. RESPIRATORY ACIDAEMIA

There is an increase in plasma carbonic acid because carbon dioxide is not expired in sufficient volume.

Causes

1. Obstruction of the respiratory passages.
2. Paralysis of the muscles of respiration.
3. Diseases of the lung causing inadequate gaseous exchange.
4. Depression of the respiratory centre by drugs, e.g. morphine, barbiturates.
5. Inhalation of excess carbon dioxide in atmosphere, e.g. in anaesthetic mishaps, industrial accidents.

---

pH: falls.
Pco_2: increased.

> *Bicarbonate:* increases at first, later fails to keep up with Pco_2 increase.

2. RESPIRATORY ALKALAEMIA

This is a reduction in carbonic acid because too much carbon dioxide is expired. The hyperventilation which causes this may be due to: fever; salicylate overdose; encephalitis; high altitude; overventilation on a respirator.

> *pH:* rises.
> *Pco₂:* falls.
> *Bicarbonate:* falls at first, later does not fall in proportion to carbon dioxide fall.

Metabolic Disturbances

1. METABOLIC ACIDAEMIA

This is a decrease in bicarbonate concentration in the plasma.
Causes:
(a) *Loss of bicarbonate*
loss of intestinal secretions, e.g. diarrhoea; or as a result of fistula or ileostomy;
renal tubular acidosis.
(b) *Inability to excrete acid*
acute and chronic renal disease;
transplanation of ureters into the colon (acidosis occurs because the intestine reabsorbs chloride and hydrogen from the urine).
(c) *Metabolic disturbance causing excess acid production*
ketosis of diabetes mellitus;
starvation.

> *pH:* falls.
> *Bicarbonate:* reduced.
> *Carbon dioxide:* falls at first due to increased respiration, later the fall is not sufficent to maintain the normal bicarbonate/carbon dioxide ratio.

2. METABOLIC ALKALAEMIA

This is an increase in the bicarbonate level.
Causes:
(a) *Intake of base*
large dose of bicarbonate or other antacid.
(b) *Retention of base*
excess reabsorption of bicarbonate, e.g. due to some diuretics.
(c) *Loss of hydrogen ions*
vomiting.
(d) *Potassium deficiency*
hydrogen ions replace the missing intra-cellular potassium ions.

> *pH:* raised.
> *Bicarbonate:* raised.
> *Pco₂:* raised at first, later its rise does not maintain the bicarbonate/carbon dioxide ratio.

CLINICAL SIGNS OF ACID-BASE DISTURBANCES

Severe acidaemia stimulates the respiratory centre so much that the patient is described as having 'air hunger'. This is seen in ketosis.

In alkalaemia there is loss of appetite, nausea and tetany. Respiration is depressed and the release of oxygen from haemoglobin to the tissues is reduced.

Chapter 9 Degenerations

Cells can have their functions impaired or can die if:
(a) they do not get enough oxygen,
(b) they do not get proper nourishment,
(c) toxic products of metabolism are not removed,
(d) they are attacked by other harmful substances.

For their functioning cells are dependent upon a series of enzyme reactions, and tampering with these enzyme is the cause of malfunctioning and death.

Some cells are less sensitive than others, e.g. fibrous tissue can withstand lack of oxygen for a long time, but nervous tissue dies within a few minutes.

Degenerations are the changes detectable in cells whose functions have been seriously impaired. If a harmful stimulus ceases without inflicting permanent damage on the enzyme system, a cell can recover its normal function; but if they cannot recover they die and necrosis sets in.

Necrosis is the series of pathological changes which occur in a cell after death:
(a) the cell absorbs fluid and swells,
(b) the nucleus of the cell either fades away or becomes dark, shrinks and is extruded from the cell either entire or in fragments.

Phagocytic cells — polymorphs and histiocytes — are attracted into the dying tissue and remove the bits of the dead cells by absorbing them. If, however, a large area of tissue dies, the phagocytic cells are too few to remove it all, and some necrotic tissue remains as a pale, structureless mass. It is firm at first but softens if it is in the brain or becomes infected.

CLOUDY SWELLING

The cells in degenerating tissue become swollen because sodium can pass freely through the cell membrane into the cell and takes water in with it. The outline of the cell become blurred. If a lot of tissue is affected, it becomes pale and swollen, and when it is cut across it tends to bulge out over the edge of any capsule that encloses it.

FATTY CHANGES

In some degenerations fat enters the cell, and it and the fat already there degenerate. Tissues become swollen, yellowish and slightly greasy.

Such fatty changes are common in the liver as a result of heart failure or infection, anaemia, poor diet. Chronic anaemia is one of the causes of fatty degeneration in the heart.

HYALINE DEGENERATION

Hyaline degeneration is the name given to the appearance of clusters of an acid-staining protein-phospholipid complex, and is particularly liable to occur in striated muscle in typhoid fever and in the liver cells of chronic alcoholics.

The same term, hyaline degeneration, is given also to a deposit of glycoprotein, fat and fibrin which develops beneath the endothelium of arterioles in hypertension and diabetes mellitus.

Ischaemia

Ischaemia means that the blood supply is inadequate to provide oxygen and other substances needed for metabolism.

Anoxia is deprivation of oxygen and may be partial or complete.

The effects of anoxia on tissues depends upon:
(a) the degree of anoxia,
(b) the duration of the anoxia,
(c) the nature of the tissue affected: some tissues (e.g. nervous tissue) are more sensitive than others.
(d) the amount of tissue involved: the anoxia may be a general one of the whole body due to anaemia, cardiac disease, respiratory disease or poisoning, or of an area of tissue supplied by a single blood vessel.

Ischaemia appears as:
infarction
replacement fibrosis.

INFARCTION

An *infarct* is an area of necrosis arising from anoxia as the result of an acute and complete obstruction of the blood supply through a particular artery. It is sharply defined and usually wedge-shaped.

The effect of such an interference with blood supply will depend upon whether or not there are other blood channels, called collateral channels, through which the tissue can get its blood when its main source is cut off. In many organs (e.g. skeletal muscle, liver, skin) there is a collateral blood supply adequate enough to take over in an emergency. The organs in which the collateral system is inadequate are:
brain   heart
kidney   spleen.
In these the obstruction of an artery is likely to cause an infarct.

Common causes of infarction are:
(a) the complete obstruction of an atheromatous artery by a clot of blood;
(b) an embolus: an embolus is any mass in the blood not normally present there;
(c) twisting of the pedicle through which run the blood vessels to an organ; this can happen to:
loop of intestine   testis
ovarian cyst   fibromyoma;
As the veins become obstructed before the arteries in this event, bleeding into the tissue is likely to occur, producing a haemorrhagic infarct;
(d) accidental tying of an artery during a surgical operation.

The pathological changes which take place in an infarct vary with the kind of tissue involved. The usual pattern is:
(a) some blood leaks back into the infarcted area from the venules; in soft tissues, such as the lungs, the blood makes the infarct dark,
(b) fluid accumulates and makes the infarct pale,
(c) phagocytes invade the area,
(d) with the breaking down of blood pigments, the infarct becomes yellowish,
(e) the infarct becomes softer,
(f) fibrosis starts at the edge and grows inwards, replacing the infarcted tissue with scar-tissue.

Infarction of a limb can occur in:
(a) old people with severe atherosclerosis
(b) diabetics with arterial degeneration
(c) Raynaud's disease
(d) people whose peripheral arteries have become blocked by large clots.

Dry gangrene is likely: the part involved becomes dry, shrinks and goes black, with usually a sharp line of demarcation between diseased and healthy tissue. *Moist gangrene* is the putrefaction which takes place if gangrenous tissue becomes infected.

REPLACEMENT FIBROSIS

Replacement fibrosis occurs in tissues which have been submitted to a mild, persistent degree of anoxia. Organs particularly liable to be affected are:
heart   kidney
brain   liver.

The normal tissue of the part dies and is replaced by fibrous tissue.

Atrophy

Atrophy is a reduction in size of an organ or tissue. It can be general or localized. It can be due to the following causes:
(a) *Starvation*. Fat is mainly affected, but other tissues can become involved. The heart and brain are little, if at all, affected, even in severe and prolonged starvation.
(b) *Pressure*. The growth of one structure may reduce the size of another, e.g. a renal tumour can flatten and shrink the adrenal gland on top of the kidney.
(c) *Reduced blood supply*. Replacement fibrosis is smaller than the healthy tissue it replaces.
(d) *Reduced functional activity*. A muscle wastes if its nerve supply is cut or a joint it acts on is immobilized. Confinement in bed for a long time produces atrophy of bone.
(e) *Reduced hormonal stimulation*. A failure of pituitary gland function produces atrophy of the endocrine glands normally stimulated by its hormones. At the menopause the ovary ceases to be stimulated by the follicle-stimulating hormone of the pituitary gland and starts to atrophy.
(f) *Old age*. A generalized atrophy sets in as a result of decreased physical activity, decreased hormonal output, reduced metabolism, and often a reduced intake of food. The height may lessen as a result of shrinking of the intervertebral discs.

Degeneration Following Exposure to Radiation

Exposure to ionizing radiation may be due to:
(a) normal background radiation from outer space, rocks, soil;
(b) diagnostic X-rays;
(c) therapeutic radiation by X-rays, radium, etc;
(d) radio-active isotopes used in medicine and industry;
(e) handling and carrying radio-active material;
(f) nuclear warfare.

Radiation affects cells most when they are undergoing mitosis, i.e. dividing into two.

The effects depend upon the dose of radiation received and length of exposure to it. The ill effects of radiation are cumulative and repeated exposure to small doses will in time produce serious damage. With small doses mitosis is temporarily checked and then renewed with excess vigour. With larger doses mitosis is completely stopped, and enzyme systems in the cells are put out of action. With still larger doses non-mitotic cells as well as mitotic ones show degeneration.

The tissues most sensitive to radiation are those whose cells are normally undergoing mitosis:

cells of fetus	red bone marrow
lymph tissue	epithelium of gastro-
squamous	intestinal tract
epithelium	malignant cells
ovary	testis

The tissues least sensitive to radiation are:
all kinds of muscle   nervous tissue.

OVER-EXPOSURE TO RADIATION

Over-exposure to radiation can cause:
chromosomal abnormalities
congenital defects
chronic myeloid leukaemia
sterility if ovaries or testes are affected.

Radiation sickness follows exposure to a large dose of radiation. The number of platelets in the blood falls, producing purpura; an aplastic anaemia follows interference with blood formation in the bone marrow; and a stopping of antibody formation reduces resistance to infection.

Chapter 10 Neoplasms

A *neoplasm* (new growth) is a mass of cells which grow continuously and apparently without restraint and without physiological or anatomical need. It is often called a *tumour*, but this term applies to any swelling, e.g. that is caused by an abscess.

A neoplasm can arise in any kind of cell. Some kinds of cell are more prone than others to develop neoplasms, and neoplasms are least likely to develop in those tissues which normally do not regenerate: striped muscle fibres and nerve cells. Usually only one type of cell is involved, but occasionally more.

Neoplasms are divided into:
I, benign neoplasms;
II, malignant neoplasms.

I. Benign neoplasms

A benign (simple) neoplasm has the following characteristics.
1. Its cells remain similar to those from which it arises, they do not show mitotic figures (the chromosome changes of a cell in the act of dividing), and they are of uniform size and appearance.
2. It usually grows slowly, over years, and remains localized in one place, not spreading to other tissues; it may stop growing or become smaller.
3. It may be enclosed within a capsule, or where there is no capsule it is clearly demarcated from normal tissue.
4. It does not usually show degenerative changes.
5. It has a supply of blood vessels and nerves similar to that of the normal tissue.
6. It produces evidence of its presence by being palpable, by pressing on adjacent tissues, or if it is composed of secreting tissue by producing an excess of that secretion, e.g. a neoplasm of the islets of Langerhans can produce an excess of insulin.

Common benign neoplasms are:
1. *Lipoma*. A lipoma is a neoplasm of fat enclosed within a capsule. The neoplasm may be lobulated and there may be more than one. They occur commonly in subcutaneous fat where they can be felt as smooth swellings.
2. *Neurofibroma*. A neurofibroma arises from the sheath of a nerve. It can cause trouble if it grows in an enclosed space or narrow canal, e.g. a neurofibroma growing from the sheath of the auditory nerve in the auditory canal in the temporal bone can press on the auditory and facial nerves.
3. *Myoma* (leiomyoma, fibromyoma, fibroid). A myoma is a neoplasm of smooth muscle and fibrous tissue. It commonly occurs in the uterus.
4. *Adenoma*. An adenoma is a neoplasm of secretory epithelial cells. They occur in the pituitary gland, thyroid gland, parathyroid gland, adrenal cortex, ovary, pancreas and intestine. Ducts are not formed and if fluid is secreted by the neoplasm a cyst forms, composed of fluid surrounded by secreting cells.
5. *Meningioma*. A meningioma arises from the meninges surrounding the brain. It is usually benign but can in time start to infiltrate the brain adjacent to it; it does not form metastases.

II. Malignant neoplasms

A malignant neoplasms has the following characteristics.
1. Its cells may not be similar to those from which they have arisen; they commonly show a reversion to a more primitive kind of cell, show

mitotic figures because they are dividing rapidly, vary in size and shape, and have nuclei which vary in size and shape and often stain heavily with dyes.

2. It grows rapidly, invading and destroying tissue locally and spreading to other parts of the body.

3. It is not enclosed within a capsule and is not clearly demarcated from normal tissue as it is growing into it at various points.

4. It has an abnormal supply of blood vessels and nerves.

5. It may produce cachexia – malaise, loss of weight, loss of strength and loss of energy.

Malignant cells invade healthy tissue by infiltrating between the normal cells and eventually destroying them.

From their original site they can spread to other parts of the body by:

1. *Lymphatic spread.* Malignant cells invade lymph vessels and grow along them into the lymph nodes draining the part. The malignant cells replace the normal cells and spread along lymph vessels from one node to another. They can break through the capsule surrounding a node and causing it to become matted to another, forming a hard mass.

2. *Blood stream spread.* Malignant cells invade capillaries and veins (and less easily arteries), and once they are in the blood stream can be transported to other parts of the body. Some are destroyed, but others start off new growths in any part they stick in. A *metastasis* (secondary neoplasm) is one of these secondary growths of malignant cells; it is composed of the same malignant cells as the primary neoplasm.

3. *Transcoelomic spread.* If malignant cells invade the peritoneum, pleura or pericardium, they can disseminate along the surface or via lymph vessels to other parts of it. An effusion of fluid into the cavity is likely to follow: the fluid may contain malignant cells.

TYPES OF MALIGNANT NEOPLASMS

Malignant neoplasms can be classified according to the cells from which they arise or which they resemble. The main types are as follows:

I. *Carcinoma*

A carcinoma (cancer) is a neoplasm that arises from epithelial tissue.

Type	Site of carcinoma

1. *Squamous cell carcinoma*
(i) Cells of stratified epithelium, such as the skin. — Skin lip mouth oesophagus pharynx larynx cervix of the uterus

(ii) Cells which have changed to a stratified appearance. — Bronchus gall bladder renal pelvis bladder

2. *Basal cell carcinoma*
Arises from stratified epithelium of skin, but has special features. — Skin (as a rodent ulcer)

3. *Transitional cell tumour*
Arises from transitional cells in the urinary tract. — Renal pelvis ureter bladder

4. *Adenocarcinoma*
Arises from secretory or glandular epithelium — Gastrointestinal tract biliary passages breast kidney ovary prostate gland pancreas thyroid gland

5. *Undifferentiated carcinoma*
Rapidly growing and very malignant neoplasms whose cells are so abnormal that their source cannot be determined.

II. *Sarcoma*

A sarcoma is a malignant neoplasm arising from connective tissue (fibrous tissue, fat, cartilage, synovial membrane, bone, muscle, blood vessels, lymph vessels, serous membranes). They are less common than carcinomas, tend to occur in younger rather than older people, may arise in a previously benign neoplasm, are very malignant, and tend to spread more via blood vessels than via lymph vessels.

Type	Site
1. *Fibrosarcoma* Connective tissue anywhere; a *myxosarcoma* is a fibrosarcoma that has undergone myxomatous, jelly-like changes.	Fascia between muscles, behind the peritoneal cavity, subcutaneous tissue, periosteum bone
2. *Leimyosarcoma* Arises from smooth muscle	Gastrointestinal tract uterus
3. *Liposarcoma* A rare neoplasm of fat cells	May arise in a lipoma
4. *Chondrosarcoma* A neoplasm of cartilage, arising in adolescence or early adult life.	Cartilage, usually in the pelvis or end of long bone.
5. *Synovial sarcoma* Arises in synovial membrane	Large joints
6. *Osteosarcoma* A neoplasm of bone, arising in adolescence or early adult life; can be a complication of Paget's disease.	Bone, usually the end of a long bone
7. *Rhabdomyosarcoma* A neoplasm in which appear striped muscle cells or cells with striations.	Infancy: bladder, prostate gland, vagina, orbit, palate. Adult life: skeletal muscle
8. *Angeiosarcoma* A very malignant neoplasm of vessels. Sarcoma of lymph vessels	Blood vessels lymph vessels

(lymphangeiosarcoma) can follow chronic lymphatic obstruction or irradiation of lymph nodes for cancer.

9. *Mesothelioma* A neoplasm of serous membrane	Pleura, peritoneum
10. *Spindle cell sarcoma* A very malignant neoplasm of spindle-shaped cells, not differentiated into special types of cell.	Connective tissue anywhere

III. *Neoplasm of nervous tissue*

Neoplasms rarely arise from nerve cells in the central nervous system (brain, spinal cord). They arise usually from glial cells, from the meninges, or from the sheaths of nerves. Outside the central nervous system, they can arise from peripheral nerves, from the adrenal medulla and from the retina.

Type	Site
1. *Glioma* Vary from benign to malignant. Classified according to cell type into: astrocytoma oligodendroglioma ependymoma medulloblastoma (from cells which have not become differentiated into nerve cells or glial cells).	Brain spinal cord
2. *Meningioma* Slowly growing, hard neoplasms, can press on brain or become locally malignant.	Meninges

3. *Neuroma*
Arise from cells in the nerve sheath, may be multiple.

Cranial and spinal nerves; *acoustic neuroma* is one arising from the sheath of the 8th cranial (auditory) nerve.

4. *Neuroblastoma*
Malignant neoplasm of childhood; quickly spreads to bone, liver and other adrenal.

Adrenal medulla, sympathetic nervous system in posterior mediastinum and abdomen.

5. *Retinoblastoma*
Malignant neoplasm of childhood; arises in primitive cells in the retina.

Retina

6. *Ganglioneuroma*
Benign neoplasm of autonomic nervous system.

Posterior mediastinum, abdomen, adrenal medulla.

7. *Phaeochromocytoma*
Neoplasm of secreting cells, with overproduction of adrenaline and noradrenaline and attacks of hypertension

Adrenal medulla

8. *Malignant melanoma*
Arises in cells which have originated in the embryo in the neural crest and migrated elsewhere.

Skin, choroid coat of eye

IV. *Mixed neoplasms*
Mixed neoplasms show a mixture of cells arising from more than one type of cell.

Type   *Site*

1. *Mixed parotid neoplasm*
Composed of a mixture of epithelial cells in a myxomatous (jelly-like) background.

Parotid gland

2. *Fibroadenoma of breast*
Firm nodule of usually benign tissue, composed of epithelial and supporting cells.

Breast

3. *Nephrobastoma*
Arises from primitive kidney tissue before it has become differentiated. A malignant neoplasm of childhood, liable to produce metastases in the lungs.

Kidney

4. *Teratoma*
A mixed neoplasm of various kinds of cells and tissues of ectodermal, mesodermal and endodermal origin (hair, bone, teeth, muscle, brain, alimentary tract, etc). Probably arises from cells which have become displaced early in fetal life. Teratoma of testis is usually malignant. Teratoma of ovary is usually benign, and forms a large 'dermoid' cyst, with bits of skin forming the outer wall.

Most commonly in testis and ovary; can occur elsewhere

Causes of malignant neoplasms

The precise cause which starts off in a cell the changes which produce a malignant neoplasm is usually unknown. Presumably it has the ability to reproduce chromosomal changes which set off a cell dividing madly. It is possible that the body may produce in a lifetime a number of potentially malignant cells, but that these cells are detected and destroyed by lymphocytes, one of their functions being the hunting out and destruction of abnormal cells which might harm the body; and the growth of a malignant neoplasm may therefore be the result of a breakdown of a normal defence mechanism.

Heredity is known to be an important factor in the production of malignant disease. There is evidence that:
(a) if one of a pair of identical twins develops a malignant neoplasm, the other is more likely to develop a similar neoplasm than would be expected by chance;
(b) there is a high incidence of cancer of the breast and uterus in relatives of a patient with either of these;
(c) there is an increased risk of cancer in some familial diseases, e.g. polyposis coli, neurofibromatosis.

ESTABLISHED CAUSES

1. Carcinoma of the bronchus (lung) and carcinoma of the larynx are caused usually by smoking. The more tobacco one smokes, especially cigarettes, the more likely is one to develop one of these carcinomas. The factor responsible has not been established but is probably a tar.
2. Carcinoma of the skin can be produced by repeated exposure to tar and shale oil, which can happen in certain industries.
3. Carcinoma of the bladder occurs in workers in plastics, rubber and aniline dyes.
4. Precancerous and cancerous lesions of the skin occur in people exposed to ionizing radiations, e.g. fair-haired people who live in bright sunlight (e.g. Australians) and people treated with X-rays or radium.
5. Leukaemia has a high incidence in radiologists, patients treated with radiotherapy for ankylosing spondylitis, and in survivors of atomic bomb explosions.
6. Carcinoma of the bronchus can occur in miners mining radio-active ores.

NOT ESTABLISHED BUT POSSIBLE CAUSES

1. *Viruses.* Some viruses can apparently cause cancer in animals. *Malignant lymphoma* (Burkitt lymphoma), which occurs in certain parts of Africa, is a human disease which may be caused by an infective agent transmitted by mosquitoes.
2. *Hormonal abnormalities.* There is some evidence that steroids play a part in the development of some cancers, but they have not been proved to be the primary cause. Stilboestrol (a synthetic oestrogen) can in some men retard or halt the progress of carcinoma of the prostate gland.
3. *Parasites.* Schistosomes, parasites of the bladder and bowel in many tropical and subtropical countries, have been thought to be a cause of cancer of the bladder.

Chapter 11   The Circulatory System

CONGENITAL DISEASES OF THE HEART AND BLOOD VESSELS

Congenital diseases of the heart and blood vessels occur in about 1 birth in 200 and are an important cause of perinatal mortality.

The development of the chambers and valves of the heart and of the great vessels is normally completed by the end of the second fetal month. Toxic factors known to interfere with normal development of them are:
maternal German measles (rubella),
other virus diseases,
irradiation,
thalidomide and possibly other drugs.
Major chromosomal abnormalities are not usually present, but some families show a high incidence of congenital heart disease, members of an affected family being liable to develop the same abnormality.

Subacute bacterial endocarditis is a common complication of any congenital heart disease.

1. FALLOT'S TETRALOGY

This is the result of a faulty development of the ventricular region of the heart.

The lesion consists of 4 abnormalities:
(a) a stenosis of the pulmonary valve,
(b) ventricular septal defect, a defect in the wall between the two ventricles: the defect can be so large that the ventricles function as one,
(c) over-riding of the aorta, which lies over the upper ends of both ventricles,
(d) right ventricular hypertrophy: the ventricle hypertrophies in order to overcome the resistance set up by the stenosed pulmonary valve.

The important lesions are the pulmonary stenosis and the ventricular septal defect. Taking the line of least resistance, deoxygenated blood passes from the right ventricle through the aperture in the septum into the left ventricle and so into the aorta without passing through the lungs and becoming oxygenated. The baby is therefore cyanosed, a 'blue baby'.

There is only a slight flow of blood through the pulmonary vessels and the pulmonary arteries are abnormally small. In about 25 per cent of cases the aortic arch lies on the right side of the thorax. Clubbing of the fingers and polycythaemia (an excess of red blood cells) can occur. Death usually occurs in childhood from a syncopal attack or from a cerebral abscess due to a spread of infection from subacute bacterial endocarditis.

2. ACYANOTIC FALLOT'S TETRALOGY

In this variant of Fallot's tetralogy the four lesions are all present but the stenosis of the pulmonary artery is slight and blood can pass through it into the lungs to become oxygenated. The patient is therefore not cyanosed.

3. PULMONARY ATRESIA

In this condition the pulmonary arteries or pulmonary valve do not develop normally and blood can get into the lungs only through the bronchial arteries (the small arteries which pass from the descending thoracic aorta to supply the lung tissue).

4. PULMONARY VALVE STENOSIS

This causes about 10 per cent of all cases of congenital heart disease. The valve is thickened and the cusps fused. The right ventricle hypertrophies to overcome the obstruction to outflow through the valve, and the right atrium has to hypertrophy to overcome the increased resistance to the filling of the right ventricle. The cardiac output is reduced by the obstruction set up to the circulation.

5. VENTRICULAR SEPTAL DEFECT

One or more holes may be present in the ventricular septum. Small defects are compatible with a full normal life and may close spontaneously in childhood. About 30 per cent of patients with the defect develop subacute bacterial endocarditis. Large defects can be fatal in infancy, and with untreated large defects the average life expectancy is 35 years.

6. ATRIAL SEPTAL DEFECT

In this condition there is a failure of development of the septum between the two atria. The foramen ovale is the large hole in the atrial wall through which during fetal life blood passes from the right into the left atrium. Normally the final development of the atrial wall with closure of the foramen occurs within a few days of birth, but a hole of varying size may persist.

With a small defect (less than 1.5 cm. in diameter) a normal life span is possible; but patients with larger holes are likely to develop atrial fibrillation in middle age and to die of cardiac failure.

A 'paradoxical embolism' can occur when there is a patent foramen ovale: an embolus (such as a piece of detached thrombus) which has arisen in the systemic side of the body and travelled up to the right atrium can pass into the left atrium and cause an infarct on the systemic side instead of in the lung.

7. DEXTROCARDIA

The heart lies with the apex pointing towards the right instead of to the left. The abdominal viscera may be in the normal position or be completely transposed with all the contents of the thorax and chest forming a mirror-image of the normal.

8. TRANSPOSITION OF THE GREAT VESSELS

In this condition the aorta develops in front of the pulmonary artery instead of behind it. The aorta can arise from the right ventricle and the pulmonary artery from the left ventricle, a condition that is incompatible with life after birth unless there is also a defect in the ventricular wall allowing blood to pass from one ventricle into the other.

9. RIGHT AORTIC ARCH

The arch of the aorta develops on the right side of the thorax instead of the left.

10. PATENT DUCTUS ARTERIOSUS

The ductus arteriosus is a short artery connecting the pulmonary artery with the arch of the aorta and remains open during fetal life to enable the deoxygenated blood from the head to pass from the right ventricle into the aorta, whence it travels to the lower part of the body and thence to the placenta to be oxygenated. With the change of pressures as the lungs inflate after birth, the ductus arteriosus should collapse and become obliterated within about 14 days.

A failure of the ductus to close may be due to fetal anoxia or be part of the rubella syndrome.

As the pressure in the aorta is higher than that in the pulmonary artery, blood passes throughout the cardiac cycle from the aorta into the pulmonary artery and so into the lungs. If the patent ductus is not closed, left ventricular failure can occur in infancy or later; subacute bacterial endocarditis is a common complication.

11. COARCTATION OF THE AORTA

This is a congenital narrowing of the aorta which in 98 per cent of cases occurs immediately below the origin of the left subclavian artery. It may be associated with:
a bicuspid aortic valve (two cusps instead of three);
congenital aneurysms on the cerebral arteries;
aortic stenosis;
other abnormalities of the cardiovascular system.

A collateral circulation is likely to develop between arteries in the upper part of the body and arteries in the lower part so that the obstruction is by-passed. There is hypertension in the arteries above the lesion and hypotension in the arteries below. The upper part of the thorax may be well developed and the legs conspicuously thin. In untreated patients, death from cardiac failure due to the hypertension is likely in childhood and the survivors of childhood rarely live beyond the age of 40, death being due to cardiac failure, cerebral haemorrhage, rupture of the aorta or subacute bacterial endocarditis (if the aortic valve is abnormal).

Infections of the Heart and Blood Vessels

1. RHEUMATIC HEART DISEASE

Acute rheumatic fever can occur about 14-21 days after infection of the throat or tonsils by *Str. pyogenes,* a haemolytic streptococcus, and is thought to be an autoimmune reaction. Streptococci cannot be found in the cardiac lesions. All parts of the heart are likely to be affected.

(a) *Endocardium*. The endocardium, especially that of the valves, shows an inflammatory reaction. *Vegetations* appear on the valves. These vegetations are clumps of inflammatory matter (mostly platelets and fibrin) which form as small, white or yellow, irregular, wart-like projections along the line of closure of the valves. Any valve can be affected, but those most likely are the mitral and the aortic.

(b) *Myocardium*. Typically, the myocardium shows numerous Aschoff nodes, which are small areas of fibrinoid necrosis surrounded by lymphocytes and giant and other cells. With a weak myocardium the heart dilates.

(c) *Pericardium*. The pericardium can be inflamed and a pericardial effusion can fill and distend the pericardial cavity.

Other lesions can be found in the joints, which are swollen and painful, in the skin as rheumatic nodules, in the lungs as an interstitial pneumonitis, and in the brain as cuffs of lymphocytes around the blood vessels, producing chorea.

Blood

White cell count: increased.
Erythrocyte sedimentation rate (ESR): increased.
Antistreptolysin antibody: a high level of antistreptolysin antibody or a rise in titre over several weeks is evidence of a recent streptococcal infection.

An acute rheumatism of the heart may heal completely and the heart become functionally normal or the patient may be left with a permanently damaged heart.

In the damaged heart:

(a) *Endocardium*. The valves may be thick, fibrotic and distorted and the chordae tendineae shortened. In consequence, the valves will function badly, being stenosed and so offering obstruction to the flow of blood through them or by being patent allow blood to pass in the wrong direction. Later in life the valve may become calcified. Mitral stenosis is the most common condition found.

(b) *Myocardium*. Healthy myocardium becomes replaced by fibrous tissue, the heart's efficiency as a pump being reduced.

(c) *Pericardium*. The two walls of pericardium may become attached to one another and fibrotic. This attachment and fibrosis impede the heart's action.

Further complications

(1) *Circulation*. As lesions occur more often on the left side of the heart than on the right, the pulmonary circulation is likely to be affected first and more gravely because of the back pressure. The heart hypertrophies to overcome the disability, but in time it can hypertrophy no more and starts to dilate, with the production of cardiac failure.

(2) *Lungs*. With chronic congestion of the lungs, there is bleeding into the alveoli and eventually thickening of the alveolar wall and impairment of alveolar function.

(3) *Pulmonary artery*. The rise of BP in the pulmonary artery and its branches produces atheromatous degeneration of the arterial wall.

(4) *Emboli*. Thrombosis may occur in the auricle of the left atrium and pieces of the thrombus may become detached, pass as emboli in the blood stream, and cause infarction of an organ or tissue.

(5) *Subacute bacterial endocarditis*. Subacute bacterial endocarditis can develop in a heart whose valves have become permanently damaged.

2. BACTERIAL ENDOCARDITIS

(a) *Acute bacterial endocarditis*

Acute bacterial endocarditis occurs as a terminal infection of the heart valves in a severe septicaemia. The organism (usually a streptococcus, a staphylococcus or a pneumococcus) invades the valves (which may previously have been healthy or diseased), and forms large vegetations, pieces of which can become detached and form septic infarction.

(b) *Subacute bacterial endocarditis*

In spite of its name this is a severe infection with about a 50 per cent mortality.

It is an infection of congenitally abnormal valves etc. or of valves damaged by rheumatism. The organisms are usually streptococci.

Parts commonly affected are:
mitral valve,
aortic valve,
ventricular defects,
persistent ductus arteriosus,
coarctation of the aorta.

The micro-organisms gain entry to the blood stream during:
(a) dental operations without antibiotic cover;
(b) hard chewing on teeth with dental caries or where there is severe periodontal disease;
(c) cystoscopy or other instrumentation of the genito-urinary tract;
(d) operations on the intestine;
(e) osteomyelitis;
(f) puerperal sepsis.

Healthy people with normal heart valves cope with any such invasion of the blood-stream by killing the micro-organisms with the usual defences of the body, but people with valvular and other structural diseases of the heart are at risk for the organisms can invade their endocardium.

When this happens, large soft vegetations appear on the valve or other tissue. These vegetations are formed of platelets, fibrin, inflammatory cells and micro-organisms. Pieces of them can break off and cause infarctions in the lungs when the lesions are in the right side of the heart or the ductus arteriosus, or elsewhere in the body when the lesions are in the mitral or aortic valves or in a coarcted aorta. These infarcts do not go septic. As a further complication, proliferative glomerulonephritis can occur as the result of the deposit in the glomerular capillaries of immune-complexes, composed of antigens and antibodies. Death is due to heart failure, severe valvular disease or renal failure.

3. SYPHILITIC AORTITIS

Syphilis can infect the aorta. The first part of the thoracic aorta, immediately above the aortic valve, is the part commonly affected.

The vasa vasorum (the small arteries supplying the walls of arteries) become surrounded by cuffs of inflammatory cells and become squashed by the inflammatory process and eventually obliterated. This cuts off the blood-supply: the elastic and muscle fibres in the wall degenerate and are replaced by fibrous tissue, which stretches with the intra-aortic pressure into an aneurysm.

An *aneurysm* is a dilatation of a vessel. An aneurysm of the first part of the thoracic aorta is almost always due to syphilis. As the aorta stretches it pulls open the ring of the aortic valve and causes the valve to become incompetent. With blood passing through the valve in the wrong direction, the left ventricle has to hypertrophy to maintain the circulation and when it can hypertrophy no more it dilates and left heart failure follows. As the aneurysm gets larger, it presses on and erodes other structures — the lungs, the oesophagus, the vertebral column, the sternum, etc. — and it may ultimately rupture with a fatal haemorrhage.

Blood

WR: positive in about 85 per cent of cases.

Endocarditis

Endocarditis is an inflammation or degeneration of the endocardium lining the heart and the valves. It occurs in:
rheumatic fever;
acute bacterial endocarditis;
subacute bacterial endocarditis;
systemic lupus erythematosus: vegetations can form on the mitral and tricuspid valves and less commonly on the aortic and pulmonary;
endocardial fibroelastosis: a fibrosis of the endocardium occurring especially in children and East African adults;
of unknown origin, thought to be due to anoxia or to a nutritional or metabolic defect;
advanced malignant or other terminal disease: vegetations can appear on the valves and thrombi form in the recesses of the ventricles and in the atrial appendices.

Myocarditis

Myocarditis is an inflammation or degeneration of the myocardium. It can occur in:
rheumatic fever;
some virus diseases (measles, mumps, influenza, etc.);
septicaemia due to any organism;
diphtheria: the exotoxin of the *B. diphtheriae* causes fatty degeneration of the myocardium;
toxoplasmosis.

Pericarditis

Pericarditis is inflammation of the pericardium. It can occur in:
infections: viral (usually Coxsackie), tuberculosis, septicaemia;
cardiac infarction;
neoplasms, e.g. spread from carcinoma of bronchus;
rheumatic fever and other collagen diseases.

An effusion of fluid into the pericardium is common. The result may be:
(a) adhesions of varying amount form between the parietal and visceral pericardium,
(b) constrictive pericarditis develops due to extensive fibrosis of the pericardium, which obliterates the pericardial sac; the pericardium becomes rigid and the filling of the heart in diastole is reduced.

Heart Failure

Heart failure is the condition in which the heart is unable to pump out an adequate amount of blood to supply the body's need.

LEFT VENTRICULAR FAILURE

Causes

Hypertension
Aortic stenosis and incompetence
Disease of the myocardium, especially coronary artery disease and myocardial infarction

The ventricle will hypertrophy first, if it can, in an attempt to cope with these conditions, but when it can enlarge no more it distends, its muscle fibres become stretched, the ventricular output is reduced, and with each contraction only a small part of the blood in the ventricle is expelled.

Consequences

Reduced cardiac output results in reduced blood flow to the kidneys and reduced glomerular filtration rate. Excessive amounts of sodium and water are retained. The failing of the ventricle causes a rise of pressure in the left atrium and pulmonary veins, which leads to an increase in pulmonary venous pressure and oedema. Respiratory tract infection can occur.

Clinically, dyspnoea, orthopnoea and paroxysmal nocturnal dyspnoea occur.

RIGHT VENTRICULAR FAILURE

Right ventricular failure is usually secondary to left ventricular failure.

Causes

Pulmonary hypersion   Pulmonary valve stenosis
Myocardial disease   Atrial septal defect
Tricuspid valve incompetence

Consequences

A raised systemic venous pressure
Oedema of the tissues (ankles, genitalia, etc.)
Pleural effusion
Ascites
Enlargement of the liver

COMBINED LEFT AND RIGHT VENTRICULAR FAILURE

This is also called congestive heart failure because the effects are a combination of those produced by individual ventricular failure with congestion of the lungs and oedema as prominent features.

Neoplasms of the Heart

Primary neoplasms are uncommon. A *myxoma,* composed of gelatinous, myxomatous tissue, can grow as a polyp (a tumour attached by a stalk to the tissue from which it grows) into one of the chambers, usually the left atrium. A myxoma there sometimes blocks the mitral valve. Fragments of the tumour can be shed and form emboli. *Sarcomas,* and *tumours of muscle, fat, fibrous tissue* or *blood-vessels* can occur.

Secondary neoplasms can occur in the heart. The most common is a spread of neoplastic tissue from a lung.

Neoplasms of Blood Vessels

A *haemangioma* is a neoplasm formed of dilated blood-vessels. Large, cavernous haemangiomata can occur in the skin, skull, meninges and brain in Sturge-Weber's disease. A *'port wine stain'* is a haemangioma of the skin formed by smaller vessels. A *stellate haemangioma* (spider naevus) is composed of a central vein and radiating capillaries; they occur in healthy children and adults and can become more numerous in pregnancy and liver disease.

An *angeiosarcoma* is a rare sarcoma of blood vessels.

Atheroma

Atheroma is a degeneration of the intima of arteries. It is a common condition. Its cause is unknown. Factors in its development are:

(a) *Age*. In general atheroma increases with age, but it can begin in childhood or adolescence.

(b) *Blood lipids*. The lipids present in atheroma are similar to those in the blood. Saturated fats (which occur in animal fat, butter, eggs) produce a high blood cholesterol, while unsaturated fats (which occur in fish, vegetables and some kinds of margarine) produce a low blood cholesterol. Patients with hypertension may have a high level of certain lipoproteins and of cholesterol in the blood. The high incidence in some societies has been attributed to the relatively large amounts of animal fat in the diet.

(c) *Hypertension*. Atheroma is sometimes associated with hypertension. It is particularly likely to occur in the pulmonary artery when there is pulmonary hypertension. But some people with hypertension have no atheroma and some people with severe atheroma have a normal BP.

(d) *Turbulence in blood-flow*. Atheroma tends to begin and be most severe at the bifurcation of large arteries and around the orifices of small arteries; these are places in which normally there is turbulence in the blood-flow.

The two principal theories of the immediate cause of atheroma are:
1. that it is due to an invasion of the intima of arteries by lipids from the blood;
2. that it is due to thrombi of platelets being deposited on the intimal surface.

The features of atheroma are:

(a) *Fatty streaks*. These are sometimes seen in the intima of children and adolescents as well as of older people and are probably the earliest signs of atheroma. They are composed of lipids, and in the connective tissue beneath them appear foamy macrophages, large scavenging cells with a foamy appearance of the cytoplasm.

(b) *Plaques*. Atheromatous plaques then develop. They appear on the surface of the intima, projecting into the lumen as yellow or cream-coloured patches, which gradually obliterate the lumen. They are composed of fibro-elastic tissue with deposits of cholesterol in the deeper layers. They have at first the consistency of putty, but they harden as they get older and may become calcified. Blood-pigment is sometimes deposited in them. Ulcerations of the surface of a plaque is likely.

Complications

1. *Reductions of blood supply*. The gradually increasing amount of atheroma gradually reduces the size of the lumen of the affected artery. Any active tissue supplied by the artery degenerates and is replaced by fibrous tissue, which requires less oxygen and nutrients to keep alive.
2. *Thrombosis*. Blood is very likely to thrombose on the ulcerated plaque and completely block the artery, causing an infarction.
3. *Aneurysm*. The reduction of blood-supply to the muscle wall of the artery itself causes degeneration of the muscle and its replacement by fibrous tissue. The fibrous tissue can stretch under arterial pressure and form an aneurysm.
4. *Cardiac infarction*. The coronary arteries which supply the heart are commonly affected with atheroma. The left coronary artery is usually more affected than the right. Fibrosis of the myocardium and attacks of angina pectoris occur.

Thrombosis in a coronary artery causes myocardial infarction. As the left coronary artery or one of its branches is the artery most likely to be affected, the infarct is likely to involve the left ventricle. The patient may die suddenly. If he survives, the following changes can occur:
(i) The myocardium involved becomes brown and surrounded by a red hyperaemic border; fibrosis of the involved muscle follows.
(ii) The pericardium may be involved; inflammatory changes in it are followed by the development of fibrous adhesions which can

bind together the two surfaces of the pericardium.
(iii) The endocardium is usually unaffected because it can get enough oxygen for its purposes from the oxygenated blood in the left atrium and ventricle.
(iv) Disturbance of cardiac rhythm can occur.
(v) The damaged myocardium may stretch to form an aneurysm, rupture into the pericardium, or rupture the interventricular wall.
(vi) Thrombi may develop in the appendix of the atrium or deep in the recesses between the papillary muscles, and pieces of them can become detached and form emboli.
(vii) Further attacks of coronary thrombosis can occur, killing the patient or further damaging the heart.

CEREBRAL ARTERY ATHEROMA

Atheroma and thrombosis of the cerebral arteries is common.

> **Blood**
>
> *Lipids, total serum:* may be raised (normal: 4.5-8.5 g/l).
> *Cholesterol, serum, total:* may be raised (normal: 3.6-7.8 mmol/l).

Aneurysm

An *aneurysm* is a permanent dilatation of an artery. It is due to the pressure of blood on an artery weakened by a congenital defect or by disease.
   An aneurysm is called:
fusiform: when the whole circumference of the artery is involved and the aneurysm has a spindle-shaped appearance.
saccular: when only part of the circumference of an artery is involved and the aneurysm projects like a pouch.
mycotic: when it is due to infection of the arterial wall (as can occur in subacute bacterial endocarditis).

At the site of an aneurysm the muscle of the artery wall has degenerated and been replaced by fibrous tissue, which stretches under the influence of the arterial pressure. An aneurysm forms a pulsatile swelling which may erode adjacent tissues (including bone) or may leak or rupture.
   There are four types of aneurysm.

(a) *Syphilitic aneurysm of the aorta*

A syphilitic aneurysm can occur in the arch of the aorta.

(b) *Dissecting aneurysm of the aorta*

This aneurysm can occur in atheroma, hypertension and Marfan's syndrome. A hole opens in the intima of the aorta and blood is forced through the hole and down inside the arterial wall itself. The wall of the aorta can rupture under the pressure or blood be forced backwards into the pericardium.

(c) *Atheromatous aneurysm*

This aneurysm is due to atheroma of the abdominal aorta, the usual site being just below the origin of the renal arteries. The aneurysm can leak or rupture.

(d) *Berry aneurysm*

This aneurysm occurs on a cerebral vessel. It can rupture and cause a subarchnoid haemorrhage.

Temporal arteritis

Temporal arteritis (giant cell arteritis) is a chronic inflammatory disease of arteries, especially the temporal and occipital arteries. The cause is unknown. It occurs in old people, has been known to follow an infection, and is considered by some to be a variant of polyarteritis nodosa.

Affected arteries show fibrosis of the intima and invasion of the muscle coat by giant cells, polymorphs, lymphocytes and plasma cells; degenerative changes follow; thromboses may form in affected arteries.

Severe headache in the temporal region is a common clinical feature. Permanent blindness can occur. The aorta and its branches are occasionally involved.

Thrombo-angiitis obliterans

Thrombo-angiitis obliterans (Buerger's disease) begins in adults under the age of 40. Its cause is unknown. By some it is thought not to be a separate disease but a condition due to the effects of atheroma and thrombosis. Sufferers are almost invariably heavy smokers.

The condition usually begins in the lower limbs, but vessels anywhere can be affected. The first signs are thought to be those of an acute inflammation of arteries and veins. Thromboses then occur and the vessels show degenerative changes. Recanalization of a thrombosis can occur and open up the vessel for blood to pass through again. Intermittent claudication and painful swellings of the calves appear; gangrene of the toes and foot can follow complete obstruction of a large artery in the leg.

Hypertension

Hypertension is a persistently raised blood pressure in adult life. At the age of 20 the average blood pressure in a healthy person is about systolic 120, diastolic 80. It rises with age and at the age of 60 is about systolic 160, diastolic 90.

Hypertension is described as:
benign; or
malignant.

Causes

1. *Essential hypertension:* in 90 per cent of patients with hypertension no cause can be found, but there is likely to be a family history of the condition.
2. *Renal disease:* glomerulonephritis; pyelonephritis; polycystic kidney; amyloidosis.
3. *Endocrine disease:* (i) Cushing's syndrome, causing an excessive glucocorticoid production; (ii) excessive aldosterone production, e.g. due to an adenoma of the adrenal cortex; (iii) phaeochromocytoma, a tumour of the adrenal medulla, causing an excess of adrenaline and nor-adrenaline.
4. *Coarctation of the aorta.*

Benign essential hypertension

The blood pressure rises gradually over many years without necessarily producing symptoms.

Complications

1. *Left ventricular hypertrophy.* The left ventricle hypertrophies because it has to act against increased resistance. In time left ventricular failure may develop.
2. *Atheroma* may develop and cause coronary artery disease.
3. *Cerebral aneurysm* may develop and by rupturing cause a cerebral haemorrhage.
4. *Malignant hypertension* develops in a minority of patients.

MALIGNANT HYPERTENSION

Malignant hypertension is a very severe form of hypertension in which the blood pressure rises rapidly to very high levels. It may arise for no known cause, be secondary to renal disease or occasionally develop in patients with benign hypertension. The predominant pathological changes in the blood vessels are:
(a) fibrinoid necrosis of arterioles, a degeneration in which fibrin or other substances are deposited in the wall;
(b) hypertrophy of the walls of arterioles and small arteries with a reduction in the size of the lumen; the walls have a layered, 'onion skin' appearance.

Complications

1. Progressive impairment of renal function because of involvement of the renal arterioles and glomerular capillaries. Renal failure is the most frequent cause of death.
2. The arteries of the retina show papilloedema, exudates and haemorrhages.
3. Left ventricular failure.

PULMONARY HYPERTENSION

Hypertension in the pulmonary arteries is not part of a systemic hypertension. It can occur in:
some congenital diseases of the heart;
mitral stenosis;
emphysema;
pulmonary fibrosis;
degeneration of the pulmonary arteries.

Chapter 12 The Respiratory System

Naso-pharynx

ACUTE TONSILLITIS

Acute tonsillitis is usually due to infection by a haemolytic streptococcus. The tonsils show the usual signs of inflammation, being enlarged, red and painful; some pus may form in the crypts.

Complications

Chronic tonsillitis
Acute otitis media
Acute rheumatic fever
Quinsy
Lung infection
Acute glomerulo-nephritis

CHRONIC TONSILLITIS

Chronic tonsillitis can be due to repeated attacks of acute tonsillitis or be secondary to chronic sinusitis and dental sepsis. The tonsils are enlarged and show signs of chronic inflammation. Cervical lymph nodes may be enlarged.

QUINSY

Quinsy (peritonsillar abscess) is an abscess between the tonsil and the muscular wall of the tonsillar fossa. A chronic abscess can develop if an acute abscess is inadequately treated.

Throat swab

Throat swabs are used to obtain specimens of secretion from which are identified the organisms responsible for a throat infection or carriers of haemolytic streptococci or the diphtheria bacillus. The organism discovered may not be the cause of the infection; but the presence of haemolytic streptococci, the spirochetes and fusiform bacilli of Vincent's angina, and the diphtheria bacillus is taken to indicate that the organism is the cause of the infection.

The swab should be sent to the laboratory as quickly as possible.

For the identification of viruses, details of special techniques for collection and transport of specimens should be obtained from the laboratory which is going to carry out the test.

ADENOIDS

Adenoids are enlarged masses of lymph tissue in the upper end of the nasopharyngeal tube. They are commonly associated with chronic tonsillitis. They may obstruct the lower end of the auditory (Eustachian) tube and the posterior nasal apertures.

Complication

Acute otitis media.

SINUSITIS

Sinusitis can involve any of the paranasal sinuses. Infection of them usually follows a common cold or other infection of the nose. A maxillary sinusitis can be due to a dental

abscess in the upper jaw. In the acute phase the mucous membrane of the sinus becomes reddened and oedematous. The activity of the cilia which project from the cells of the mucous membrane is diminished, pus tends to collect, and a chronic sinusitis develops as a result of an inadequate drainage of a sinus. Inadequate drainage is due to blocking of the sinus orifices by:
oedema of the nasal mucous membrane;
deviation of the nasal septum;
nasal polyps.

TUMOURS

Various types of malignant neoplasms can occur in the naso-pharynx:
squamous carcinoma;
adenocarcinoma;
lymphadenoma.
They can invade the deep cervical lymph nodes, the base of the skull, and the auditory (Eustachian) tube.

Larynx

ACUTE LARYNGITIS

Acute laryngitis occurs as part of an acute upper respiratory tract infection. Predisposing factors are:
nasal obstruction   sinusitis
tonsillitis   dusty occupations.

The membrane of the larynx, vocal cords and epiglottis becomes swollen and reddened, and there may be an excessive secretion of mucus. In young children oedema and muscular spasm produce respiratory obstruction.

CHRONIC LARYNGITIS

Chronic laryngitis is due to repeated attacks of acute laryngitis and associated with the same predisposing factors. The vocal cords lose their normal lustre, become congested and develop a thick edge. There may be an excessive secretion of mucus from the mucous membrane. Areas of excessive keratinization occasionally develop and occasionally become malignant.

Singer's nodes are small projections which develop on the vocal cords and can become polyps. They are the result of tiny haemorrhages caused by excessive use of the voice, especially by attempting to sing or shout while suffering from acute laryngitis.

TUBERCULOSIS OF THE LARYNX

Tuberculosis of the larynx is one of the complications of pulmonary tuberculosis. Having gained entry to the tissues, the micro-organisms produce a typical tuberculous reaction, which can go on to ulceration.

OEDEMA OF THE LARYNX

Oedema of the larynx can be due to:
acute infection (especially in young children);
angioneurotic oedema;
irritating gases;
inhalation of steam;
drinking corrosive poisons.

The mucous membrane becomes oedematous and respiratory obstruction occurs.

NEOPLASMS OF THE LARYNX

Squamous carcinoma of the larynx occurs usually in middle-aged or old men. The growth appears on a vocal cord as a warty or ulcerated mass. Cervical lymph nodes are invaded.

Trachea and Bronchi

ACUTE TRACHEITIS

Acute tracheitis occurs as part of an infection of the upper respiratory tract.

ACUTE TRACHEO-BRONCHITIS

Acute tracheo-bronchitis is due to infection by:
viruses — *measles, rhinovirus, influenza, enteroviruses*, etc;
Bord. pertussis;
pneumococcus;
staphylococcus.

The degree of inflammation varies from slight to severe. In severe infections, ulceration can occur. If ulceration leads to fibrosis, deformation or blockage of a tube can occur.

CHRONIC BRONCHITIS

Chronic bronchitis is characterized by:
(a) hypertrophy of the bronchial mucous glands, with a continuous or intermittent oversecretion of mucus,
(b) impaction of mucus in the smaller airways,
(c) infection by various organisms, especially: viruses; streptococci; staphylococci,
(d) narrowing of airways,
(e) interference with respiratory function,
(f) right ventricular hypertrophy and ultimately failure.

Contributing factors are:
(a) smoking, especially smoking cigarettes,
(b) atmospheric pollution by smoke and sulphur dioxide,
(c) dusty occupation, e.g. mining, quarrying.

Chronic bronchitis is more common in men than women. The incidence and mortality are higher in smokers than non-smokers, in town-dwellers than country-dwellers, and in members of the lower socio-economic groups than in members of the upper socio-economic groups.

Sputum

Sputum is a mixture of:
(a) fluid produced in the alveoli and bronchioles,
(b) mucus secreted by the epithelial cells of the respiratory tract,
(c) saliva.

The amount produced by healthy people is so small that coughing is not necessary to clear the respiratory passages. Any excess of sputum has to be removed by coughing, and coughing up sputum is an indication that there is something, slight or serious, wrong with the respiratory tract.

Sputum is examined in the laboratory for:
(a) micro-organisms which may be producing a respiratory tract infection,
(b) the sensitivity of these organisms to drugs,
(c) the presence of cells, especially malignant cells,
(d) the presence of other significant structures, e.g. asbestos bodies.

The best specimen for laboratory examination is the first one coughed up in the morning. About 5 ml should be sent in a sterile container with a screw cap. Wax cartons are not suitable as they can be contaminated, cannot be sterilized, and cannot be sent through the post. If an examination for viruses or malignant cells is required, the laboratory in which tests are to be carried out should be consulted about the method of collection and transport.

Bronchial Adenoma

A bronchial adenoma is a benign neoplasm or one of limited malignancy. There are two main kinds:
(a) *Carcinoid tumour.* These form 90 per cent of adenomata of the bronchus, grow from the walls of large bronchi, and are composed of small cells. Degeneration, calcification and ossification can occur in them. Rarely they form metastases.

(b) *Cylindroma*. These are formed of darkly staining cells, spread in the bronchi and trachea, can invade other tissues, and can spread to lymph nodes and the liver.

Carcinoma of the Bronchus

Carcinoma of the bronchus is more commonly known as carcinoma of the lung.

FACTORS IN ITS CAUSATION

1. *Smoking*. Cigarette smoking is the most important cause of carcinoma of the bronchus. The more cigarettes one smokes, the more likely is one to die of this disease. The death rate of heavy smokers from the disease is 20 times greater than that of non-smokers. The incidence is less in pipe-smokers and cigar-smokers, but higher than in non-smokers. The precise agent in tobacco has not been identified but is probably a tar.
2. *Atmospheric pollution*. Carcinogens in the air are a possible cause as the incidence of carcinoma of the bronchus is higher in people who dwell in large towns than it is in people who live in the country.
3. *Radiation*. There is an increased incidence of carcinoma of the bronchus in people who have been exposed to big doses of radiation.
4. *Scar tissue*. The carcinoma seems in some patients to begin in scar tissue, e.g. of healed tuberculosis.
5. *Dust diseases*. Some dust diseases, e.g. asbestosis, predispose to carcinoma of the lung.

PATHOLOGICAL FEATURES

Carcinoma of the bronchus arises in the epithelium of mucous glands of the bronchi. The commonest site of origin is one of the large primary divisions of the bronchi. The cells of which one is composed vary. The neoplasm may be (in order of frequency):
a squamous carcinoma,
an oat-cell carcinoma,
an adeno-carcinoma.

The first appearance of the growth is as a rough area in a bronchus. It can block the bronchus and cause collapse of that part of the lung supplied by the bronchus. The growth then spreads into lung tissue and pleura. Some neoplasms appear as spherical masses in the lungs. The centre may degenerate and form a cavity.

Secondary effects in the lungs are:
congestion   oedema   consolidation
collapse   abscess   bronchiectasis
emphysema   pleural effusion

The neoplasm can spread into other tissues:
hilum of the lung   mediastinum
hilar lymph nodes   pericardium
cervical and axillary lymph nodes
In these places it can cause obstruction of the great vessels and press on nerves.

Metastases are common, occurring usually in:
skin   brain
bone   liver
adrenal glands   kidney

ASSOCIATED SYNDROMES

Various syndromes can be found in association with carcinoma of the bronchus, but the precise reasons for their occurrence are not known. They include:
Cushing's syndrome   cerebellar
peripheral   degeneration
  neuropathy   over-secretion of anti-
                                diuretic hormone

Sputum

Slide: fresh specimens are stained and examined for malignant cells. The first morning specimen is the best. The patient must not eat anything, have a drink or clean his teeth with toothpaste before producing a specimen as the specimen must not contain particles of food, fat droplets or toothpaste. The laboratory may ask for several specimens on successive days. Cancer cells may be

found in the sputum up to 3 years before it is possible to identify the site of the carcinoma. In about 30 per cent of patients with carcinoma of the bronchus no malignant cells can be found in the sputum.
Biopsy
Tissue is obtained by bronchoscopy or mediastinoscopy, by pleural biopsy or from enlarged lymph nodes, and examined for malignant cells.
Pleural fluid
Fluid may contain red cells, inflammatory cells, mesothelial cells, and rarely malignant cells.

Lungs

The lungs of infants and country-dwellers are a pinkish-grey colour. The lungs of town-dwellers become progressively grey or black with a deposit of soot particles from the atmosphere.

CONGESTION

Congestion of the lungs is usually due to:
acute inflammation;
mitral stenosis;
left ventricular failure.
The capillaries around the alveoli are distended with blood. In acute congestion the lungs are purplish-red and in chronic congestion brownish-red.

OEDEMA

Oedema of the lungs is usually due to:
acute infection of the lungs;
left ventricular failure;
generalized oedema of the body;
inhalation of a chemical irritant;
injury of the brain.
The lungs are more solid than usual, feel like a wet sponge, and when cut and squeezed exude a clear fluid.

COLLAPSE

Collapse is due to an inability to replace air absorbed from the alveoli. It is the result of:
obstruction of a bronchus by a foreign body,
undrained bronchial secretion,
neoplasm, compression by a pneumothorax or pleural effusion.
The part of the lung involved shrinks, is more solid than normal, and has a purple-grey colour.

FIBROSIS

Fibrosis of the lung is an excess of fibrous tissue in lung and often in overlying pleura. It is a result of:
chronic bronchitis   bronchiectasis
tuberculosis   pneumonia
pneumoconiosis   carcinoma of lung
sarcoidosis
Fibrosis interferes with respiratory function, and can cause respiratory failure and right ventricular failure.

Congenital Diseases of the Lungs

AGENESIS

Agenesis of a lung can occur. The lung is absent. There is a shift of the mediastinal contents to the affected side. Other congenital abnormalities may be present. In some cases part of a lung is small or absent.

CYSTIC LUNG

Cystic lung is a rare condition in which a number of small cysts are present either throughout the lung or in part of it.

ATELECTASIS

Atelectasis is the state produced when a lung does not expand after birth and remains totally or partly airless. It is due to:
aspirated amniotic fluid;
birth injuries to the brain;
hyaline membrane disease.

HYALINE MEMBRANE DISEASE

Hyaline membrane disease is a condition in which the distal air passages of newly-born infants are lined with a membrane which prevents gaseous exchanges. It occurs in:
premature babies;
babies of mothers with diabetes mellitus.
It may be due to an absence of surfactant, a substance normally present in the lungs of newborn infants and necessary for the expansion of alveoli to take place.

Pneumonia

Pneumonia is an acute inflammatory condition of the lungs in which the alveoli and smaller bronchioles are filled with an inflammatory exudate. It may be a primary disease or secondary to bronchitis, carcinoma of the bronchus or other diseases of the lung.

Pneumonias can be classified by:
(a) the infecting micro-organisms or other agent, usually:
Pneumococcus
Staphylococcus pyogenes
Myco. tuberculosis
virus: influenza, measles, adenovirus, picornavirus.
Several other micro-organisms, some protozoa and some yeasts and fungi occasionally cause pneumonia.
(b) the site in which the inflammation occurs:
lobar pneumonia: when the pneumonia is limited to one or more lobes
bronchopneumonia: when the pneumonia is scattered in various parts of the lung or of both lungs, with consolidation occurring around the terminal bronchi.

PATHOLOGICAL CHANGES

Pathological changes vary with the type of micro-organisms, the degree of resistance of the patient to the organism, the age of the patient (the very young and the very old being liable to suffer bronchopneumonia severely), and the speed with which chemotherapy is begun.

Pneumonia is thought to be precipitated by the aspiration of some infected mucus and its lodging in a small peripheral branch of the bronchial tree and with a failure of the ciliary mechanism to remove the infected particles from the smaller air-spaces.

The first changes are those of congestion and oedema. Then a fluid exudate, containing fibrin, red cells and polymorphs, fills up the alveoli and adjacent air-spaces. The pulmonary capillaries dilate. In an untreated patient red hepatization develops: this is a consolidation of the lung that is red because of the red cells and dilated capillaries in it and looks, cut across, like a cut surface of liver (hepar). Red hepatization is followed by grey hepatization, in which the colour change is due to an increase in the number of polymorphs and a decrease in the number of red cells and dilated capillaries. In the patient who recovers the tissues return gradually to normal, the debris being broken up by enzymes and absorbed by scavenger cells and the exudate absorbed or coughed up.

Some influenzal pneumonias are marked by very haemorrhagic exudates. Staphylococcal pneumonia is usually severe, with a high death rate.

Complications

Pleurisy: inflammation of the pleura
Pleural effusion: fluid in the pleural cavity
Empyema: pus in the pleural cavity
Spontaneous pneumothorax: air in the pleural cavity; can be due to rupture of a cyst formed in staphylococcal pneumonia
Lung abscess: single or multiple; can form in staphylococcal pneumonia
Fibrosis of lung: can occur with pneumonias that clear up slowly
Pericarditis: inflammation of the pericardium
Congestive heart failure: due to toxic effects on myocardium
Jaundice: due to toxic effect on liver cells

Anuria: failure of secretion of urine, due to toxic effects on kidneys

Bacteraemia: invasion of blood by micro-organism; can cause endocarditis, meningitis, suppurative arthritis

---

Sputum

Culture: for identification of micro-organism and its drug-sensitivity.

Blood

Blood count: increase in polymorphs in bacterial pneumonia.

Pulmonary Tuberculosis

Pulmonary tuberculosis is due to infection of the lung by the human strain of *Myco. tuberculosis*.

The pathological changes are the same as those of tuberculosis elsewhere in the body. Infection is most likely to occur in the superior and posterior parts of a lung.

Primary complex.

The primary complex is composed of a Ghon focus and associated lymph nodes in the hilum of the lung. A Ghon focus is the first sign of infection. It is composed of tubercles and in most people its heals with fibrosis and sometimes years later calcification. The organisms spread along the lymph vessels to infect the lymph nodes in the hilum, and there too the lesions usually heal.

If, however, the patient's degree of immunity is inadequate to prevent further infection, the inflammatory changes become worse with the development of a secondary complex.

Secondary complex.

This is any further development of tuberculosis in a lung after the primary complex. It may take the form of:

(a) Direct spread from the Ghon focus into neighbouring lung tissue and the formation of more and more tubercles. A tubercular pneumonic process may start. If the patient's resistance is inadequate, areas of caseation and cavitation develop.

(b) Spread via the broncial tree to other parts of the same lung or to the other lung. There the same kind of pathological changes take place.

In *chronic pulmonary tuberculosis* the patient is likely to show both advancing disease and attempts to heal or limit it by fibrous reactions. Abscesses can form and burst into the bronchi or pleural cavity. Haemoptysis is caused by the rupture into the bronchial passages of blood vessels involved in the inflammation.

Complications

(a) *Pleurisy*. The pleura is often involved and tubercles develop on its surface.

A *pleural effusion* of clear fluid is likely. It may be eventually completely absorbed, but fibrous attachments can bind one layer of pleura to the other.

(b) *Blood-borne infection*. The micro-organisms may get into the blood-stream. A *miliary tuberculosis* is the result of such a general infection. Tubercles form in several organs and tissues, especially:

lungs   brain
bones   meninges
joints   adrenal glands
genito-urinary tract

(c) *Tuberculosis of the larynx*

(d) *Amyloidosis* can occur in chronic tuberculosis of many years duration.

(e) *Carcinoma of lung* appears to develop sometimes in the scar of a healed tuberculous lesion.

Sputum

Smears: stained with Ziehl-Neelsen stain and examined for *Myco. tuberculosis*. Several smears may have to be examined as the organisms may be excreted intermittently and in small numbers; at least 3 specimens should be sent at intervals of a day or more.

Blood

Erythrocyte sedimentation rate (ESR): raised in active disease. Repeated measurements are made to check progress and the effects of treatment.
Red cells: number usually reduced.
White cells: number and appearance often normal. In miliary tuberculosis various abnormalities can occur.

Pleural effusion

Fluid: clear, contains lymphocytes; is cultured to grow organisms.

Sarcoidosis

Sarcoidosis is a disease of unknown origin characterized by a chronic granulomatous invasion of tissues, especially:
lungs (in almost all cases)
lymph nodes   liver   uveal tract of eye
spleen   kidney   skin
bone   heart   pancreas.
Microscopically the lesions look very much like those of tuberculosis, but they do not caseate and *Myco. tuberculosis* cannot be demonstrated in them. It is thought that sarcoidosis is possibly an immunologically determined alteration in tissues, precipitated by certain agents, of which one may be *Myco. tuberculosis*. The condition can heal spontaneously; and when a generalized invasion of a lung has occurred and healed, the result is a 'honeycomb' lung.

Kveim test

A saline suspension of sarcoid tissue (obtained from the spleen or lymph nodes of a patient with sarcoidosis) is injected intradermally. 70 per cent of patients with sarcoidosis will develop within 6 weeks a nodule with sarcoid histology at the site of injection.

Metastases in the Lungs

Many malignant neoplasms form metastases in the lungs. Common sites of origin are:
breast   gastro-intestinal tract
pancreas   prostate gland
thyroid gland   bone
genito-urinary tract
Metastases may be single or multiple. If the pleura is involved, a pleural effusion is likely.

Pneumoconioses

Pneumoconioses are lung diseases produced by the inhalation of a harmful dust during an industrial process. They vary with the kind of dust inhaled.

1. SILICOSIS

Silicosis is due to the inhalation of silica dust. Among the industrial processes in which silica is inhaled are:
(a) coal mining in mines where there is a high proportion of silica-containing rock;
(b) quarrying and trimming granite, slate, etc;
(c) sand-blasting;
(d) pottery manufacture;
(e) boiler scaling.

Particles of silica are absorbed by macrophages in the lungs, but the macrophages are killed in the process and the particles remain in the lungs. A reaction to them is set up, a reaction that in part may be an immunological reaction. Silica nodules up to 1 cm in diameter are formed, partly of collagen fibres with particles of silica at the periphery. Calcification of the nodules can occur.

Complications

(a) fibrosis of lung, which will in time cause a gross interference with respiratory function.
(b) pulmonary tuberculosis in a slowly developing form.

2. ASBESTOSIS

Asbestosis is due to the inhalation of dust containing asbestos. Asbestos is a mineral composed of various silicates of magnesium, iron, etc., and is mined in various parts of the world. It is stronger than steel and resistant to fire, water, acid and alkalis, and is used in many industries. Asbestosis can arise as a result of working in:

asbestos mining	electrical insulation
pipe lagging	brake lining
ship building	refrigeration, etc.

Microscopic fibres are inhaled and penetrate as far as the smaller bronchioles. In the lungs 'asbestos bodies' are formed of a tiny asbestos fibre enclosed in protein material, and have a characteristic shape.

Asbestosis causes:
(a) fibrosis of the lung,
(b) plaques of hyaline tissue in the lung.

It has been suggested that it is also responsible for: some cases of carcinoma of the lung; mesothelioma, a tumour of pleura and peritoneum.

Lung

Smears and *sections:* examined for the presence of asbestos bodies.

Bronchiectasis

Bronchiectasis is a dilatation of the bronchi. It can occur as a result of:
(a) Some congenital diseases of the lung in which the walls of the bronchi do not fully develop
(b) Obstruction to a bronchial tube by:

a foreign body	neoplasm
stricture	pressure by enlarged lymph nodes.

The obstruction causes collapse of the part of the lung supplied by the bronchus or bronchiole; mucus accumulates in the tubes; and if the obstruction is not relieved and the lung does not re-expand, bronchiectasis is likely to develop.
(c) Infection of the lung in childhood by bronchiolitis, measles, whooping cough, pneumonia, tuberculosis.
(d) Fibrosis of the lung in any chronic lung disease.

Bronchiectasis may be diffused through one or both lungs or limited to a segment or lobe. The bronchial wall, weakened by disease, expands into a number of saccular, cylindrical or fusiform enlargements. Infection is likely to follow, and the spaces are likely then to fill with stagnant, offensive pus.

Complications

Pneumonia, due to the aspiration of pus;
Pleurisy, pleural effusion;
Infected nasal sinuses;
Pericarditis, due to direct spread of infection;
Abscess of brain, due to a septic embolus;
Amyloidosis, in chronic cases.

Emphysema

Emphysema is a condition in which the alveoli and the air-spaces next to them are enlarged. It may be:
(a) rarely, a congenital condition;

(b) a primary emphysema of unknown origin, affecting middle-aged men and women in about equal numbers;
(c) associated with chronic bronchitis, and therefore more common in men.

The lungs become enlarged, with visible air-spaces and sometimes bullae (a bulla in this sense is an emphysematous space greater than 1 cm diameter). The amount of dead air-space in the lung is increased and respiratory function is accordingly impaired.

Complications

Spontaneous pneumothorax, due to rupture of a subpleural bulla.
Pulmonary hypertension and atheroma.
Right ventricular hypertrophy and failure.

Infarction of Lung

An *infarct of a lung* is an area of necrosis produced by cutting off the blood-supply to part of a lung. The causes are:
(a) thrombosis superimposed upon atheroma of the pulmonary artery;
(b) embolism of a pulmonary artery by a piece of thrombus detached from a thrombus in a vein or from the right atrium during atrial fibrillation;
(c) fat embolism following severe injury;
(d) polycythaemia and sickle cell anaemia;
(e) contraceptive pills.

It is most common in middle-aged or elderly people. Drug addicts can develop septic thrombi by injecting themselves intravenously.

A wedge-shaped area of necrotic lung is produced. Some infarcts heal up, leaving small scars.

Complications

Pleurisy, pleural effusion;
Abscess in the infarcted area.

Loeffler's syndrome

Loeffler's syndrome is a condition or group of conditions in which there is an increase in the number of eosinophils in the blood up to 500-10,000 per mm^3. and an infiltration of the lungs by eosinophils.

Respiratory Failure

Respiratory failure is present when as a result of a disorder of respiration or of the nervous control of respiration the blood-gases are abnormal at rest.

There are two types.

TYPE I

In this type the arterial carbon dioxide tension (P_{CO_2}) is normal or low and the arterial oxygen tension (P_{O_2}) is low. It is due to a defect in gas-transfer in the lungs as a result of an uneven distribution of inspired air and pulmonary bloodflow. It occurs in:
(a) fibrosis or oedema of the lungs,
(b) severe asthma,
(c) acute bronchial infection,
(d) disease of the pulmonary blood-vessels, especially thrombo-embolic disease in them.

TYPE II

In this type the arterial carbon dioxide tension (P_{CO_2}) is high, there is a respiratory acidosis, and the arterial oxygen tension (P_{O_2}) is low. It occurs in:
(a) emphysema, asthma, chronic bronchitis;
(b) disorders of respiratory control produced by drugs, anaesthesia, chest injury, polyneuritis, poliomyelitis, myasthenia gravis;
(c) the terminal stage of a Type I respiratory failure.

Pleura

PLEURISY

Pleurisy is an inflammation of the pleura. It is usually secondary to disease of the lung, chest wall or subphrenic region, especially:

pneumonia
bronchiectasis
carcinoma of bronchus
subphrenic abscess
pulmonary tuberculosis
pulmonary infarction
injury of chest wall

In the area of inflammation the pleura loses its lustre and becomes hyperaemic and roughened. Fibrin is deposited on its surface. Adhesions may form between the visceral and parietal pleura. The inflammation may clear up completely or the pleura may be left permanently thickened.

PLEURAL EFFUSION

A *pleural effusion* is a collection of fluid in the pleural cavity. It may be an exudate or a transudate.

An *exudate* is caused by a neoplasm or inflammation and can occur in:
1. Carcinoma of the bronchus,
2. Inflammatory diseases of the lung, e.g. tuberculosis, pneumonia,
3. Systemic infection or infection outside the chest, e.g. subphrenic abscess,
4. Collagen diseases.

A *transudate* is due to the same mechanisms which cause oedema:
1. reduced osmotic pressure of plasma due to lack of plasma proteins, as in nephrotic syndrome and liver disease, especially cirrhosis;
2. increased venous pressure, as in cardiac failure.

A pleural effusion due to an infection is usually absorbed. Sometimes pleural fibrosis with adhesions between visceral and parietal pleura may form and impair lung function.

A *haemothorax* is a pleural effusion stained with blood or composed of blood (as after a chest injury). A *chylothorax* is a pleural effusion containing chyle, which gets into it from a thoracic duct damaged by disease or injury.

Pleural fluid

Exudate. Amber or straw-coloured. May clot quickly. Specific gravity (SG): greater than 1015. Protein content: greater than 30g per litre.

Transudate. Yellow. Specific gravity (SG): less than 1015. Protein content: less than 30g per litre.

EMPYEMA

Empyema is pus in the pleural cavity. It may be generalized or local. It is usually due to disease of a lung, especially,

pneumococcal pneumonia
tuberculosis
lung abscess
perforating wound.
staphylococcal pneumonia
bronchiectasis
carcinoma of lung

Non-pulmonary causes are:
mediastinal infection
carcinoma of oesophagus
amoebic abscess
osteomyelitis of rib
subphrenic abscess
perinephric abscess
septicaemia.

The fluid is green, yellow or grey, opaque, and sometimes foul-smelling. The pleura is covered with a fibrinous exudate. Adhesions can form, and pockets of pus can be enclosed within fibrous walls. Any permanent fibrosis of the pleura will interfere with lung expansion.

Fluid

Fluid: thick, contains pus, has a high protein content.

PNEUMOTHORAX

A *pneumothorax* is a collection of air in the pleural cavity. It can be:
(a) *Spontaneous*. This is most commonly the result of the rupture of a subpleural bulla in a

lung. The bulla can be the result of a congenital defect, and rupture of one is common in apparently healthy young men. A spontaneous pneumothorax can also be the result of asthma, bronchial carcinoma, staphylococcal pneumonia, pulmonary tuberculosis, pneumoconiosis, etc.

(b) *Traumatic*. The pneumothorax can be the result of a penetrating or non-penetrating wound of the chest wall.

Mediastinum

MEDIASTINITIS

Mediastinitis is infection of the mediastinum and can be due to:

trauma;
perforation of the oesophagus by a cancer, injury or foreign body;
tuberculous lymph nodes.

MEDIASTINAL NEOPLASMS

Mediastinal neoplasms are primary or secondary. Many of the primary neoplasms are benign. They can cause symptoms by pressing on the great vessels, nerves and other structures in the mediastinum.

Chapter 13 Blood

Iron Deficiency Anaemia

As iron is an essential part of haemoglobin a deficiency of it reduces the amount of haemoglobin that can be formed and so the amount in each red blood cell. An average daily diet contains 10-20 mg of iron, mostly in meat and vegetables, but only about 5-10 per cent of this is absorbed by healthy people with normal stores of iron in the body. The amount absorbed will increase to 50 per cent if tissues have become depleted or if there is a special demand for it.

The causes of iron deficiency anaemia are:
(a) deficient intake of iron due to poverty, food fadism, special 'light' diets;
(b) deficient absorption after partial gastrectomy and in steatorrhoea;
(c) increased loss of iron due to chronic bleeding from the gastro-intestinal tract, which can occur with:
oesophageal varices,
frequent aspirin ingestion,
peptic ulcer,
hiatus hernia,
ulcerative colitis,
carcinoma of the gastrointestinal tract,
haemorrhoids.

Iron deficiency anaemia can occur at any age, but is most common in young children, women of child-bearing age and old people.

Young children. About one-third of the iron in store in a newly-born infant is deposited there during the last months of fetal life. A premature baby is therefore likely to be short of iron. In a healthy infant fed on milk only the iron in store at birth is used up in the first 6 months of life, and if he is not by this time given iron-containing food in adequate amounts he will develop an iron deficiency anaemia.

Women of child-bearing age lose iron in menstruation, pregnancy (due to loss to the fetus and placenta) loss of blood at childbirth, and lactation.

Old people tend to become anaemic if they cannot afford to buy meat or cannot chew it because they are edentulous or have badly fitting dentures.

Associated abnormalities

Tongue: redness and loss of papillae
Nails: flat or spoon-shaped
Mucous membrane of mouth: inflamed
Spleen: enlarged

Blood

Film: red cells are small and pale and may vary in size and shape.
Haemoglobin: reduced below normal. Normal for men: 13.0-18.0 g/dl; for women: 11.5-16.5 g/dl; for children at 1 year (mean): 11.2 g/dl; for children at 10 years (mean): 12.9 g/dl.
Mean corpuscular haemoglobin concentration (MCHC): reduced. Normal 30-35 per cent.

Chronic Hypochromic Anaemia

A chronic hypochromic anaemia can occur in:
chronic infections of any kind,
rheumatoid arthritis,
malignant growths,
renal failure.

The anaemia that occurs in these conditions is the result of:
(a) a failure to release iron from iron-stores for the production of new red cells
(b) a failure of erythropoietin production; erythropoietin, a hormone produced by the kidney, stimulates the release of red cells from the bone marrow
(c) a reduction of the life-span of red cells in the circulating blood below the normal of 120 days.

Anaemia due to these conditions does not respond to the administration of iron.

Blood

Film: red cells are small and pale.

Megaloblastic Anaemias

In megaloblastic anaemia there is an abnormality of the red cell precursors in the bone marrow. These abnormal precursors are called megaloblasts. Normal precursors are called normoblasts. In these anaemias the mature red cells in the blood are macrocytic, i.e. larger than normal.

The causes of megaloblastic anaemias are:
vitamin B_{12} deficiency;
folic acid deficiency.
In both deficiencies the changes in the bone marrow and circulating blood are identical.

Vitamin B_{12} Deficiency

Vitamin B_{12} contains cobalt. It is necessary for the synthesis of cells, particularly the blood-forming cells, and for the health of cells of the nervous system. It is present in all animal food (meat, eggs, milk, cheese) and more than average requirements are present in an ordinary diet. It is stored mainly in the liver. Minute amounts are excreted daily in the bile and urine, and the amount in a healthy body at any one time should be sufficient to last for about 4 years. For it to be absorbed into the body intrinsic factor is necessary.

Intrinsic factor is a mucoprotein secreted by the fundus and body of the stomach. It combines with vitamin B_{12} to make a form in which the vitamin can be absorbed. This absorption takes place in the ileum. Without the intrinsic factor little vitamin B_{12} is absorbed.

The causes of vitamin B_{12} deficiency are:
lack of intake of vitamin B_{12};
lack of intrinsic factor;
malabsorption of vitamin B_{12};
increased requirement for vitamin B_{12}.

Lack of intake of vitamin B_{12}

This is rare as there needs to be lack of intake of all animal products, e.g. eggs, milk, butter, as well as of meat. It is likely to occur only in strict vegetarians (vegans) and chronic alcoholics.

Lack of intrinsic factor

1. FAILURE OF SECRETION OF INTRINSIC FACTOR

This causes pernicious anaemia.

Congenital pernicious anaemia is rare. It occurs in infancy. There is no gastric atrophy.

Classical pernicious anaemia occurs mainly between 50-70 years. It is due to atrophy of the gastric mucous membrane. The atrophy can be due to:
(i) an autoimmune factor. The majority of patients have an antibody to gastric parietal cells. Half of them have an antibody to intrinsic factor
(ii) a genetic factor. The incidence of pernicious anaemia in relatives of a patient with pernicious anaemia is about 20-30 per cent, the incidence in the population as a whole being only 0.1 per cent.

2. LACK OF INTRINSIC FACTOR DUE TO GASTRECTOMY

The parts of the stomach which secrete intrinsic factor may be removed in gastrectomy. Vitamin B_{12} cannot then be absorbed and a megaloblastic anaemia occurs as in pernicious anaemia.

Malabsorption of vitamin B_{12}

This can occur in sprue, coeliac disease and idiopathic steatorrhoea, and after resection of the ileum.

Increased requirements of vitamin B_{12}

1. PREGNANCY

Vitamin B_{12} deficiency is rare. Megaloblastic anaemia in pregnancy is more likely to be due to folic acid deficiency.

2. OTHER CONDITIONS

Some parasites of the intestine (e.g. the fish tapeworm) absorb vitamin B_{12}. When anatomical abnormalities cause stasis of the intestinal contents, the partly digested food is invaded by bacteria, some of which are capable of absorbing all the vitamin B_{12}, leaving none to be absorbed by the body.

Clinical features of vitamin B_{12} deficiency

1. ANAEMIA

The usual features of anaemia are present. Particular features are:
'lemon-yellow' colour of the skin which results from a combination of the paleness of anaemia and slight jaundice;
sore tongue — may be deep red and atrophic;
diarrhoea.

2. NEUROLOGICAL DISEASE

Combined degeneration of the spinal cord occurs. The term 'combined degeneration' refers to involvement of both lateral and posterior columns of the spinal cord. This may occur with or without anaemia. Peripheral neuritis causes tingling of hands and feet.

Tests in Vitamin B_{12} Deficiency

Plasma B_{12} level: measured by microbiological methods; is below normal of 300-1000 ng/l.

Film

Megaloblasts may be present in 'buffy coat' (the layer which forms over red cells after centrifuging).
Red cells: count low. Macrocytosis is present — red cells are enlarged in volume and diameter; diameter 8-9μm (normal: 6-8μm) M.C.V. (Mean Corpuscular Volume) increased. Anisocytosis: big variation in size of red cells. Morphological abnormalities are present.
Polymorphs: count low; large number of hypersegmented nuclei, with 5 or more lobes.
Platelets: count low.

Bone marrow

Megaloblasts and giant metamyelocytes are present, up to 2-4 times normal size, often with abnormal nuclei.

Tests for Pernicious Anaemia

Hydrochloric acid in gastric juice

The presence of hydrochloric acid in gastric juice can be tested (p. 116).

In pernicious anaemia hydrochloric acid is absent, except in the rare cases of congenital intrinsic factor deficiency.

Schilling test

A small dose of vitamin B_{12} with a radio-active tracer is given by mouth. 2 hours later a larger dose is given intramuscularly. The urine is examined. In normal people 5-40 per cent of the vitamin appears in the urine. In patients with no intrinsic factor less than 3 per cent appears, showing that the vitamin was not absorbed. The test is then repeated in them, with intrinsic factor being added to the dose of vitamin; the amount of vitamin in the urine then reaches the normal level.

Folate Deficiency

Folic acid is necessary for the life of many plants, bacteria and animals, and is essential for the formation of RNA and DNA and therefore of red blood cells. It is present in animal food products and fresh green vegetables, is absorbed in the upper half of the small intestine, and is stored in the liver. An ordinary diet contains about twice as much as the necessary intake. As the folic acid store in the body is sufficient for about 4 months, any deficiency of it becomes apparent earlier than a deficiency of vitamin B_{12}, the store of which at any one time is sufficient for about 4 years.

The *causes* of folic acid deficiency are:
1. *Dietary deficiency:* can occur with a poor diet and in chronic alcoholism, as a result of both a poor diet and a need for folic acid in the metabolism of alcohol.
2. *Defective absorption:* occurs in malabsorption syndrome due to coeliac disease or idiopathic steatorrhoea.
3. *Increased requirement:* in pregnancy and with malignant neoplasms and haemolytic anaemias. In pregnancy, folate deficiency is due to:
   inadequate diet, anorexia, vomiting
   increased red cell volume of mother with demands for a bigger production of cells
   demands of fetus, placenta and uterus for more DNA and RNA.
4. *Decreased utilization:* in ascorbic acid deficiency and when the patient is taking folic acid antagonist drugs, especially anticonvulsants and methotrexate.

Clinical features of folate deficiency are due to anaemia and similar to those of B_{12} deficiency. Neurological complications do not occur.

Blood

Film: similar to that seen in pernicious anaemia. Red cells may show iron deficiency characteristics, being small and low in haemoglobin.
Red cell folate level: below normal. Normal: 150-640 µg/l.
Serum level: tested by microbiological assay. Normal: 1.9-14 µg/l.
Film from 'buffy coat' (the layer of white cells which forms on top of a packed red cell column after blood has been centrifuged in a narrow tube): megaloblasts may be present.

Bone marrow

Film: similar to that seen in pernicious anaemia, megaloblasts being present; may be similar to marrow in iron deficiency anaemia.

HAEMOLYTIC ANAEMIAS

Haemolysis is the rupture of the red cell membrane with release of haemoglobin. In the haemolytic anaemias the red cells have a shortened life and are destroyed in less than the average of 120 days. Haemolytic anaemias may be intrinsic or extrinsic.

Intrinsic Haemolytic Anaemias

Intrinsic haemolytic anaemias are due to an inherent defect in the red cell, a defect which may be congenital or acquired.

1. *Congenital haemolytic anaemias*

(a) Sickle cell anaemia
Thalassaemia
Spherocytosis
(b) Enzymatic defect: glucose–6–phosphate–dehydrogenase deficiency

2. *Acquired haemolytic anaemia*

Paroxysmal nocturnal haemoglobinuria

Extrinsic Haemolytic Anaemias

In these anaemias the haemolysis is due to external factors which destroy the red cells. The anaemia can be:
1. A haemolytic anaemia due to antibodies.
2. A haemolytic anaemia due to other causes.

CHARACTERISTICS OF HAEMOLYTIC ANAEMIA

Haemolytic anaemias due to different causes show similar results.
1. *Anaemia* occurs when the bone marrow cannot replace red cells at the rate at which they are being destroyed.
2. *Bone marrow* shows erythroid hyperplasia, i.e. an increased production of erythroid cells, the precursors of red cells.
3. *Reticulocytosis.* — The presence of reticulocytes in the circulating blood. Reticulocytes are immature red cells which can be seen with staining to contain still a few threads of nucleoprotein. Normally only 0.5 per cent of red cells are reticulocytes. A raised reticulocyte count indicates a rapid production of red cells.
4. *Morphological abnormalities.* The shape and size of the red cells are often abnormal.
5. *Raised serum bilirubin.* The increased breakdown of haem causes more bilirubin to be produced. In consequence the serum bilirubin is usually raised, jaundice may occur, and pigment gallstones may form.

Sickle Cell Anaemia

This is an inherited defect of the globin portion of the haemoglobin molecule. The patient must be homozygous for the gene, i.e. receive a gene for HbS from each parent. (Normal Hb is HbA — adult haemoglobin.)

The disease occurs in negroes in tropical Africa, the majority dying in childhood. 20 per cent of negroes in better economic circumstances survive to adult life.

The haemoglobin molecule is fragile, particularly in conditions of low oxygen tension. The erythrocytes lose their normal shape and become sickle-shaped.

The disease presents in infants and young children with anaemia, pallor, jaundice and a palpable spleen. Collections of sickled cells in the blood cause thromboses and severe pain, particularly abdominal pain and pains in the joints. Thromboses occur in the kidneys and brain. Marrow hyperplasia in infants causes radiological changes in bone. Periosteal thickening causes swellings, especially of the hands and feet.

Older patients. Ulcers on the malleoli are common in older patients. The spleen becomes shrunken due to infarcts caused by blocking of the blood vessels by red cells. Gallstones are common.

Bone marrow

Erythroid hyperplasia is present; sickled red cells can be seen.

> **Blood**
>
> *Haemoglobin:* about 90 per cent is HbS (the abnormal sickle cell haemoglobin); the rest is HbF (fetal Hb). (Normal adult Hb is HbA.)
> *Red cells:* usually severe anaemia. Hb 3-9 g/dl. Sickle cells can be seen in a wet preparation treated with a reducing agent; cells are of abnormally varied shape and size.
> *Reticulocytes:* increased to 10-20 per cent. Normal: 0.5 per cent in circulating blood.
> *Serum bilirubin:* raised to 20-40 μmol/l. Normal: 2-17 μmol/l.
> *Erythrocyte sedimentation rate* (ESR): low.

Thalassaemia

Thalassaemia occurs particularly around the Mediterranean. It is inherited through a dominant gene. If it is inherited from both parents, the patient has thalassaemia major. If it is inherited from one parent, the patient has thalassaemia minor.

THALASSAEMIA MAJOR

The abnormal gene interferes with the production of normal adult haemoglobin, and a large proportion of the haemoglobin formed is fetal haemoglobin (HbF). This causes a defect of red cell production, the red cells being small, abnormally shaped and with a shortened life. The disease presents in infancy with anaemia, jaundice, splenomegaly and retarded growth, and death in infancy is common. Adult patients are liable to develop ulcers around the malleoli and gallstones.

> **Bone marrow**
>
> *Film:* erythroid hyperplasia occurs; cells are normoblastic.

> **Blood**
>
> *Film:* red cells are small, hypochromatic, abnormally shaped. Nucleated red cells are present. Reticulocytes are increased up to 10 per cent (normal: 0.5 per cent).
> *Haemoglobin:* large proportion of HbF.
> *Serum bilirubin:* increased to 20-60 μmol/l. Normal: 2-17 μmol/l/

THALASSAEMIA MINOR

Patients have mild or moderate anaemia, but otherwise show few clinical symptoms.

Spherocytosis (Acholuric Jaundice)

This condition is usually transmitted as a dominant genetic defect from either parent. Red cells are swollen into spheres which are trapped and destroyed in the spleen.

It can be present at any age — severe cases in infancy, mild cases not until adult life. Clinical features are anaemia, jaundice and splenomegaly. Crises occur with more severe anaemia, fever, tachycardia and abdominal pain; these are probably 'aplastic crises' due to a temporary failure of bone marrow, not haemolytic crises. Pigment gallstones are common.

In patients without biliary obstruction due to gallstones, there is no bilirubinuria, i.e. the jaundice is 'acholuric'.

The precise nature of the defect is not known, but it is thought to occur because: 1, as the red blood cell ages, the sodium pump fails and sodium ions enter the cell at an increased rate; 2, there is a defect of lipid in the cell membrane, and the cell may become a sphere in order to compensate for this defect.

Bone marrow

Film: simple hyperplasia of erythroid precursors is present, i.e. the precursors of red cells are not abnormal.

Blood

Film: spherocytes and reticulocytes are present.
Red cells: moderate or mild anaemia. Haemoglobin 8-13 g/dl. Red cell count low. Red cells show increased osmotic fragility, rupturing in higher concentration of hypotonic saline than normal cells.
Serum bilirubin: raised — 17-85 μmol/l. (Normal: 2-17 μmol/l).
Erythrocyte sedimentation rate (ESR): low.

Glucose-6-Phosphate-Dehydrogenase Deficiency

The inheritance of this condition is sex linked. Two types occur — a negro type and a Mediterranean type.

NEGRO TYPE

The deficiency of glucose-6-phosphate-dehydrogenase causes no symptoms until certain drugs are taken. These drugs cause metabolic changes which require extra glucose-6-phosphate-dehydrogenase if the iron in haemoglobin is to be maintained in its normal state. Lack of glucose-6-phosphate-dehydrogenase causes red cells to degenerate, haemoglobin to be liberated, and a mild or moderate anaemia to occur. Drugs likely to cause haemolysis include some in the following groups: antimalarials sulphonamides analgesics anticonvulsants anti-tuberculosis drugs.

MEDITERRANEAN TYPE

In this type the haemolysis is more severe, the anaemia worse, and the condition precipitated by a greater number of drugs and by infection and chronic diseases.

Paroxysmal Nocturnal Haemoglobinuria

This is a defect of red cells which makes them susceptible to destruction by certains factors in the plasma and in an acid pH. Haemolytic episodes occur, mainly during sleep, and the first morning specimen of urine may be red or black.

Ham's test: red cells placed in normal serum which has been acidified undergo rapid haemolysis.
Red cells: show abnormal shapes and sizes. Reticulocytes increased to 10-20 per cent. Haemoglobin reduced, 9 g/dl.
Serum bilirubin: increased to 20-60 μmol/l. Normal: 2-17 μmol/l.

Extrinsic Haemolytic Anaemias

These anaemias may be due to:
circulating antibodies
other causes.

1. CIRCULATING ANTIBODIES

(a) *Idiopathic:* the patient acquires antibodies to his own red cells. It is not known why these antibodies develop.
(b) *Secondary to other diseases:* antibodies to red cells can occur during some illnesses, particularly malignant lymphoma, carcinoma and connective tissue diseases, and as a reaction to some drugs.

The clinical features are chronic anaemia or haemolytic episodes with abdominal pain, pyrexia and haemoglobinuria.

2. DUE TO OTHER CAUSES

(a) Infections by bacteria, especially *Clostridium welchii*, and protozoa, especially of malaria.
(b) Chemicals, drugs, lead poisoning.
(c) Burns.

Excessive Bleeding

Bleeding is stopped by:
1. A contraction of the wall of the blood vessel.
2. The formation of a plug of platelets over the hole in the vessel, the platelets adhering to the damaged wall and to one another.
3. The formation of a clot of fibrin which forms around the platelet plug and eventually replaces it.

Excessive bleeding can be due to:
1. Disease of the blood vessel which prevents contraction of a cut vessel.
2. A deficiency of platelets.
3. A failure of the normal blood-clotting mechanism.

In a number of cases of excessive bleeding, no abnormalities of vessels, platelets or the clotting mechanism can be found by the methods at present available.

Tests Used in the Investigation of Haemorrhagic Disorders

1. Platelet count

The normal count is $150\text{-}400 \times 10^9/l$. Thromboplastin formation is deficient if the platelets number less than $100 \times 10^9/l$. In some rare bleeding diseases the number may be normal or raised, but the platelets are abnormal in shape and function.

2. Bleeding time

The lobe of the ear is punctured and a piece of blotting paper applied to the blood drop every 30 seconds. In normal people bleeding stops after 1-4 minutes. The time is prolonged in thrombocytopenia (platelet deficiency) and in defects of the capillary wall.

3. Clot retraction test

Clot retraction is the process by which the soft clot formed first squeezes out serum and becomes a firmer clot. In normal blood 40 per cent of serum is expressed after incubation for 2 hours at 37°C.

4. Tourniquet test

A sphygmomanometer cuff is placed around the upper arm and inflated to the point midway between the systolic and diastolic pressures. After 5 minutes the number of petechial spots in the antecubital fossa is counted. The normal count is 0-4 in an area of 3 cm diameter. The number is raised in states of platelet deficiency or functional abnormality in which the capillaries are abnormally fragile.

5. Whole blood coagulation time

Venous blood is placed quickly in a glass tube at 37°C and the tube repeatedly inverted. Time taken for the blood to clot is measured. Normal time: 5-11 minutes. In this test blood will coagulate when there is as little as 5-10 per cent of the normal amount of factor VIII present. Therefore moderate or mild defects are missed and only gross clotting defects detected.

6. Prothrombin consumption test

This test measures the amount of prothrombin in the serum after coagulation has taken place. If the conversion of prothrombin to thrombin has been defective, a large amount of prothrombin will still be present after clotting has taken place. Results are abnormal in haemophilia and with deficiency or abnormality of platelets.

7. Thromboplastin generation test

This test is used to:
(a) determine the amount of thromboplastin formed; (b) detect the factor which is deficient in the thromboplastin formation. Prothrombin is removed from a specimen of the patient's blood so that the coagulation process cannot go further than the formation of thromboplastin. Small quantities of the patient's thromboplastin mixture are added to a prepared blood mixture at regular time intervals. The amount of thromboplastin present can be determined by the speed of clotting. By adding the patient's plasma to blood preparations with known deficiencies, the factor which is defective can be determined. The results are abnormal when there is a deficiency in the factors required for thromboplastin formation, i.e. platelets, factors V, VII, VIII, IX. Qualitative measurements of the defect can also be carried out.

8. More specialized tests

Tests to determine precise deficiencies are carried out in the specialized laboratories attached to Haemophilia Centres.

Platelet Deficiency

Platelets are formed in the bone marrow by the breaking up of the cytoplasm of large cells called megakaryocytes.
Normal count in blood: $150\text{-}400 \times 10^9/l$.
Life: usually 10 days. Where they are destroyed is not known.

FUNCTIONS OF PLATELETS

Platelets are important in several stages of haemostasis (arrest of bleeding).
1. They clump together to form a plug over a hole in a capillary wall.
2. After clumping they break down and release a substance necessary for the formation of thromboplastin.
   (Some of the other blood clotting factors are involved in both these reactions).
3. In the final stages of coagulation they form a focus for the fibrin threads which form the clot.
4. Possibly (this has not been proved) they strengthen capillary walls by being continuously incorporated into the capillary endothelium.
   Thromboplastin formation is deficient if the platelet count is less than $100 \times 10^9/l$. If the number of platelets falls to between $20\text{-}100 \times 10^9/l$, small haemorrhages appear as purpura, bruises and nose-bleeds. If the number falls below $20 \times 10^9/l$, bigger haemorrhages occur from the gastro-intestinal tract, urinary tract and uterus. Spontaneous bleeding may be the result of:
1. possibly, a weakness of the capillary wall due to not enough platelets being incorporated into it

2. a failure to form a platelet plug.
Bleeding may then be due to ordinary muscle movement or to minimal trauma.

Acetylsalicylic acid (aspirin) interferes with the ability of platelets to clump to form a plug, and taking it can cause bleeding from the gastric mucosa or from a peptic ulcer.

CAUSES OF PLATELET DEFICIENCY (THROMBOCYTOPENIA)

Thrombocytopenia may occur because platelets are not being produced by the bone marrow or because they are being destroyed in the circulation.

1. *Deficiency of megakaryocytes in the bone marrow*

This can be due to:
(a) other diseases of the blood, e.g. aplastic anaemia, leukaemia;
(b) invasion of bone marrow by carcinomatous deposits, myelofibrosis, malignant lymphoma, etc;
(c) agents causing a depression of platelet production or of all marrow function, e.g. radiation, drugs and chemicals (e.g. gold salts, nitrogen mustards).

2. *Shortened platelet life span*

This can be due to:
(a) antibodies destroying the platelets, e.g. (i) in idiopathic thrombocytopenic purpura agglutinins against the platelets can often be discovered; the cause of this is not known; (ii) some drugs and infections cause the development of agglutinins which destroy the platelets, e.g. sedormid, quinine;
(b) hypersplenism, in which platelets are destroyed;
(c) some infections, e.g. rubella, chickenpox.

Platelet count: below $100 \times 10^9/l$.
In some rare bleeding diseases the count may be normal, but the platelets are abnormal in shape and function.
Bleeding time: prolonged.
Clot retraction: defective.
Tourniquet test: abnormal.
Prothrombin consumption test: reduced.
Bone marrow: the marrow picture varies with the cause of the platelet deficiency. If the platelets are being destroyed in the circulation, the marrow may be normal or hyperplastic. The megakaryocytes may be normal.

Coagulation of Blood

The clotting of blood is a complex sequence of events by which fibrinogen, a soluble plasma protein, is converted to a stable fibrin clot. The factors necessary for coagulation are platelets and the following factors I-XIII.

Factor I	Fibrinogen
Factor II	Prothrombin
Factor III	Tissue thromboplastin
Factor IV	Calcium ions
Factor V	Prothrombin accelerator (labile factor)

There is no Factor VI

Factor VII	Proconvertin (stable factor)
Factor VIII	Anti-haemophilic globulin (AHG)
Factor IX	Christmas factor
Factor X	Stuart-Prower factor
Factor XI	Plasma thromboplastin antecedent
Factor XII	Hageman factor
Factor XIII	Fibrin stabilizing factor

Some of these factors are normally present in the plasma; others (thromboplastin, thrombin, fibrin) are formed by the interaction of those occurring earlier in the sequence. As a result of complex interactions thromboplastin is released and then thrombin is formed, which together with fibrinogen forms fibrin.

The process can be summarized simply:

Prothrombin (in plasma) + thromboplastin + calcium ions → thrombin
Fibrinogen (in plasma) + thrombin → fibrin

The sequence is complicated and several interactions occur at each stage.

Thromboplastin is formed by the operation of two systems, known as intrinsic and extrinsic. In the intrinsic system thromboplastin results from the breakdown of platelets interacting with other factors. In the extrinsic system thromboplastin is released as a result of tissue being damaged. Some of the factors are necessary for both systems. In natural blood coagulation after injury both systems operate.

Defects of coagulation

Defects of coagulation may be congenital or acquired.

1. CONGENITAL DEFECTS

(a) *Haemophilia*

Haemophilia (factor VIII deficiency) occurs mostly in males, being transmitted as a sex-linked recessive condition due to a genetic defect on the X chromosome. A woman with the defect on one of her chromosomes will transmit the disease to half her sons, and half her daughters will become carriers. On theoretical grounds the disease could happen in women, and in practice about 1 in 200 patients with haemophilia is a woman. A family history of the disease occurs in about 75 per cent of cases; in others the disease may have arisen as a result of a maternal gene mutation.

Patients usually fall into two groups: (a) a group with severe haemophilia who bleed spontaneously or after mild trauma, and (b) a group with mild haemophilia who bleed excessively only after injury, tooth extraction or surgical operation. Spontaneous bleeding occurs into muscles, joints, the gastrointestinal tract, the urinary tract and under the periosteum. Repeated bleeding into a joint leads to ankylosis and muscular contractures. Haemorrhagic cysts follow subperiosteal haemorrhages.

> *Platelet count:* usually normal unless there has been a recent haemorrhage.
> *Red and white cell counts:* usually normal.
> *Coagulation time:* may be prolonged to 1 hour (normal: 5-11 minutes). The coagulation time may be normal if there is only a slight or moderate deficit of factor VIII, AHG (anti-haemophilic globulin).
> *Thromboplastin generation time:* result is abnormal due to deficiency of factor VIII, AHG (antihaemophilic globulin).

(b) *Christmas disease*

This disease (factor IX deficiency) gets its name from the family in which it was discovered. The clinical features are similar to those of mild haemophilia.

> *Thromboplastin generation test:* the result is abnormal due to a deficiency of factor IX (Christmas factor).
> The results of other tests are similar to those in haemophilia.

(c) *Von Willebrand's disease*

Von Willebrand's disease is inherited but not sex-linked. There is a combination of two faults – a capillary defect and a coagulation defect leading to a slight deficiency of factor VIII. It seems that some factor is present in both normal and haemophilic blood which is missing in patients with von Willebrand's disease. There may be bleeding from the umbilical cord at birth: bleeding into joints is rare. Otherwise the clinical features are similar to those of haemophilia.

> *Bleeding time:* usually prolonged.
> *Tourniquet test:* positive
> *Thromboplastin generation test:* often abnormal due to a deficiency of factor VIII.
> *Capillaries:* may show abnormalities.

2. ACQUIRED DEFECTS

Vitamin K is necessary for the synthesis in the liver of factors II, VII, IX and X. Deficiency of vitamin K occurs in:
premature babies,
liver disease,
malabsorption syndrome,
patient taking heparin (which is a vitamin K antagonist).

In these conditions abnormal bleeding occurs as a result of a failure of synthesis of one or more of the factors.

Blood Groups

The different blood groups have arisen because mutations have occurred in the genes responsible for the constituents of the surface of the membrane on the outside of the cells. These changes do not affect the functioning of the cells. As a result of the mutations different blood groups systems have developed. The two important systems clinically are:
ABO system
Rhesus system.

ABO groups

Three genes known as A, B and O determine the substances present on the red cells. These substances are capable of stimulating antibody formation and are known as antigens. There are also naturally occurring antibodies to these substances.
• Group AB blood has A and B antigens on the cells, but antibodies to neither in the serum
• Group A blood has A antigen on the cells and anti-B antibody in the serum
• Group B blood has B antigen on the cells and anti-A antibody in the serum
• Group O blood has neither antigen on the cells, but has anti-A and anti-B antibodies in the serum.

Because of the presence of antigens on the cells and of antibodies in the serum, the blood transfused has to be of the same ABO group as the recipient's blood. If blood of a wrong group is transfused, the antibodies in the recipient's serum may cause the donor cells to clump. These clumped cells block the smaller blood vessels, producing incompatibility reactions.

Group O particularly may have antibodies so potent that they destroy the cells of group A, B or AB.

People are divided into 4 groups – AB, A, B and O – in the following proportions (in Britain):
group AB   3 per cent
group A   42 per cent
group B   9 per cent
group O   46 per cent

Rhesus groups

This system gets its name from the Rhesus monkeys which were used in the original investigations.

It is thought that 3 pairs of genes are responsible for producing antigens (C and c, D and d, E and e) on the surface of red cells. Of these the clinically important one is D.

People with D on their red cells are called Rhesus positive (Rh positive).

People without D on their red cells are called Rhesus negative (RH negative).

About 85 per cent of people are Rh positive and about 15 per cent are Rh negative.

Antibodies against the Rhesus factor do not occur naturally (as do antibodies against A and B in the ABO system). A Rh negative person can develop anti-D antibodies in 2 ways:

1. By being given a transfusion of Rh positive blood. If a second transfusion of Rh positive blood is given, a haemolytic reaction is likely to occur when the antibodies agglutinate the donated red cells.
2. A Rh negative woman who has a Rh positive baby is likely to be sensitized by the feto-maternal leak of red cells which usually occurs during birth when the placenta separates from the uterus. As little as 0.5 ml of fetal blood is enough to sensitize the mother.

Other blood groups

Other blood groups (e.g. Kell, Duffy and Kidd groups) exist, but occur less commonly in the population. They can cause haemolytic disease and incompatibility reactions. Antibodies to their antigens do not usually occur naturally.

Tests to Ensure Compatible Blood

1. The ABO group of the recipient is determined by:
(a) adding agglutinating anti-A and anti-B to his red cells;
(b) adding the recipient's serum to known group A and group B cells. The Rh group of the recipient is determined by using the appropriate antisera and examining for agglutination.
2. Donor blood of the right ABO and Rh group is selected. These groups should have been determined by the organization collecting the blood.
3. *Cross-matching*. Blood is not examined for every possible antigen as over 100 exist. Therefore direct tests are performed to ensure that the actual blood to be given is compatible with that of the patient.
(a) Plasma or serum of the patient is incubated with cells from the donor's blood.

(b) *Indirect Coombs test*. This is a very sensitive test for Rh antibodies in the patient's serum.

The blood should not be transfused unless both these tests are negative.

Dangers of blood transfusion

1. INCOMPATIBLE TRANSFUSION

Haemolytic reactions occur due to destruction of donor red cells by antibodies in the recipient's plasma. Occasionally, donor's plasma may clump recipient's cells. The severity of the reaction depends on the strength of the antigen-antibody reaction. In mild cases there may be no symptoms at all, but the transfused red cells are removed quickly from the patient's circulation. In extreme cases there is an immediate reaction, which may be fatal. Circulatory collapse and haemorrhages can occur. Renal failure can be caused by hypotension and the toxic effect on the kidney of lysed cells in a hypotensive patient. There is particular danger in an emergency when the patient is likely to be hypotensive and shocked before transfusion.

2. SENSITIZATION

This means the development of antibodies when red cells with a certain antigen are given to a recipient without that antigen. The hazards of Rhesus positive blood being given to Rhesus negative patients are described above.

Other blood groups can sensitize. A patient who lacks a very common antigen is likely to be given a blood with that antigen. Antibodies develop, and if a subsequent transfusion is necessary only blood from the small number of people who do not have the antigen will be compatible.

If a rare antigen is given to a patient the development of antibodies is less important, because at any subsequent transfusion blood from the majority of people will be compatible (as the rare antigen occurs rarely).

3. INFECTION

(a) *Disease transmitted in the blood from the donor*
(i) *Viral hepatitis* (see p. 33). A post-transfusional viral hepatitis is the commonest of the dangers of transfusion. About 1 in 20 donors in some parts of the world are carriers of virus A (the cause of infectious hepatitis) or of virus B (the cause of serum hepatitis). Blood should not be used from would-be donors who have had jaundice or are carriers of Australia antigen (see p. 33).
(ii) *Syphilis.* Would-be donors should be serologically tested. The spirochete dies within a few days in blood stored at 40°C.
(iii) *Malaria.* People who have had malaria should not be used as donors.
(iv) *Brucellosis.*

(b) *Disease transmitted by contamination of the blood after it has been taken.*
(i) *Staphylococci* from the skin may infect the blood. They die in blood stored at 4°C.
(ii) *Cryophilic organisms* are organisms which grow in the cold. Some Gram-negative organisms (bacilli) can contaminate blood at 4°C.

4. OVERLOADING OF THE CIRCULATION

Too rapid transfusion can overload the circulation, especially of old people or patients with severe anaemia. Signs of overloading are dyspnoea, cough, rales heard at the bases of the lungs, and a rise of pressure in the jugular veins.

5. CITRATE TOXICITY

This is due to the reduction of ionized calcium in the blood. Signs of it are gross tremors and a lengthening of the QT interval in the electrocardiogram. Death has occurred after too rapid a transfusion. It is prevented by adding calcium gluconate 1 g to each litre of blood.

6. PYROGEN REACTIONS

Pyrogens are soluble polysaccharides produced by bacteria, and are liable to occur in distilled water, dextrose, sodium chloride and citrate. Strict control in the manufacture of anticoagulants have made these reactions rare. Signs are chills and pyrexia 30-60 minutes after beginning the transfusion.

Haemolytic disease of the newborn

The commonest cause of haemolytic disease of the newborn is RhD incompatibility. This occurs when a Rhesus negative woman already sensitized (i.e. having anti-D antibodies) has a Rh positive baby. Anti-D antibodies pass across the placenta into the fetal circulation and coat the fetal Rhesus positive erythrocytes, which are destroyed. This causes:
- *either* the death of the fetus and its stillbirth;
- *or* in a live baby anaemia, jaundice soon after birth and congestive heart failure. Jaundice may not be present at birth, but develops 24-36 hours later. If the condition is not treated by exchange transfusion, anaemia and jaundice become worse.

Kernicterus may develop. If the serum unconjugated bilirubin reaches 400 μmol/l or more, deposition of it in the basal ganglia and cerebral cortex causes spasticity and mental retardation.

Tests on Baby with Haemolytic Disease of the Newborn

Results of tests show a progressive haemolytic anaemia.
Red cell count: reduced.
Haemoglobin: low.
Reticulocytes: increased up to 70 per cent of the red cells.
Normoblasts: large number in peripheral blood.
Erythropoiesis: increased in tissues.
Platelets: number reduced.
Direct Coombs test: positive. This

test detects the presence of anti-D antibodies on Rhesus positive cells. The test is usually carried out on umbilical cord blood at birth.
Bilirubin: raised above 60 μmol/l. The amount continues to rise if the baby is not treated by exchange transfusion.

Tests During Pregnancy

1. The *ABO and Rh groups* of a pregnant woman are determined early in pregnancy. If she is Rhesus negative:
2. *Indirect Coombs test.* The mother's serum is investigated for the presence of anti-D antibodies at 12 weeks and at 28 weeks.
3. If the woman's anti-D has increased between 12 and 28 weeks, an amniocentesis is performed to obtain a specimen of amniotic fluid. The amount of bilirubin in the fluid is estimated as this gives an indication of the amount of red cell damage in the fetus.
4. If there is evidence of haemolysis of fetal red cells: (a) before 32 weeks: an intrauterine infusion of red cells into the peritoneal cavity of the fetus is carried out; (b) after 32-34 weeks: premature induction of birth may be advisable.

PREVENTION OF HAEMOLYTIC DISEASE BY IMMUNIZATION OF MOTHER.

Kleihauer test

This is carried out on the maternal blood to determine whether a feto-maternal leak has occurred. Because of chemical difference between adult and fetal haemoglobin, the maternal cells are denatured in an acid solution and the fetal cells look normal.

If the mother has not previously been sensitized and the Kleihauer test is positive, she should be given human gamma globulin containing anti-D antibodies within 36 hours of the birth. This destroys the fetal cells in the circulation and prevents her from developing antibodies against Rhesus positive blood. The antibodies injected are destroyed before the next pregnancy.

Erythrocyte Sedimentation Rate (ESR)

Erythrocyte = red cell.
5 ml of blood taken with a dry sterile needle and syringe are necessary. The blood is mixed with EDTA (ethylene-diamine-tetra-acetic acid), an anticoagulant, a dry deposit of which coats the bottle into which the blood is put. The bottle should be turned upside down several times to mix the blood with the anticoagulant. The test must be set up within 6 hours of taking the blood.

The test measures the rate at which red cells fall down a narrow glass tube. Red cells fall because their density is greater than that of plasma, but the formation of rouleaux increases the rate of fall (the sedimentation rate). Rouleaux are columns of cells, one on top of another, which form in certain conditions, such as when blood comes into contact with glass. A rouleau has the same mass but a lower surface area than the same number of separate red cells; the spaces between descending cells are therefore increased and descent is quickened. The ESR is higher when rouleaux are long. Rouleaux length determines the ESR. Factors favouring rouleaux formation are: (1) the normal biconcave shape of red cells, (2) an increase in fibrinogen content in plasma.

The result is the meniscus (top level) of red cells at the end of 1 hour. The extent of the fall is visible as the height of the column of plasma at the top of the tube.

Normal (Westergren method)

Males: 3-5 mm.
Females: 4-7 mm.

Physiological increase

In pregnancy.

Pathological increase

Falls greater then normal occur when tissue-destroying disease is present. They occur in:
infections (except influenza, cystitis and sometimes infections of the central nervous system)
myocardial infarction
fractures   burns   acute gout
some malignant and degenerating neoplasms

Pathological decrease

1. Polycythaemia: because the cells are so close to each other that there is more resistance to the plasma being forced upwards.
2. Conditions which increase the viscosity of the plasma, e.g. hyperproteinaemia.
3. Conditions which reduce rouleaux formation because abnormal cells do not form rouleaux: spherocytosis, sickle cell disease, iron deficiency anaemia when cells are of abnormal size and shape.

The ESR is used to assess the course of a disease, e.g. tuberculosis, connective tissue disease, rheumatic fever.

Aplastic Anaemia

Aplastic anaemia is an anaemia in which the number of red cells, white cells and platelets in the circulating blood is reduced as a result of a breakdown in supply from the bone marrow.

Some agents invariably cause aplastic anaemia if given in large enough doses:
radiation
some drugs given for malignant disease, e.g. nitrogen mustards and methotrexate

Other known causes are:
1. *Drugs:* chloramphenicol, hydantoin (Epanutin) and possibly other anticonvulsants, phenylbutazone, gold salts, antibiotics, antithyroid drugs, antihistamines.
2. *Industrial chemicals:* benzene.

In about half the cases no cause can be found.

In some cases the red bone marrow is acellular and turns out an inadequate number of cells. In other cases the bone marrow appears normal or is hypercellular, but the cells are destroyed before they get into the circulating blood.

Blood

Count: the number of red cells, white cells and platelets is much below normal, and repeated counts show that the anaemia is becoming worse.

Polycythaemia Vera

Polycythaemia vera is a disease characterized by an excessive number of red cells in the circulating blood. The cause is unknown. The disease is a chronic one from which the patient ultimately dies.

The blood shows an excessive number of red cells in all cases, an excessive number of leucocytes in about 70 per cent of cases, and an excessive number of platelets in about 50 per cent. There is an overgrowth of red bone marrow into the yellow marrow. The spleen is often enlarged. The patient's face, hands and feet are duskily cyanosed. Thrombosis in a blood vessel is common, being due to the increased viscosity of the blood and the increased number of platelets when present. Haemorrhages can occur, but their cause is uncertain.

After several years the blood picture changes: red bone marrow is replaced by fibrous tissue, red cell production falls, and the patient becomes anaemic. Acute myeloblastic leukaemia develops as a terminal event in about 10 per cent of patients with the disease.

Secondary polycythaemia can develop in people with severe chronic cardiac or respiratory disease and in people who live at high altitudes.

Blood

Red cell count: increased up to $6.0\text{-}8.0 \times 10^{12}/l$.
Haemoglobin concentration: above 17 g/dl in women and 18 g/dl in men.
Packed cell volume (PCV): increased to 55-80 per cent. Normal: men 40-54 per cent, women 35-47 per cent.
Leucocyte count: may be increased up to $10\text{-}30 \times 10^9/l$. Marked rise in percentage of neutrophils. Later myeloblasts may appear.
Platelet count: may be increased. Normal $150 \times 10^9/l$.

Erythrocyte sedimentation rate (ESR): low.

Bone marrow

Film: hyperplasia of all elements; later myelosclerosis or leukaemia.

Leukaemia

Leukaemia is a neoplastic disease in which there is abnormal proliferation of white cells and of the leucopoetic tissues from which white cells develop. The main leukaemias are:

1. Acute leukaemias — Acute myeloblastic leukaemia
   Acute lymphoblastic leukaemia
2. Chronic leukaemias — Chronic myeloid leukaemia
   Chronic lymphatic leukaemia

AETIOLOGY

(a) *Ionizing radiations*

Ionizing radiations are known to be capable of producing myeloid leukaemia. Leukaemia may develop 5-10 years after exposure to radiation from an atomic bomb explosion or after frequent exposure to smaller doses. It is an occupational hazard of radiologists and radiographers. Children of women exposed to X-rays during pregnancy may have a higher incidence of leukaemia than average.

(b) *Genetic factors*

Leukaemia has been reported as occurring in several members of the same family, which suggests that a genetic factor is involved. A chromosomal abnormality is present in about 95 per cent of patients with chronic myeloid leukaemia: it consists of a loss of part of chromosome no. 22 (a short one, known as the Philadelphia chromosome). An increase or decrease in the number of chromosomes can occur in both kinds of acute leukaemia.

(c) *Virus infections*

A virus infection may initiate the neoplastic changes or cause a genetic mutation which leads to leukaemia.

Acute leukaemias

An acute leukaemia usually runs a rapid course, but with modern treatment life may be prolonged beyond the 6-12 months that was usual. There are peaks of incidence in childhood and old age. Both acute leukaemias present the same clinical pattern: fever, anaemia, purpura, enlargement of liver, spleen and lymph nodes. Leukaemic tissue (of primitive polymorphs or primitive lymphocytes) can invade the skin, bone and nervous system, and haemorrhages into the nervous system and eye can occur. Infection by bacteria, viruses or fungi is common.

The predominating feature in the blood in acute leukaemias is the high number of 'blast' cells circulating. Normally 'blast' cells occur only in the bone marrow. The total white cell count may be high, but it is not always so. About one-third of all patients have a normal or below normal white cell count at some stage of the disease.

(a) ACUTE MYELOBLASTIC LEUKAEMIA

This leukaemia may occur at any age; it is the most common type to occur in middle age. The characteristic feature of the blood is the high count of myeloblasts, which may form 20-70 per cent of the total white cell count. Myeloblasts are the earliest form of polymorphonuclear cells, and are not normally present in circulating blood. The count increases as the disease progresses.

> **Blood**
>
> *Leucocytes*: total count may be $20-50 \times 10^9/l$, but may be below average (average $5-10 \times 10^9/l$.)
> *Myeloblasts*: high count forming 20-70 per cent of all leucocytes, according to stage of the disease.
> *Red cells*: count low. Haemoglobin reduced.
> *Platelets*: count low, becoming lower as disease progresses.

> **Bone marrow**
>
> Hyperplasia is present, the majority of cells being myeloblasts.

(b) ACUTE LYMPHOBLASTIC LEUKAEMIA

This is the most common leukaemia of childhood and occurs most often below 15 years.

The majority of leucocytes in the blood are lymphoblasts (the earliest form of lymphocyte), but other early forms are also present in large numbers.

> **Blood**
>
> *Leucocytes*: total count usually raised. Majority of cells are lymphoblasts and other early forms. Neutrophils are low.
> *Red cells*: count low. Haemoglobin reduced.
> *Platelets*: count low.

> **Bone marrow**
>
> Hyperplasia is present, the majority of cells being lymphoblasts.

Chronic leukaemia

Chronic leukaemias begin with slight symptoms and run a course of several years before proving fatal.

(a) CHRONIC MYELOID LEUKAEMIA

This leukaemia occurs mainly between 30-60 years. The spleen is very much enlarged, and patients often present with symptoms resulting from this. The symptoms of anaemia are also common presenting symptoms.

In contrast with acute leukaemia, the total leucocyte count is very high. At the beginning of the disease the majority of cells are mature polymorphs, but as the disease progresses the proportion of polymorph precursors increases. Terminally the disease may change to an acute myeloblastic leukaemia with the highest number of cells being myeloblasts.

> **Blood**
>
> *Leucocyte count:* grossly raised, may be 100-500×10⁹/l. Normal: 5-10 ×10⁹/l.
> *Differential count:* the majority of white cells are neutrophils and myelocytes. Terminally myeloblasts usually predominate.
> *Red cells:* count low. Haemoglobin slightly reduced. The degree of anaemia is at first moderate; terminally it becomes severe.
> *Platelets:* count raised in early stages, very low in terminal stages.
>
> **Bone marrow**
>
> Proliferation of myeloid series of cells.

(b) CHRONIC LYMPHATIC LEUKAEMIA

This leukaemia occurs in people of 55 onwards. The presenting feature is often enlargement of the lymph nodes. Enlargement of the spleen is slight.

The characteristic feature of the blood is the high number of lymphocytes, which look normal.

> **Blood**
>
> *Leucocytes:* raised count of 30-300 ×10⁹/l, but in early stages the count may not be raised.
> *Differential count:* high proportion of lymphocytes, which may form 90 per cent of the total.
> *Red cells:* count slightly low. Haemoglobin slightly low. Anaemia becomes more severe as the disease progresses.
> *Platelets:* low in terminal stages.
>
> **Bone marrow**
>
> Marked increases in cells of the lymphoid series.

Agranulocytosis

This is a rare disease in which there is a disappearance complete or almost complete of polymorphs (granulocytes) from the blood.

Causes: The agents which cause aplastic anaemia always cause granulocytopenia (a reduction in the number of granulocytes), which may go on to agranulocytosis; these agents are ionizing radiations and drugs used in the treatment of malignant disease, e.g. nitrogen mustards and methotrexate. The effects of other drugs seems to be related to the sensitivity of the patient to the drug rather than to the total amount of drug received by him. These drugs include: amidopyrine, thiouracil and other antithyroid drugs, chloramphenicol, chlorpromazine and other tranquillisers.

In about half the cases no cause can be found.

Patients develop a severe and often fatal illness, with severe infection and ulceration of the mouth and throat.

> **Blood**
>
> *Count:* total leucocyte count is very low. Differential count show polymorphs absent or forming 2-3 per cent of the total (normal 60-70 per cent.

Chapter 14 The Alimentary Tract

LIPS, MOUTH AND TONGUE

The lips, mouth and tongue are frequently involved in the same pathological process.

Lip

A *squamous cell carcinoma* can develop on either lip but is more common on the lower. It occurs especially in pipe-smokers, and in fair skinned people exposed for years to strong sunlight, and can be preceded by leukoplakia, a premalignant warty growth of squamous epithelium. The carcinoma infiltrates local tissues, can ulcerate and then become infected, and is likely to spread into lymph nodes draining the site.

Mouth

STOMATITIS

Stomatitis is any infection of the mucous membrane of the mouth. It can be a viral, bacterial or fungal infection.

(a) *Aphthous stomatitis*

The cause of this is unknown; it may be a viral infection, but the virus has not been identified. It occurs usually during the first half of adult life and in women more than men. Small raised vesicles surrounded by a red areola form in the mucous membrane, burst and leave grey ulcers. In about 10 per cent of affected women similar lesions appear on the vulva and vagina. The condition heals spontaneously, but further attacks can occur.

(b) *Vincent's angina*

This appears to be the result of a double infection – by a spirochete and a fusiform bacillus. It occurs usually in children and adolescents and is associated with dental caries and poor dental hygiene. All parts of the mouth and pharynx can be affected, particularly the gum margin. The mucous membrane is inflamed and swollen, bleeds easily, and may ulcerate.

Swab

Smear: examined for *Borrelia vincenti,* a spirochete, and *B. fusiformis fusiformis.*

(c) *Thrush*

This is an infection of the mouth and fauces by *Candida albicans,* a fungus. It occurs in debilitated children and adults with poor oral hygiene and as a complication of treatment with corticosteroids and oral antibiotics. Greyish-white spots and patches appear on the mucous membrane.

Swab

Smear: examined for spores and filaments of the fungus.
Culture: fungus grows on blood agar and Sabouraud's medium.

Retention cysts are small cysts in the mucous membrane due to blockage of the ducts of small salivary glands in the mucous membrane.

Pigmentation of the mouth. A brown pigmentation of the mucous membrane can occur in:
Addison's disease   haemochromatosis
poisoning by arsenic, bismuth, gold, silver and other metals.

Tongue

Atrophy of the mucous membrane is liable to occur in:
iron deficiency
vitamin B$_{12}$ deficiency
riboflavine deficiency
The papillae become flattened and the surface of the tongue is smooth and shiny. In iron deficiency the tongue is pale; in the other deficiencies it is likely to be very red.

Squamous cell carcinoma of the tongue occurs in both sexes. It may be preceded by leukoplakia. It can ulcerate, become infected, and spread into adjacent lymph nodes.

Geographic tongue (erythema migrans) is a condition of unknown causation which occurs mostly in children and young women. Irregularly shaped areas on the surface of the tongue lose their papillae and become bright red. The condition clears up spontaneously.

Salivary Glands

INFECTIONS

Mumps

Mumps is caused by a virus of the myxovirus group. The parotid and other salivary glands become inflamed. The glandular and surrounding tissues become oedematous and infiltrated by lymphocytes.
Complications:
orchitis   oophoritis
meningitis   meningo-encephalitis

Parotitis

This is an inflammation of the parotid gland usually due to an infection spreading upwards from the mouth through the parotid duct to the gland. It can occur in apparently healthy people or in:
dehydration and the absence of chewing and salivation;
obstruction by a calculus in the parotid duct;
Sjögren's syndrome;
diabetes mellitus;
septicaemia.

In acute attacks *Staphylococcus pyogenes* is the usual infecting organism; in subacute and recurrent attacks *Streptococcus viridans* and *pneumococci* are the usual organisms.

CALCULI

Calculi can form in the parotid and submandibular ducts. They are composed of calcium oxalate mixed with dried mucus and cell debris, and cause swelling of the gland.

NEOPLASMS

A *mixed parotid neoplasm* is composed of glandular and squamous epithelium in a stroma resembling cartilage. It is usually lobulated and poorly encapsulated; occasionally one becomes malignant. *Carcinoma* can develop in the parotid and submandibular glands. Neoplasms of the sublingual and smaller salivary glands in the mouth are rare.

OESOPHAGUS

Achalasia

Achalasia is a disturbance of the function of the oesophagus as a result of degenerative and sometimes inflammatory changes in the autonomic nerves which lie between its muscle coats and control its movements. The cause is unknown. In time the oesophagus becomes dilated and elongated, sometimes developing an S-shaped curve. Carcinoma of the lower end of the oesophagus develops in about 5 per cent of cases.

Diverticula

Diverticula of the oesophagus can be present:
(a) at the junction of pharynx and oesophagus,
(c) opposite the bifurcation of the trachea,
(c) at the lower end of the oesophagus.
Food can stagnate in them.

Oesophagitis

Oesophagitis is an inflammation of the oesophagus due to:
(a) fungus infections of the mouth and pharynx spreading downwards,
(b) a reflux of gastric contents into the lower end of the oesophagus,
(c) swallowing hot or corrosive liquids or solids.

Severe or chronic inflammation can produce ulceration of the mucous membrane, and fibrosis of an ulcerated area can produce stenosis.

Carcinoma of the oesophagus

A *squamous cell carcinoma* can develop in the oesophagus. It is:
(a) more common in men than women (except when it is associated with iron-deficiency),
(b) associated with heavy drinking.

It usually occurs about the middle third. It can project into the lumen of the oesophagus, infiltrate the oesophageal wall and adjacent parts of the mediastinum, and invade lymph nodes draining the site.

An *adenocarcinoma* of the oesophagus can develop:
(a) at the lower end of the oesophagus, which is lined with gastric mucous membrane,
(b) in islands of ectopic (i.e. out of place) gastric mucous membrane which have developed higher up in the oesophagus as a developmental error.

Biopsy

Specimens of a growth can be removed at oesophagoscopy and examined for malignant cells.

STOMACH AND DUODENUM

Gastritis

Acute gastritis is an acute inflammation of the mucous membrane of the stomach due to the ingestion of alcohol, acetylsalicylic acid (aspirin), corrosive liquids, etc. The mucous membrane becomes hyperaemic, swollen and invaded by polymorphs and other cells, and the surface may be shed. With removal of the irritant the mucous membrane regenerates.

Chronic gastritis takes several forms, about which there is no general agreement. Two types which have been described are:
(a) *chronic superficial gastritis* which occurs in chronic alcoholics and in which the superficial layers of the mucous membrane degenerate;
(b) *chronic atrophic gastritis* which can occur in pernicious anaemia and in which the mucous membrane and deeper layers become atrophic and there is decreasing secretion of hydrochloric acid.

Peptic Ulcer

A *peptic ulcer* is an ulcer of the gastrointestinal tract due to the action of hydrochloric acid and pepsin on the wall.

An ulcer occurs:
(a) commonly in the stomach and duodenum,
(b) less commonly at the lower end of the oesophagus, in a Meckel's diverticulum (where gastric mucosa is sometimes present), and in the jejunum after gastro-enterostomy or partial gastrectomy.

A peptic ulcer can be:
an acute peptic ulcer;
a chronic peptic ulcer.

Acute peptic ulcer

An acute peptic ulcer is a common condition, but the full incidence of them is unknown as many do not produce symptoms. Gastroscopy shows that some people have small haemorrhagic lesions of the mucous membrane of the stomach, most of which heal up without leaving a scar, but some of which ulcerate. Acute ulcers can be up to 1 cm in diameter.

The cause of most ulcers is unknown. Some are known to follow:
surgical operations;
severe burns;
lesions of the base of the brain.

The lesion may be the result of:
spasm of a small blood-vessel;
a thrombus or embolism in a small blood-vessel.
Following interruption of the blood supply an area of mucous membrane would degenerate and an ulcer could be produced.

Chronic peptic ulcer

A chronic peptic ulcer or the scar of an old one is found in about 10 per cent of all autopsies.

A peptic ulcer looks the same wherever it occurs. It:
(a) is a sharply defined ulcer of the mucous membrane and sometimes deeper layers of the gastrointestinal wall,
(b) varies in size from a few millimetres to about 4 cm in diameter,
(c) has a floor formed of a purulent exudate, a layer of necrotic tissue, a layer of granulation tissue and a layer of fibrous tissue,
(d) may have arteries visible in the floor, the lumen of the artery often being partially or completely blocked by endarteritis obliterans,
(e) can heal, leaving a scar.

DIFFERENCES BETWEEN GASTRIC AND DUODENAL ULCERS

	Gastric ulcer	Duodenal ulcer
1. *Situation*	lesser curvature and adjacent part of posterior wall of stomach	first part of duodenum
2. *Age of onset*	commonly 40–50 years	commonly 30–40 years
3. *Male/female ratio*	3:2	10:1
4. *Social class of patient*	most common in lowest social class	equally distributed in all social classes
5. *Blood group of patient*	no association	blood group O likely
6. *Acid secretion in stomach*	lower than normal	higher than normal
7. *Malignant disease*	develops in about 5 per cent	does not develop

COMPLICATIONS

1. *Haemorrhage* may be slight when due to oozing from the surface of the ulcer and severe when due to ulceration of a large vessel.
2. *Perforation* of the wall of the stomach or duodenum with the production of a generalized or localized peritonitis.
3. *Scarring* can produce (according to the site of the ulcer) an hour-glass deformity of the stomach, pyloric stenosis or duodenal stenosis.
4. *Malignant diseases* occurs on the edge of the ulcer in about 5 per cent of chronic gastric ulcers.

Carcinoma of the Stomach

Carcinoma of the stomach is a common disease and responsible for about 10 per cent of all deaths from malignant disease. It occurs in middle and old age, is more common in East Asians than Europeans and in people of blood group A.

The cause is unknown. Predisposing factors appear to be:
gastric atrophy
chronic gastric ulcer

adenoma of stomach (a rare condition).

The site of the carcinoma is:
pylorus and antrum: 50 per cent
lesser curvature: 25 per cent
cardiac orifice: 10 per cent
elsewhere in stomach: 15 per cent.

The carcinoma is an adeno-carcinoma, but its cells vary considerably in different tumours, and it contains a variable amount of fibrous tissue.

The neoplasm may be:
(a) an ulcerative lesion. This is the commonest form. The neoplasm projects into the interior of the stomach and its surface becomes ulcerated. In some cases the ulceration involves all the coats of the stomach and perforates into the peritoneal cavity.
(b) a polypoidal lesion. The neoplasm forms a large irregular polyp projecting into the interior of the stomach.
(c) an infiltrative lesion in which the growth spreads through the wall of the stomach thickening it and tending to narrow the stomach into a 'leather-bottle stomach'.

Spread of the neoplasm is into:
lymph nodes draining the site;
lower end of the oesophagus.

Metastases can occur in:
liver   peritoneum (causing ascites)
lung   brain
bone   ovary (producing a Krukenberg tumour)
left supraclavicular lymph gland (reaching it via the thoracic duct).

Pyloric Stenosis

Pyloric stenosis can be:
(a) *congenital pyloric stenosis*. This condition appears to develop during the first three weeks of life and not to be truly congenital. The cause is unknown. There is a familial incidence and there is a preponderance of boys to girls 5:1. The pyloric muscle becomes hypertrophied and can be felt as a small rubbery-hard lump; and the mucous membrane is often oedematous and infiltrated by inflammatory cells. The obstruction causes vomiting, and the vomiting causes dehydration.
(b) *acquired pyloric stenosis*. This is due to a peptic ulcer in the duodenum or less commonly in the prepyloric region or antrum of the stomach, or to a carcinoma of the stomach.

Maximal Gastric Secretion Tests

These tests depend on the aspiration of gastric juice and its analysis. The volume and acidity are measured. The tests are performed by producing maximal secretion of gastric juice by either (a) histamine diphosphate given as a single intravenous injection or as a continuous intravenous infusion, or (b) pentagastrin given as a single intramuscular injection. Histamine has unpleasant side effects, which can be prevented by giving mepyramine maleate (Anthisan) 100 mg by mouth; mepyramine maleate does not interfere with gastric acid secretion.

Total basal acid output (BAO) is measured in hydrogen ions and in normal people is less than 5 mmol/hour. Maximum acid output (MAO) in 1 hour after injection of pentagastrin is about 20 mmol in a man and 10 mmol in a woman.

Patients with gastric ulcer usually have a normal acid secretion.
Patients with duodenal ulcer may have a high BAO and/or a high MAO.
Patients with carcinoma of stomach have achlorhydria or may have normal secretion.
Patients with pernicious anaemia have absolute achlohydria (none of the specimens have pH less than 7).

Tubeless tests

Tubeless tests (e.g. Diagnex Blue) are designed to determine the presence or absence of free acid in gastric juice without submitting the patient to the discomfort produced by the passing of a gastric tube. The reagent is swallowed; if hydrochloric acid is present in gastric juice, a dye is released and can be seen in the urine in which it is excreted. Renal function must be normal. The tests are unreliable. A positive reaction suggests that there is an adequate secretion of hydrochloric acid, but false positive reactions can occur, and a negative reaction has to be checked with a histamine or pentagastrin maximal secretion test.

Examination for malignant cells

Saline lavage of the stomach is carried out and the fluid examined for malignant cells detached from a carcinoma of stomach.

Hernia

A *hernia* is a protrusion of an organ or part of any organ out of the cavity in which it is normally contained. An abdominal hernia can be:
(a) *congenital:* as a result of a failure of normal development in a part of the abdominal wall;
(b) *acquired:* as a result of a muscular or fibrous weakness of part of the abdominal wall due to:

obesity	pregnancy
old age	nerve injury or disease

infection or haematoma of a wound.

A hernia can be precipitated by:
straining to lift a heavy object
straining at stool or micturition
chronic cough

An abdominal hernia is composed of:
(a) a sac of peritoneum,
(b) often part of an abdominal organ within the sac:

omentum	small intestine
large intestine	Meckel's diverticulum
stomach	appendix.
bladder	

A hernia is:
(a) *reducible,* when the contents of a hernial sac can be pushed back into the abdominal cavity;
(b) *irreducible,* when the contents cannot be pushed back because they have become swollen or formed adhesions with the sac;
(c) *obstructed,* when the movement of intestinal contents in a loop of intestine within the sac is stopped, usually as a result of narrowing of the neck of the sac;
(d) *strangulated,* where the blood supply (veins first, then arteries) to the hernial contents is interrupted and gangrene sets in.

TYPES OF HERNIAS

1. *Inguinal hernia*

An inguinal hernia occurs through the inguinal canal, the oblique narrow passage in the lower abdominal wall through which passes the spermatic cord in males and the round ligament in females.

An *indirect inguinal hernia* enters the canal at the deep inguinal ring; it may extend the whole length of the canal only, or in the male as far as the top of the testis or down into the scrotum. It can occur at any age, is more common in males than females, and may be bilateral.

A *direct inguinal hernia* bulges through the posterior wall of the medial third of the inguinal canal. It occurs usually in middle-aged or old men, is small, and does not enter the scrotum.

2. *Femoral hernia*

A femoral hernia enters the femoral canal in the upper inner aspect of the thigh, lying be-

between the femoral vein laterally and a ligament called Gimbernat's ligament medially. Because of this ligament strangulation is not uncommon. A femoral hernia is more common in women who have had children than in men and women who have not had children.

3. *Umbilical hernia*

Most umbilical hernias are no more than a small peritoneal sac which bulges through a weak spot in the umbilical scar.

An *exomphalos* is a large congenital umbilical hernia due to a failure of the midgut to return to the abdominal cavity during fetal life as it should, and may contain a large part of the abdominal contents.

4. *Para-umbilical hernia*

A para-umbilical hernia is a hernia through a weak spot in the linea alba near the umbilicus. It is a result of obesity or pregnancy. The coverings of the hernia may become thin and break down, and a faecal fistula can develop.

5. *Incisional hernia*

An incisional hernia is a hernia through a surgical operation wound or scar and is due to:
clumsy surgery   infection of the wound
haematoma of the   post-operative cough
  wound
track left by a drainage tube
damage to a motor nerve producing paralysis of muscles in the abdominal wall.

6. *Diaphragmatic hernia*

A diaphragmatic hernia can be:
(a) congenital: as a result of failure of normal development of the diaphragm which is formed from several different muscle masses;
(b) acquired: due to a penetrating wound, a crush injury or a subphrenic abscess.

In a common type the abdominal part of the oesophagus and the upper part of the stomach pass through the oesophageal opening of the diaphragm into the thoracic cavity. There is no peritoneal sac. The lower oesophageal valve is weak and allows gastric juice to enter the oesophagus. This can cause an oesophagitis, which can ulcerate, and the ulcer can heal with fibrous tissue which forms a stricture.

Meckel's Diverticulum

Meckel's diverticulum is a pouch 2-6 cm long which in 2 per cent of people projects from the ileum about 1 metre from the ileo-caecal junction. It is a congenital abnormality due to a persistence of the intestinal end of the vitello-intestinal duct, and is sometimes connected to the umbilicus by a fibrous band formed from the degenerated duct. It is composed of the same layers as the small inestine except occasionally the mucous membrane contains some ectopic gastric mucous membrane or pancreatic tissue.

Complications

Inflammation   peptic ulcer in gastric mucous
                  membrane
ulceration   perforation, peritonitis
intestinal obstruction due to compression by the fibrous band
volvulus (the diverticulum being the start of it)
involvement in a hernia

Hirschsprung's Disease

Hirschsprung's disease (true megacolon) is a dilatation of part of the colon and hypertrophy of its walls due to a congenital absence of nerve cells from the plexuses in the muscular part of the wall of the colon. The cause is unknown; it is more common in boys than girls, and there is a familial incidence.

The extent of colon involved varies. The most common site is a small area at the junction of the pelvic colon and rectum, but in severe cases the transverse, descending and pelvic colon are affected. Peristalsis does not occur in the affected zone, and the dilatation and hypertrophy build up above it.

In a few cases there may be a similar lack of innervation in the bladder, which enlarges.

Diverticulosis and Diverticulitis

Diverticulosis is a condition in which multiple pouches of mucous membrane project through the muscular wall of the colon. The condition begins in middle life and affects usually the descending and pelvic colon. The cause is unknown. It is thought that pockets of high intestinal pressure may force the pouches through weak spots in the muscle wall at the points where the nutrient arteries pass through it. The condition appears to be associated with a low-roughage diet. Faeces may become impacted in a diverticulum.

Diverticulitis is inflammation of a diverticulum. It can cause:
a pericolic abscess;
adherence to other viscera (bladder, vagina, small intestine) with ulceration and the formation of a fistula between the colon and the other organ;
rupture into peritoneal cavity, peritonitis;
erosion of a blood vessel and haemorrhage.

Peridiverticulitis is a chronic inflammatory state around a diverticulum. It can cause fibrosis and contractures of the colon.

Volvulus

Volvulus is a rotation of part of the gastrointestinal tract around its mesenteric axis, with the production of intestinal obstruction.

(a) *Large intestine.* This is the commonest site for a volvulus. The rotation occurs usually in an anti-clockwise direction. The pelvic colon is the part usually involved; less common is a volvulus of the caecum or transverse colon. It occurs most commonly in constipated old men. The loop of intestine becomes enormously dilated.

(b) *Small intestine.* A volvulus of the small intestine can occur, sometimes as a result of a fixation of part of it by peritoneal adhesions.

(c) *Stomach.* The stomach can rotate, usually at right angles to its long axis. A volvulus here is associated with a diaphragmatic hernia, an hour-glass stomach, adhesions following a peptic ulcer, or a carcinoma of stomach.

Complications

obstruction of blood supply   gangrene
perforation   peritonitis

Intestinal Obstruction

Intestinal obstruction is an obstruction to the onward movement of the intestinal contents. It may be mechanical or paralytic.

1. MECHANICAL OBSTRUCTION

Mechanical obstruction causes blockage of the lumen. The cause may be:
(a) *in the lumen of the intestine,* e.g. a gallstone or foreign body
(b) *in the wall of the intestine:* any process which results in thickening of the wall and obliteration of the lumen, e.g. neoplasm, Crohn's disease, ulcerative colitis
(c) *outside the wall of the intestine,* e.g. neoplasms in other organs pressing on the wall, fibrous adhesions, volvulus.

2. PARALYTIC OBSTRUCTION

Paralytic obstruction is a cessation of peristalsis without a mechanical obstruction. It occurs:
(a) *post-operatively.* After abdominal operations paralytic ileus is common during the first 24 hours. The causes include handling of the intestine, traction on the mesentery, and an overactivity of the sympathetic nervous system.
(b) *in peritonitis.* The paralysis is due to toxic effects on the nerve plexuses in the intestinal wall.

(c) *in severe biochemical disturbances,* e.g. uraemia.

In *simple obstruction* the part distal to the obstruction collapses and the part proximal dilates. The walls of the dilated part become oedematous and congested; the part becomes filled with a fluid composed of bile, pancreatic juice, intestinal juice and partly digested food; the fluid becomes brown as blood oozes out of the mucous membrane into it, and gas accumulates as a result of bacterial fermentation of the intestinal contents.

In *strangulated obstruction* the veins and then the arteries become compressed, and with the cutting off of its blood supply the length of intestine involved starts to go gangrenous.

In a *closed loop obstruction* a loop of bowel obstructed at both ends by a fibrous band or at the neck of a hernia becomes grossly dilated, its veins become thrombosed, and it goes gangrenous.

COMPLICATIONS

Perforation of intestine   peritonitis
fluid and electrolyte loss into the intestine
regurgitation of intestinal contents into the stomach.

Intussusception

Intussusception is the invagination of part of the intestine into the adjacent distal part. It arises as a result of peristalsis acting upon a mass in the intestinal wall which it treats as a foreign body and tries to push along. The mass can be:
(a) in infants, a patch of enlarged lymph tissue,
(b) in later life, a neoplasm.
   The usual types are:
(a) an ileo-ileal type, in which ileum is pushed into ileum,
(b) an ileo-colic type, in which ileum is pushed into colon,
(c) an ileal-caecal type, in which the ileo-caecal valve, thickened by a ring of lymph tissue, is pushed into the caecum,
(d) a primary colic type, in which colon is pushed into colon; an uncommon type, can be produced by a tumour of colon in adult life.

The invaginated part becomes oedematous, its blood-supply is cut off, and gangrene and peritonitis follow.

Haemorrhoids

Haemorrhoids (piles) are varicosities of the superior rectal vein, which arises from a plexus in the rectal wall and transmits blood to the inferior mesenteric vein, which is part of the portal system.
Predisposing factors in their production are:
(a) there may be a familial incidence of haemorrhoids,
(b) the superior rectal vein lies relatively unsupported in the loose submucosal coat of the rectum,
(c) the inferior mesenteric vein contains a long column of blood which when the body is in the erect position puts pressure on the superior rectal vein,
(d) the superior rectal vein lies at one of the sites of connection between the portal and systemic systems and is subject to rises of pressure in either.

   Precipitating factors are those conditions which cause a rise of pressure in the vein:
constipation   straining at stool
cough   difficulty in micturition
pregnancy   neoplasm of rectum
pelvic tumour   portal hypertension

Complications

Haemorrhage   anaemia
irreducibility due to spasm of anal sphincter
thrombosis   infection
ulceration   gangrene
portal pyaemia.

Acute Appendicitis

Acute appendicitis is an acute inflammation of the appendix. In most cases no cause can be found. Possible factors in its causation are:
(a) *age:* it is most common at 10-30 years and may be associated with the prevalence of lymph tissue at that time,
(b) *diet:* it has been thought to be associated with a low roughage, high meat diet,
(c) *stagnation of faeces:* faeces may stagnate in it and form a faecolith, a hard pellet which can go on to calcification.

E. coli and *Strept. faecalis* are the usual infecting micro-organisms.

The appendix becomes oedematous and inflamed. A fibrinous or fibropurulent exudate may form on its surface. In some cases the inflammation is limited to the distal half of the appendix. If the blood supply is obstructed by the oedema, the appendix becomes gangrenous. Perforation can occur. The omentum may seal off the infected area and limit the peritonitis to an abscess in a small area.

Complications

Appendix abscess   peritonitis
pelvic abscess   subphrenic abscess
adhesions to other organs
faecal fistula following drainage of an abscess through the skin
portal pyaemia (spread of infection through the portal system of veins).

Subphrenic Abscess

A *subphrenic abscess* is an abscess immediately below the diaphragm; the usual site is between the diaphragm and the right lobe of the liver.

It can be a complication of:
acute appendicitis   acute cholecystitis
perforated peptic ulcer   gastrectomy

E. coli and *Strept. faecalis* are the usual infecting micro-organisms. The condition is difficult to diagnose and has a high mortality.

Complications

Toxaemia
empyema (by spread of the infection through the diaphragm)
diaphragmatic hernia.

Ulcerative Colitis

Ulcerative colitis is a chronic inflammation of the large intestine. Its cause is unknown. It is thought that it might be an auto-immune disease; some of its complications (erythema nodosum, episcleritis of eye, arthritis) would suggest this. There is a familial incidence. In some cases there appears to be an allergy to milk. It usually begins in early adult life and runs a chronic course with remissions and relapses which occur for no obvious reason. Stress may be a factor in prolonging attacks.

The inflammation almost always involves the rectum and also a variable amount of colon above the rectum. The mucous membrane of the infected area becomes oedematous, hyperaemic and infiltrated with lymphocytes, eosinophils and plasma cells. In severe cases the mucous membrane is shed, leaving ulcerated bleeding areas. The ulcer can perforate the wall of the intestine. In acute fulminating cases the whole colon is acutely inflamed and the patient seriously ill. In course of time the lumen of the colon becomes narrowed.

Complications

Haemorrhage from ulcers   anaemia
dehydration   electrolyte loss
hypoprotinaemia (low blood protein due to loss of protein into the bowel)
oedema, due to hypoproteinaemia
perforation
ano-rectal fistula   stricture
liver degeneration and dysfunction, hepatic cirrhosis
polypoid granulation tissue in large intestine
carcinoma of colon (after years of disease)
erythema nodosum   episcleritis of eye
arthritis of large joints.

> **Blood**
>
> *Red cells:* reduced in number.
> *Haemoglobin:* reduced.
> *Erythrocyte sedimentation rate (ESR):* raised.
>
> **Rectal biopsy**
>
> *Specimen* of rectal mucous membrane and submucosa is removed for microscopic examination; inflammatory cells and fibrosis of wall are present.

Idiopathic Steatorrhoea

Idiopathic steatorrhoea (non-tropical sprue; coeliac disease in children) is a disease of the mucous membrane of the small intestine due to a sensitivity to a fraction of gluten, a protein present in wheat and rye. The jejunum is more affected than the ileum because gluten reaches it in greater concentration. The surface of the mucous membrane is flattened, its villi deformed or absent. In coeliac disease the amount of lymph tissue in the body is reduced. As the mucous membrane cannot absorb essential food stuffs, a malabsorption syndrome is produced.

> **Biopsy**
>
> A specimen of mucous membrane from the small intestine is examined microscopically.

Crohn's Disease

Crohn's disease is a chronic inflammatory disease of the intestine of unknown origin. It affects men and women in equal proportions and usually begins in middle life.

Any part of the gastro-intestinal tract can be involved from the stomach to the anus, but the ileum is most commonly affected (hence the old name of regional ileitis). Lengths of the gastro-intestinal tract become oedematous and infiltrated with lymphocytes and other cells while intervening parts appear unaffected. In the affected parts the mucous membrane can ulcerate or fissures can appear in the wall. Loops of intestine can become matted together and fistulae develop between them or with other organs such as the bladder or vagina. Stenosis of the intestine can occur and cause intestinal obstruction.

Complications

Malabsorption syndrome   iron-deficiency anaemia
megaloblastic anaemia (due to malabsorption of vitamin B_{12})
hypoprotinaemia (low blood protein due to loss into bowel)
dehydration and electrolyte loss
polyarthritis, iritis of eye, erythema nodosum.

Malabsorption Syndromes

A *malabsorption syndrome* is one due to a failure of absorption of essential foodstuffs from the small intestine. The syndrome varies with the cause of the failure and the types of foodstuffs not absorbed. It can be the result of:
(a) *disease of the small intestine*
Crohn's disease   coeliac disease
fistula of intestine   stricture of intestine
infestation by hookworms, giardiasis
(b) *surgical removal of large part of small intestine for:*
Crohn's disease   volvulus
(c) *deficiency of pancreatic juice or bile*
cystic fibrosis of pancreas   pancreatitis
carcinoma of pancreas   hepatic cirrhosis
cholecystitis   gallstones
(d) *interference by drugs with absorption*
large doses of neomycin
The type of deficiency produced can be:

(a) *protein deficiency:* failure to absorb essential aminoacids causes muscle degeneration, diminished growth in children;
(b) *fat deficiency:* causes large fatty stools, vitamin D deficiency;
(c) *iron deficiency:* iron deficiency anaemia;
(d) *vitamin deficiency:*
megaloblastic anaemia
pellagra, beri-beri;
(e) *calcium deficiency:* osteomalacia.

Various combinations of these deficiencies occur.

Neoplasms of the Intestine

Small intestine

Neoplasms of the small intestine are rare. Adenomata, lipomata, adenocarcinomata and lymphosarcomata can occur and cause obstruction and intussusception.

Appendix

A yellow 'carcinoid' tumour can occur, usually near the tip of the appendix. It has a low malignancy, sometimes spreading along lymph vessels or forming metastases in the liver.

Large intestine

Polyps and papillomata

Polyps of various kinds can occur in the colon and rectum. *Adenomatous polyps* are small pedunculated tumours, up to 2 cm in diameter. A *villous papilloma* is a larger, broad-based papilloma with multiple finger-like projections, occurring usually in the rectum. Both these kinds of neoplasm can become malignant.

Familial polyposis coli is inherited as a Mendelian dominant. Multiple adenomatous polyps develop during adolescence or early adult life and become malignant.

Carcinoma of colon and rectum

Carcinoma of the large intestine is a common disease. The usual sites are the rectum and pelvic colon. They are adenocarcinomata, but the types of cell in them vary. They occur in 3 forms:
(a) an ulcerated mass: the commonest type in the rectum,
(b) a polypoid or proliferating tumour, which forms a fungating, cauliform mass,
(c) a scirrhus or annular growth, which forms a ring in the wall of the intestine and is likely to cause obstruction.

Complications

Direct spread into bladder, ovary, small intestine, etc.
direct spread into peritoneum
spread into lymph vessels and nodes draining the part
perforation   peritonitis
haemorrhage   iron-deficiency anaemia
intestinal   metastases in liver, lungs,
  obstruction   etc.

Faeces

Faeces are examined for fresh and occult blood

Biopsy

Specimen is removed at sigmoidoscopy for microscopic examination.

Carcinoma of anus

Squamous cell carcinoma of the anus occurs. Spread is into the inguinal lymph nodes and into lymph nodes along the line of the inferior mesenteric vein.

> **Biopsy**
>
> Part of growth is taken for microscopic examination.

Peritoneum

Acute peritonitis

Acute peritonitis can be a result of:
1. perforation of an appendix, of a peptic ulcer, of a diverticulum, of a malignant ulcer, of ulceration through a Peyer's patch in typhoid fever;
2. spread of infection from appendicitis, cholecystitis, infection of a uterine (Fallopian) tube, etc.;
3. ischaemia due to interference with blood supply of bowel, e.g. by a volvulus or intussusception, causing gangrene of bowel;
4. septicaemia, especially one due to a staphylococcal or streptococcal infection;
5. a perforating wound of the abdomen or as a post-operative complication.

The peritoneum or part of it becomes acutely inflamed. A peritoneal exudate forms and may contain pus. A localized abscess can form at the site of infection (e.g. around an acute appendicitis), being sealed off by fibrous tissue and sometimes rupturing into an internal organ or through the skin. Paralytic ileus is a common complication. A peritonitis may heal completely, but sometimes abdominal organs become matted together or fibrous bands form, extending from one organ to another. Death can occur from circulatory failure or toxaemia.

> **Peritoneal fluid**
>
> Smears are examined for cells and the fluid is cultured for organisms, which are usually *E. coli* or *Str. faecalis*.

Tuberculous peritonitis

Tuberculous peritonitis is the result of either (a) spread of infection from the intestinal wall and the mesenteric lymph nodes, in which case the type of organism is the bovine one, or (b) a generalized miliary tuberculosis due to the human or bovine organism.

Miliary tubercles form on the peritoneum and there is an exudate of fluid into the peritoneal cavity. Areas of peritoneal cavity can be obliterated by fibrous tissue and chronic abscesses can form.

> **Peritoneal fluid**
>
> *Fluid:* Straw coloured; contains more than 25 g of protein per litre; contains lymphocytes and a few polymorphs. On culture, *Myco. tuberculosis* can be grown in only about one-third of cases.

MESENTERIC LYMPHADENITIS

Mesenteric lymphadenitis is an inflammation of mesenteric lymph nodes. It can occur:
(a) as a complication of an acute viral or upper respiratory tract infection, the nodes showing signs of acute inflammation;
(b) in abdominal tuberculosis, the nodes showing the usual tuberculous reaction, sometimes becoming matted together and breaking down into chronic abscesses.

Retroperitoneal fibrosis

Retroperitoneal fibrosis is a disease of unknown origin in which a thick mass of firm grey adherent tissue forms on the posterior peritoneal surface and can press on and constrict the structures lying retroperitoneally – the ureters, inferior vena cava, biliary tract, duodenum, colon, nerves of the lumbar plexus. Some patients have a similar fibrosis in the mediastinum. Spontaneous remission can occur.

Ascites

Ascites is an accumulation of fluid within the peritoneal cavity. It is a transudate which can occur in:
cirrhosis of the liver
nephrotic syndrome
cardiac failure
malignant disease.

A *chylous ascites* is one in which chyle is present as a result of pressure (usually by a neoplasm) on the thoracic duct or a large abdominal lymph vessel.

Meigs' syndrome is a combination of ascites with a fibroma of the ovary.

Ascitic fluid

Protein content: low in nephrotic syndrome and liver disease; high in neoplasm.

Malignant cells: may be present when ascites is due to neoplasm.

Faeces

Specimens should be sent to the laboratory in a screw-capped container. A waxed plastic carton must not be used. About a teaspoonful of faeces is required; any blood or mucus should be included. As pathogenic organisms are excreted intermittently specimens should be sent from three consecutive bowel-actions or three consecutive days. Specimens should not be sent by post as faecal micro-organisms are likely to die during the transit.

A rectal swab is not satisfactory as it is liable to produce a misleading negative culture. If one is taken, it must be from the rectum and not from the anal canal.

Macroscopic examination: for fresh blood, melaena, mucus, worms.

Microscopic examination: for blood, pus, amoebae, *Giardia lamblia,* ova of intestinal worms, undigested meat fibres, excess of fat globules.

Occult blood: various reagents are used to detect the presence of haemoglobin.

Cultures: on appropriate media for the detection of pathogenic micro-organisms.

Chapter 15   Pancreas, Liver, Biliary Tract

PANCREAS

Fibrocystic Disease

Fibrocystic disease (mucoviscidosis) is an inherited disease in which there is a disorder of mucus-secreting glands in the ducts and wall of various organs, especially:
pancreas   lungs   liver
sweat glands   salivary glands   intestine
The mucus secreted by these glands is excessively viscid and is retained in the glands and forms cysts. Normal pancreatic tissue is replaced by fibrous tissue, and the organ shrinks.

Complications

Malabsorption and failure to thrive in infancy,
intestinal obstruction in infancy due to inspissated mucus in the intestine (meconium ileus)
pulmonary infections, bronchiectasis, emphysema
biliary cirrhosis of the liver.

Acute Pancreatitis

Acute pancreatitis is a disease of uncertain origin in which areas of pancreatic tissue and adjacent fatty tissues are destroyed, apparently by the pancreas's own enzymes. It may follow a large meal or an abdominal operation, and is especially common in alcoholics. In some cases it is associated with gallstones or disease of the biliary tract, and then it may be due to reflux of bile into the pancreatic duct.
The pancreas becomes swollen and inflamed, and there may be bleeding into the inflamed tissue. Pancreatic tissue is destroyed and the areas is invaded by polymorphs. There is a high mortality. A pseudocyst − of fluid, blood and debris − may form in a patient who survives the attack.

Blood

Serum amylase: raised. A figure of over 500 I.U./1 likely to be due to acute pancreatitis; may rise to 1000 I.U./1 or more. Normal: 148-333 I.U./1.

Chronic Pancreatitis

Chronic pancreatitis is a disease of uncertain origin. It can follow an attack of acute pancreatitis, occur in chronic alcoholics, or be possibly a result of obstruction of the pancreatic duct by a neoplasm or calculus.
    The glandular tissue of the pancreas degenerates and is replaced by fibrous tissue, causing the organ to become shrunken and firm. The islets of Langerhans are spared at first, but they too in time degenerate.
    Pancreatic function is impaired with the production of a malabsorption syndrome first and later of diabetes mellitus.

Secretin test

The functioning of the pancreas can be investigated by stimulating it and then aspirating pancreatic secretion from the duodenum. Secretin (a hormone produced in the small intestine) is injected intravenously.

In patients with chronic pancreatitis the bicarbonate concentration may not reach 60 m.mol/l (normal: 90 m.mol/l and above), and the pH does not become as alkaline as normal (normal: pH rises above 8).

Faeces

Steatorrhoea may be present (i.e. more than 6 g of fat excreted per day. *Undigested muscle fibres* may be present.

Urine

Glucose: present when islet function is impaired.

Glucose tolerance test

Diabetic curve likely.

Carcinoma of the Pancreas

Primary *carcinoma of the pancreas* occurs in middle or old age and more often in men than women.

The growth is an adenocarcinoma, develops from the cells which secrete pancreatic juice or from the smaller ducts, and forms a hard grey mass. In about 75 per cent of cases the neoplasm develops in the head of the pancreas and causes jaundice by pressing on and invading the common bile duct as it traverses the head of the pancreas. The growth can develop in the ampulla (the joint opening of the common bile duct and the pancreatic duct into the duodenum), quickly producing jaundice.

Local spread is into:

common bile duct   duodenum   vertebral bodies

Metastases form in:

liver   peritoneum   lungs

Complications:

Jaundice   ascites
portal vein thrombosis
multiple venous thromboses, usually in the lower limbs.

These results are found when the carcinoma is in the head of the pancreas and causing obstructive jaundice.
Serum bilirubin. Mainly conjugated. Levels rise with increasing obstruction and may reach 500 μmol/l or more. (normal: 2-17 μmol/l).
Urine. Bilirubin present. Urobilinogen absent if obstruction is complete.
Faeces. Stools pale. Urobilinogen reduced (absent if obstruction is complete).
Alkaline phosphatase. Raised. Likely to be more than 250 I.U./l. (Normal 30-125 I.U./l.)

LIVER

Infections of the Liver

Virus infections of the liver are common. Among them are:
infective hepatitis   serum hepatitis
yellow fever   rubella
herpes simplex   infective mononucleosis

The degree of infection varies from slight to severe. The tissues around the lobules are invaded by inflammatory cells (polymorphs, lymphocytes, plasma cells, etc.) and the liver cells show degenerative changes. Bile becomes stagnant in the biliary canaliculi. In severe cases the whole liver is involved. *Acute yellow atrophy* is the name given to the appearance of the liver after a massive infection, the liver being shrunken, its capsule wrinkled and its cut surfaces appearing yellow and structureless. In less severe cases chronic hepatitis can follow. In mild cases there is recovery, structurally and functionally, with the development of new liver cells.

Other infections are:
(a) *Weil's disease*. This is an infection by *Leptospira icterohaemorrhagiae*, a spirochete, which invades the body through the skin, invades many tissues and causes a severe and sometimes fatal hepatitis.
(b) *Abscesses*. Single or multiple abscesses can form in the liver as a result of a spread of infection from some septic focus in the body. The spread may be via the portal viens, the hepatic artery, the bile ducts or directly. The original septic focus may be:

appendix abscess empyema
osteomyelitis perinephric abscess
subphrenic abscess suppurative cholangitis
(c) *Amoebic abscess*

Jaundice

Jaundice is the yellow colour of the conjunctivae, mucous membranes and skin produced by an excess of bilirubin in the blood. Bilirubin is the bile pigment derived from haemoglobin. For jaundice to be visible the amount of bilirubin in the plasma has to be above 35 μmol/l.

BILE PIGMENTS IN NORMAL PEOPLE

Haemoglobin breaks down into iron and bilirubin bound to albumin. Bilirubin in this form is called unconjugated and is not soluble in water.

This unconjugated bilirubin passes to the liver where it is conjugated (joined) with glucuronic acid and becomes soluble in water.

Conjugated bilirubin is excreted in the bile into the intestine. In the large intestine bacterial action breaks it down into urobilinogen and other substances. Most urobilinogen is excreted in the faeces. Air alters it to urobilin, which is partly responsible for the colour of faeces. A little urobilinogen is reabsorbed into the portal circulation. Most of this is excreted again into the bile, but a small amount reaches the systemic circulation and is excreted in the urine.

Normal bile pigments	
Serum:	
total bilirubin	present
excess conjugated bilirubin	absent
Urine:	
bilirubin (conjugated)	absent
urobilinogen	trace
Faeces:	
urobilinogen	present

Jaundice can be classified as:
pre-hepatic jaundice
post-hepatic jaundice (obstructive jaundice)
hepatic jaundice (cellular jaundice).
An absolutely clear distinction cannot be made between hepatic and post-hepatic jaundice: for example, a liver tumour may cause obstruction of the biliary system, and a gallstone may damage liver cells. These two kinds may exist together and the laboratory results may be similar.

1. PREHEPATIC JAUNDICE

Prehepatic jaundice is due to an excessive breakdown of red blood cells to such a degree that the liver cannot cope with the amount of bilirubin delivered to it for excretion. It occurs in:
haemolytic anaemias

haemolytic disease of the newly born
malaria
after an incompatible blood transfusion.

The jaundice is mild. Biliary calculi can form in the smaller liver ducts and there may be interference with liver function. The liver and spleen are sometimes enlarged.

> *Blood serum:* bilirubin (unconjugated) increased.
> *Urine:* bilirubin is absent because unconjugated bilirubin is not water soluble. Urobilinogen is increased.
> *Faeces:* dark in colour. Urobilinogen is increased.
>
> Urobilinogen is increased in urine and faeces because a large amount of bilirubin is excreted into the gut.

2. POST-HEPATIC (OBSTRUCTIVE) JAUNDICE

Obstructive jaundice is due to an obstruction to the discharge of bile into the duodenum. The bile is therefore reabsorbed from the liver into the blood stream. The cause may be:
(a) *in the lumen of the common bile duct*
gallstones
mucoviscidosis
(b) *in the wall of the common bile duct*
neoplasm of the bile duct
stricture of the bile duct
(c) *compression outside the wall*
carcinoma of the head of the pancreas
carcinoma of the ampulla of Vater
chronic pancreatitis
malignant lymph nodes.

The jaundice varies in intensity according to the degree of obstruction. In malignant disease it becomes progressively deeper. The liver is enlarged, and in chronic cases the spleen also.

> *Serum:* bilirubin is mainly conjugated and the level is high. The levels become very high in malignant disease, up to 500 μmol/l.
> *Urine:* bilirubin appears in the urine because conjugated bilirubin is soluble in water. Urobilinogen is absent if obstruction is complete as no bilirubin then passes into the intestine.
> *Faeces:* the stools are pale. Urobilinogen is reduced when obstruction is partial and absent when obstruction is complete (because no bilirubin passes into the intestine).

3. HEPATIC (CELLULAR) JAUNDICE

Liver damage causes a failure of the cells to excrete conjugated bilirubin into the bile. The causes are:
(a) hepatitis
(c) cirrhosis of the liver
(c) the action of some drugs and chemicals:
chlorpromazine and similar drugs
halothane   chloroform
arsenic   gold
alcohol   carbon tetrachloride.

The patient becomes jaundiced rapidly. The liver and spleen may be enlarged.

> The bile pigment findings may be similar to those in post-hepatic (obstructive) jaundice.
> *Serum:* total bilirubin level is raised (both conjugated and unconjugated).
> *Urine:* bilirubin may appear in the urine (because much of the serum bilirubin is conjugated). Urobilinogen is variable.
> *Faeces:* stools may be pale due to low or absent urobilinogen if bile is not being excreted into the intestine.

Chapter 15

Cirrhosis of the Liver

Cirrhosis of the liver is a chronic disease in which occurs widespread damage to the liver cells, fibrosis, necrosis, and the growth of nodules of regenerated liver cells. It is classified in two ways.

1. CAUSE

Cirrhosis of the liver can be due to:
alcoholism   viral hepatitis
haemochromatosis   stagnation of bile in the
                      bile ducts
cardiac failure   hepato-lenticular
                      degeneration.

Cryptogenic cirrhosis is a cirrhosis for which no cause can be found. Cases of cryptogenic cirrhosis form the largest group.

2. PATHOLOGICAL CHANGES

There are several ways of classifying cases of cirrhosis by the pathological changes in the liver. One method is to divide them into:
(a) *Micro-nodular cirrhosis*. The regenerated liver nodules are small (up to 4 mm diameter). All the liver lobules are affected, and the liver is large and uniformly granular. This type is common in alcoholism.
(b) *Macro-nodular cirrhosis*. The regenerated liver nodules are large (up to several cm in diameter). Some liver lobules are unaffected, and the liver shows scars and is usually small.

Microscopic changes

The microscopic changes in the liver vary with the cause and duration of the disease. In general the changes are:
(a) the liver cells degenerate,
(b) inflammatory cells appear around them,
(c) some liver tissue dies and is replaced by fibrous tissue,
(d) nodules of regenerated tissue grow and are functional.

When the cirrhosis is due to biliary to obstruction, necrotic bile-stained debris is found in the degenerated areas. In haemochromatosis (in which there is an abnormally large absorption of iron by the small intestine) iron is deposited in large amounts in liver cells, in the Kupffer cells lining the sinusoids, and in the walls of the portal tracts. In hepato-lenticular degeneration (in which there is an abnormality of copper metabolism) copper is deposited in liver cells.

RESULTS OF CIRRHOSIS

I.   Liver cell failure
II. Portal hypertension

I. *Liver cell failure*

There is a progressive failure of liver function as more and more liver cells degenerate, although to some extent the loss of cells is compensated by the growth of nodules of functioning cells.
1. A failure to synthesize albumin. This causes hypoproteinaemia (a reduction of the amount of protein circulating in the blood), which leads to fluid retention, oedema and ascites.
2. A failure to synthesize some of the factors necessary for the clotting of blood, especially prothrombin and Factor VII. This causes excessive bleeding.
3. A failure to detoxify ammonia, which could be converted into urea. This interferes with normal cerebral functioning and causes confusion and coma.

II. *Portal hypertension*

Fibrosis and regenerating liver nodules cause obstruction and obliteration of the normal blood channels, so that pressure in the portal vein rises. Portal hypertension results in:
1. Hypersplenism, a condition in which the spleen destroys too many red cells, white cells or platelets.
2. Enlargement of porta-caval anastomoses. The normal anastomoses between the portal system and tributaries of the inferior vena cava

become larger. Varicosities develop around the oesophageal-gastric junction and can burst and bleed profusely. Veins at the umbilicus can become enlarged.

Complications

1. *Ascites* occurs for the following reasons:
(i) hypoproteinaemia due to failure of the liver to produce albumin,
(ii) raised blood pressure in the capillaries of the hepatic venous system,
(iii) sodium retention due to an increase in aldosterone.
2. *Encephalopathy.* Attacks of confusion, drowsiness and coma occur and are probably due to the raised blood ammonia level.
3. *Hepatoma.* A hepatoma is a malignant neoplasm arising in a regenerated nodule and occurs in some patients with cirrhosis. Multiple neoplasms are common.
4. *Vascular changes.* Spider naevi and 'liver palms and soles' (a dusky erythema due to enlarged vessels) can occur. Their cause is unknown.
5. *Gynaecomastia* amd *testicular atrophy* can occur in men. Their cause is unknown.

Death is due to a total failure of liver function or to the development of a neoplasm in the cirrhotic liver.

Results of tests may be confusing as three separate processes are occurring in cirrhosis — damage to the liver, regeneration of the liver, and impairment of circulation.

Serum

Serum enzymes. Transaminases raised; the levels are higher when necrosis is occurring. Alkaline phosphatase likely to be raised.
Serum proteins. Albumin level lowered. Gamma globulin level raised.

Bromsulphthalein excretion

Bromsulphthalein excretion is impaired.

Neoplasms of the Liver

Benign neoplasm

A *cavernous haemangioma* is a congenital growth formed of grossly dilated blood vessels.

Malignant neoplasms

(a) *Primary malignant neoplasms* can be: a *hepatoma*, which arises in regenerated liver tissue in cirrhosis of the liver and is often multiple; a *cholangioma*, which arises from a bile duct within the liver; or a *hepatoblastoma*, a rapidly growing neoplasm arising in infancy.
(b) *Secondary neoplasms* are the commonest tumours of the liver. They are commonly metastases from primary growths in:

stomach	intestine
lungs	gall bladder
breast	adrenal gland
skin	

They may reach the liver by the portal vein, the hepatic artery, by lymph vessels, or by direct spread. Multiple growths are likely. They may appear as separate grey nodules which are liable to become necrotic at the centre, or as an infiltration along the portal tracts.

Tests Used in Investigating Liver Disease and Jaundice

1. Serum bilirubin

Normally there is a small amount of bilirubin in the circulating blood en route to the liver for excretion. It builds up if the liver cannot cope with it.

Less than 17 μmol/l plasma: normal
Above 35 μmol/l plasma: jaundice visible.

Bilirubin is in two forms: conjugated with glocuronic acid or not conjugated with it.

VAN DEN BERGH REACTION

Conjugated bilirubin rapidly gives a purple colour when it reacts with certain chemicals: this is the *direct Van den Bergh reaction. Unconjugated bilirubin* does not give the colour *(negative direct Van den Bergh reaction.)* If unconjugated bilirubin is treated with alcohol, the protein to which it is bound is removed, the bilirubin dissolves, and the purple colour appears; this is the *positive indirect Van den Bergh reaction.*

Normal serum does not contain sufficient conjugated bilirubin to give a direct Van den Bergh reaction.

In *haemolytic jaundice:* serum bilirubin may be up to 85 μmol/l and higher if liver damage is also present. The retained pigment is all unconjugated.

In *liver cell jaundice* and *obstructive jaundice,* serum bilirubin is usually in the range 50-500 μmol/l; the higher levels occur in obstructive jaundice and particularly when the obstruction is due to malignant disease. In liver cell jaundice a high proportion of the bilirubin is likely to be conjugated. In obstructive jaundice 90 per cent or more of the bilirubin is likely to be conjugated.

2. Serum alkaline phosphatase

Alkaline phosphatase is an enzyme produced in liver, bone, intestinal mucous membrane and placenta. Normal: 30-125 I.U./l. It is normal in haemolytic jaundice. In liver cell jaundice it may be up to 250 I.U./l. In obstructive jaundice the level is likely to be over 250 I.U./l. The alkaline phosphatase is also raised in some bone diseases.

3. Other serum enzymes

When liver cells are damaged, some enzymes are liberated into the blood and the amount in the blood is a measure of liver damage. The ones usually estimated are:
serum glutamic oxaloacetic transaminase (SGOT, aspartate transaminase): normal: 5-15 I.U./l.
Serum glutamic pyruvic transaminase (SGPT, alanine transaminase): normal: 4-12 I.U./l.

The two enzymes can be considered together. In severe liver disease, the rise is high (over 150 I.U./l.); the levels are particularly high in acute hepatitis. In obstructive jaundice there is a moderate rise.

4. Serum proteins

The total serum protein is estimated and separated into its albumin and globulin fractions.

In prehepatic jaundice the serum proteins are normal.

In hepatic jaundice the serum albumin falls and the albumin/globulin ratio is reversed, i.e. there is more globulin than albumin. In cirrhosis there is a high gamma globulin and low albumin. In hepatitis there is high gamma but low alpha[7] globulin.

In obstructive jaundice alpha 2 globulin may be raised.

Serum
   proteins: normal: 60-80 g/l.
   albumin: normal: 35-55 g/l.
   globulin: normal: 25-35 g/l.

5. Bromsulphthalein excretion

Bromsulphthalein (BSP) is a dye which when excreted into the blood is removed from it by the liver and excreted into the bile. In impaired liver function the dye is not removed. In the *simple method*, 5 mg in solution per kg body weight is injected intravenously. A blood sample is taken 45 minutes later from the other arm. More than 7 per cent retention of the dye is an indication of impaired liver function. The test is not performed if the patient is jaundiced as some retention of the dye occurs in all cases of jaundice.

Urine

Ictotest: used to detect bilirubin in the urine. The tablet turns purple if bilirubin is present.
Ictostix: a strip test for detecting bilirubin in urine.
Urobilistix: a strip test for detecting normal or raised levels of urobilinogen in urine.

Faeces

Faeces are pale and fatty when urobilinogen is not present, as in obstructive jaundice.

Gallstones

Gallstones (biliary calculi) are stones which develop in the gall bladder and biliary tract. *Cholelithiasis* is another name for the condition.

Gallstones cause symptoms in about 10 per cent of people over the age of 40. They are three times more common in women than men.

There are three types: mixed stones, pigment stones, cholesterol stones.

1. *Mixed stones*

Mixed stones are so-called because they are composed of a mixture of bile-pigment, cholesterol, calcium salts, protein, etc. They are the commonest types of stone. They are shiny and deep greenish brown and have several facets because they have developed in contact with other stones, for they are almost always multiple. They are associated with inflammation of the gall bladder. The calcium in them makes them radio-opaque.

2. *Pigment stones*

These are stones composed of bilirubin. They are small, dark brown and usually multiple.

3. *Cholesterol stones*

These are stones composed of cholesterol. They usually occur singly, each stone being oval, pale brown and with a slightly granular surface.

The precise reasons for the development of gallstones are obscure. Among the factors in their development and growth are:

1. *High concentration*

(a) *Cholesterol concentration in the bile.* An increase in the concentration of cholesterol in the bile or a decrease in the amount of bile salts (which hold the cholesterol in solution) are factors in the development of gallstones. An increase in the concentration of cholesterol occurs in:
obesity   high fat diet
pregnancy   diabetes mellitus
A decrease in the amount of bile salts occurs in:
liver disease   biliary stasis
cholecystitis.

(b) *Blood destruction.* Excessive blood destruction causes an excess of bilirubin to be excreted into the bile and is a factor in the development of pigment stones, but not of the others.

2. *Biliary stasis*

Stones are likely to develop when the flow of bile into and out of the gall bladder and along the ducts is slowed.

3. *Infection*

Inflammation of the gall bladder produces within it small accumulations of mucus, pus, micro-organisms and cell debris. Bile pigments, cholesterol and calcium can form around these accumulations and start a stone.

Complications

1. *Acute cholecystitis.* An acute inflammation of the gall bladder is occasionally precipitated by gallstones. It can follow blocking of the neck of the gall bladder by a stone.
2. *Empyema of the gall bladder.* Pus in the gall bladder can follow acute cholecystitis. The gallbladder wall can become gangrenous and perforate, with the development of a local abscess (if the area is sealed off by fibrous tissue) or a generalized peritonitis.
3. *Chronic cholecystitis.* Chronic cholecystitis may follow acute cholecystitis or be a chronic inflammation from the start.
4. *Mucocele of the gall bladder.* This is an accumulation of mucus in the gall bladder with a reabsorption of pigment and can occur when the neck of the gall bladder is obstructed by a stone.
5. *Fistula.* A fistula can develop between the gall bladder and adjoining organs, especially a loop of small intestine.
6. *Obstruction in the small intestine.* A large stone passed through a fistula into the small intestine sometimes causes intestinal obstruction.
7. *Obstruction of the common bile duct.* A stone may obstruct the common bile duct, causing an obstructive jaundice and sometimes an ascending cholangitis (infection of the biliary ducts).
8. *Carcinoma of the gall bladder.* A carcinoma of the gall bladder can develop after years of irritation by stones.
9. *Pancreatitis.* Pancreatitis is sometimes associated with stones in the common bile duct.

Acute Cholecystitis

Acute cholecystitis is an acute inflammation of the gall bladder. It occurs:
(a) following obstruction in the cystic duct or the neck of the gall bladder, by a gallstone or neoplasm,
(b) as a complication of chronic cholecystitis,
(c) in septicaemia.

Inflammatory changes occur in the wall of the gall bladder. In severe cases gangrene and ulceration of the wall can occur, with a perforation causing either a local abscess or a generalized peritonitis. An *empyema of the gall bladder* is pus in the gall bladder.

Chronic Cholecystitis

Chronic cholecystitis is more common than acute cholecystitis. Gallstones are present in 80-90 per cent of cases.

The gall bladder becomes white and opaque. It shrinks and may be attached to the intestine by adhesions. The mucous membrane is flattened and often in some places absent, and there is fibrosis of the wall. A mucocele can be produced. Arteries in the wall of the gall bladder may have their lumen obliterated by endarteritis obliterans.

Acute Cholangitis

Acute cholangitis is an acute inflammation of the biliary tract, both within and without the liver. It follows:
(a) impaction of a gallstone in the common bile duct,
(b) obstruction of the common bile duct by a neoplasm,
(c) rarely obstruction of the common bile duct by *Ascaris* or by liver fluke infestation,
(d) surgical operations (e.g. cholecyst-enterostomy) which allow a reflux of intestinal contents into the biliary tract.

The bile ducts above the obstruction are inflamed and dilated and fill with pus. Multiple abscesses can occur in the liver from the infection and dilation of the intra-hepatic ducts. *E. coli* is the usual infecting micro-organism.

Carcinoma of the Gall Bladder and Biliary Tract

Carcinoma of the gall bladder is uncommon. When it does occur, it is usually as a complication of gallstones. It is an adenocarcinoma and spreads into the liver either directly or via lymph vessels.

Carcinoma of the biliary tract can occur in any of the major ducts of the biliary tract, but it usually begins in the ampulla of Vater or at the junction of the two major ducts. It is not associated with gallstones. It is an adenocarcinoma and by blocking the duct causes a progressively severe jaundice. The liver and spleen become enlarged.

Chapter 16   The Urinary System

Congenital Abnormalities of the Kidney

Congenital abnormalities of the kidney can be:
(a) one kidney is smaller than the other or absent;
(b) a kidney may remain in the early fetal position in the pelvis and not move as it should higher in the abdomen;
(c) a *horse-shoe kidney:* the kidneys are joined together at their lower poles by renal tissue, with the ureters passing downwards in front of the union;
(d) a solitary *cyst* may be present, containing a clear yellow fluid, which can become haemorrhagic or infected.
The above abnormalities do not usually affect renal function.
(e) *polycystic disease of the kidneys.* This is a congenital familial condition in which a large number of cysts is present in both kidneys. The cysts contain fluid which may be clear, turbid or haemorrhagic, and are lined with a layer of flattened cells. With enlargement of the cysts renal tissue is destroyed, but renal failure or hypertension may not appear until 40-50 years. Similar cysts may be present in other organs.

Tests of Renal Function

Tests of renal function fall mainly into 2 groups:
1. Test of glomerular function
2. Tests of tubular function.
Some advanced tests used in research are unsuitable for clinical work.

---

1. Tests of glomerular function

(a) *Estimation of glomerular filtration rate* (GFR). The GFR is an indication of the efficiency of the renal glomeruli. Serial determination of the GFR is an accurate method of detecting changes, for the better or worse, in renal function.
Endogenous creatinine clearance is the method often used clinically. It requires: (i) the collection of urine over two consecutive 24-hour periods, and (ii) a sample of 5-10 ml of blood taken on the morning of the second day. Normal range: men, 95-140 ml/min (= 140-200 litres/24 hours); women about 10 per cent lower than men. The rate of creatinine clearance almost equals the glomerular filtration rate.
(b) *Blood urea.* The blood urea can be estimated. It is partly dependent on the amount of protein in the diet and on the breakdown of protein already in the body. Persistently high levels indicate impaired glomerular function. Normal: 2.5-6.5 mmol/l.

2. Tests of tubular function

These tests measure the concentrating power of the renal tubules. A *urine concentration test* is the one usually performed. As the test can be dangerous, a preliminary test is carried out to see if the full test is really necessary.

The *preliminary test* consists of taking a random early morning specimen of urine. If it has a SG of 1020 or higher and does not contain albumin or sugar, concentration by the tubules is almost certainly normal.

Urine concentration test

The patient must be carefully observed throughout the test. He is either (a) deprived of all fluids after 16.00 hours or (b) given 5 ml of pitressin tannate in oil intramuscularly. Any urine passed during the night is discarded. Three specimens of urine are taken: on awakening, 1 hour after waking, 2 hours after waking. The SG of each specimen is measured. If concentration is normal, the SG of at least one of them will be 1025 or higher.

Acute Proliferative Glomerulonephritis

This condition can occur at any age but is most common in children and young adults. It is an acute immunologico-inflammatory reaction, which occurs:
(a) usually as a complication of an acute infection by beta haemolytic streptococci, e.g. tonsillitis
(b) less commonly in other infections
(c) occasionally in bacterial endocarditis and collagen diseases.

The kidneys become swollen and congested.
Microscopic examination shows:
glomeruli: an overgrowth of endothelial and epithelial cells (i.e. proliferative glomerulonephritis) in the capillary walls and infiltration by polymorphs. The glomerular tuft is swollen and obliterates the capsular space. Immunoglobulin and complement are deposited in the capillary walls.

tubules: cloudy swelling is present because of impaired blood flow from the efferent arteriole of the glomerulus.

Renal function is impaired. Urine output is reduced or stopped altogether. The patient has haematuria, hypertension, and some oedema of the tissues, especially the face.

Course

(a) The majority of children and about 80 per cent of the adults make a complete recovery. The kidneys return to normal with full function. Second attacks are rare.

(b) About 5 per cent die without recovering from the acute stage. Most of these die within a few weeks because of (i) renal failure, (ii) cardiac failure or cerebral haemorrhage due to hypertension.

A few run a progressive course and die from renal failure after a few months. In them the proliferation of cells continues with the formation of crescents due to epithelial cells building up in Bowman's capsule. The glomerular tufts become sclerosed and the tubules atrophy.

(c) About 10-15 per cent run a slowly progressive course. Patients are clinically better, but show persistent mild proteinuria. After an interval of 5-20 years they develop renal failure or nephrotic syndrome followed by renal failure. In them the kidneys become small and granular. The proliferation of cells continues. The glomerular tuft becomes adherent to Bowman's capsule; the glomerulus becomes avascular; the dead tissue is replaced by fibrous tissue. The tubules atrophy because their blood supply is lost.

Complications

Acute heart failure;
acute pulmonary oedema due to heart failure;
hypertensive encephalopathy: attacks of constriction of the cerebral vessels, cerebral oedema, and severe hypertension;
infections: pyelonephritis is common;
renal failure.

Tests in Acute Phase

Urine

Small amounts or none. Can contain blood, which makes it 'smoky' with small amounts, bright red or dark red. Contains albumin, epithelial cells, epithelial and later granular casts, leucocytes. Cultures are usually negative.

Blood

Serum: antistreptococcal antibody titres are high in the majority of patients.
Erythrocyte sedimentation rate (ESR): raised. Normal: 3-5 mm in males, 4-7 mm in females.
Urea: raised. Normal: 2.5-6.5 mmol/l.

Membranous Glomerulonephritis

This is less common than proliferative glomerulonephritis, occurs mainly in adults, and does not follow an acute streptococcal infection. It is thought to be possibly an immunological process.

The kidneys become large and pale, with a smooth external surface. Later they may become small and granular.

Microscopic examination shows:
glomeruli: a thickening of the basement membrane (which is the middle layer in the wall of the capillaries, lying between endothelium and epithelium); the thickening is due to a deposit which stains with silver and is possibly an antigen-antibody complex. There is fusion of the foot processes, small projections from the surface of the epithelial cells. (Unlike proliferative glomerulonephritis there is no increased cellularity and no polymorph infiltration.)

tubules: there is a deposit of lipid in the epithelium of the tubules.

The results of these changes are:
glomerulosclerosis from avascularity.
tubular atrophy.

Clinical course

This condition is one of the causes of nephrotic syndrome. There is a severe loss of protein. Death occurs from renal failure. Hypertension can occur as a late complication.

Urine

Urine: amount increased at first, then reduced. SG normal. Albumin present in large amounts. In severe cases: red cells, white cells and granular casts are present.
Renal biopsy
Renal biopsy is sometimes performed to establish the diagnosis.

Nephrotic Syndrome

The *nephrotic syndrome* is a condition characterized by:
excessive excretion of plasma proteins by the kidney;
hypoproteinaemia (low protein level in the blood);
generalized oedema (an osmotic oedema due to lack of plasma protein);
raised blood cholesterol.
It occurs in several renal diseases and some other diseases as a result of damage to the glomeruli:
commonly in: membranous glomerulonephritis
less commonly in: proliferative glomerulonephritis
    diabetic glomerulo-sclerosis
    amyloid disease of the kidney
    collagen disease, especially systemic lupus erythematosus

The basic fault in the kidney is an excessive permeability of the glomeruli which allows protein, especially albumin, to leak from the kidney into the urine. In some cases the condition appears to be functional and reversible. Often no change can be seen in the kidney with the naked eye, but microscopic examination reveals glomerular abnormalities of various kinds. In patients who do not recover the glomeruli and tubules degenerate and death follows renal failure.

The amount of protein lost can be as much as 30 g a day, most of it as albumin. The results of this loss are:
reduction in plasma proteins;
lowered plasma volume, because of reduced osmotic pressure;
sodium retention, because there is an increase of aldosterone, which is possibly due to the decreased blood volume;
oedema, because of hypoprotinaemia and sodium retention;
gross wasting, masked by oedema.

Complications

Rise in blood urea, because the low plasma volume leads to a reduced glomerular filtration rate;
hypertension;
renal failure.

Blood

Serum cholesterol: raised, may be up to 25 mmol/l. (normal: 3.6-7.8 mmol/l).
Urea: raised. (Normal: 2.5-6.5 mmol/l).
Serum proteins: low.
Albumin may drop to 10 g/l or even lower. (Normal: 35-50 g/l).
Oedema occurs when level drops below 20 g/l.
Electrophoresis shows a typical pattern of proteins.

Urine

Protein: present in large amounts, up to 30 g in 24 hours, mostly as albumin. (Normal: 1-5 g in 24 hours). If proteinuria is higher than 10 g in 24 hours, oedema is likely to occur.
Red cells: may be present.
Casts: granular casts may be present.

Pyelonephritis

Pyelonephritis is an infection of the pelvis of the kidney spreading into the kidney itself, and can be acute or chronic.

The common infecting micro-organisms are those which normally inhabit the intestine and manage to invade the urinary system.
The commonest micro-organism is: *E. coli.* Less common are: *Str. faecalis, Proteus vulgaris, Staph. albus, Staph. aureus.*

Acute pyelonephritis can occur in previously healthy people, or as a complication of disease of the urinary tract and stasis of the urine due to:
obstruction at the bladder-neck
urinary calculus   enlarged prostate gland
urethral stricture
neoplasm obstructing the urinary tract
dilation of ureters in pregnancy.

Both kidneys are infected unless the cause is unilateral. Infection begins in the pelvis of the kidney, which becomes congested and swollen, and spreads into the medulla, where yellow streaks formed of inflammatory and pus cells can be observed. The cortex can also be involved. In severe cases abscesses form in the kidney.

Urine

Specimens are examined for micro-organisms, white cells, red cells. A bacterial count is made: a count of over 100 000 colonies per ml. is an

> indication of infection. Cultures are made.
> Suprapubic aspiration is a method of obtaining uncontaminated urine.
>
> **Blood**
>
> White cells: number increased.

Chronic pyelonephritis is liable to develop after several attacks of acute pyelonephritis have occurred. Repeated virus infection of the kidney is a possible cause. The pelvis of the kidney shows chronic inflammation. The kidney substance shows degenerative changes in the tubules and to a lesser degree in the glomeruli, and scar tissue and cysts develop. Degenerative changes take place in the smaller renal arteries. The kidneys become small. The condition is a progressive one which leads to hypertension and renal failure.

> **Urine**
>
> *Leucocyte excretion count:* higher than 400 000 per hour.
> *Micro-organisms:* exceed 100 000 per ml.
> *Albumin* present or absent.
> *Urine concentration test:* shows low SG and an inability to concentrate urine because of damage to the tubules.

Virus Infection of the Kidney

The role of viruses in the production of diseases of the kidney is not clear. Viruria (the presence of viruses in the urine) occurs in several virus infections, e.g. mumps, measles, Coxsackie infections; but it is thought that the kidneys are getting rid of viruses without necessarily being infected by them. When virus infection of the kidney does take place it is slight and only occasionally is it possible to detect even minimal impairment of renal function.

Viral antigens are suspected of being involved in precipitating an attack of acute nephritis. Recurrent viral infections are a possible cause of some cases of chronic pyelonephritis.

Tuberculosis of the Kidney

Tuberculosis of the kidney is secondary to tuberculosis of the lungs or lymph nodes. Tubercles appear in the kidney and can develop into tuberculous masses and abscesses, and calcification can occur in the wall of an abscess. Infection can spread into the ureters, where a tuberculous pyonephrosis can develop, and bladder. Haematuria can occur.

> **Urine**
>
> Specimen should be obtained from each kidney at cystoscopy. Albumin, pus and blood may be present. *Myco. tuberculosis* may be demonstrated by Ziehl-Neelsen stain or a specimen of urine sent for culture.

Urinary Calculi

Urinary calculi are stones formed in the urinary tract. They form in the pelvis of the kidney, staying there and getting bigger or moving down the ureter into the bladder, or they may form in the bladder itself. They may be single or multiple, unilateral or bilateral, and are of varied chemical composition.

Composition

Urinary stones vary in composition, colour and shape. They can be composed of:

(a) *calcium oxalate*. About 60 per cent of all urinary stones are composed of calcium oxalate. They form in acid urine and are hard, white and radio-opaque.
(b) *triple phosphate* (calcium, magnesium and ammonium phosphate) and *calcium phosphate*. Phosphate stones form in alkaline urine and are white and crumbly. In the renal pelvis, a stone can grow into a 'staghorn calculus', occupying the renal pelvis and taking its shape, and gradually destroying renal tissue.
(c) *uric acid* and *urate*. Uric acid and urate stones form in acid urine and are usually in the bladder. They are yellowish or purple.
(d) *cystine*. Cystine stones are found in congenital cystinuria, have the consistency of candle-wax and are radio-opaque.

Causes

The causes of many calculi are obscure. Among the known causes and contributing factors are the following:

(1) STASIS OF URINE

A stone is liable to form in a hydronephrosis or in a bladder when there is prostatic obstruction.

(2) INFECTION OF URINE

A stone is liable to form around a nucleus of cellular and bacterial debris produced by an infection of the urinary tract.

(3) ALKALINITY OF URINE

An alkaline urine predisposes to the precipitation of calcium phosphate and triple phosphates. This can occur particularly in infections where organisms split urea (causing an alkaline urine) and in renal tubular acidosis (causing an alkaline urine).

(4) EXCESS OF NORMAL CONSTITUENTS IN THE URINE

(a) *Excess calcium*

(i) *Hyperparathyroidism:* the excretion of calcium in the urine is raised when there is a parathyroid tumour and the amount of calcium in the blood is raised.
(ii) *Prolonged immobilization* for a fracture or disease of the spine: calcium is lost from bones when they are not subject to muscular activity and weight bearing, and is excreted in the urine.
(iii) *poliomyelitis and other muscle paralysis:* lack of muscular activity causes decalcification.
(iv) *idiopathic hypercalciuria:* a congenital disorder in which calcium excretion is high but the blood level normal, which suggests that there is a defect of calcium reabsorption by the renal tubules.

(b) *Excess serum uric acid*

Gout: urate stones form in about 20 per cent of people with gout because of excessive amounts of uric acid in the blood and so in the urine.

(c) *Excess cystine*

Congenital cystinuria: cystine stones form.

Complications

Infection of urinary tract: chronic pyelonephritis, pyonephrosis, perinephric abscess, cystitis;
hydronephrosis;
obstruction in the ureter by the stone attempting to move down the ureter;
renal failure;
anuria: total failure of urine production can follow obstruction if the other kidney is absent or non-functioning for any other reason;
impaction of urethra: by a stone attempting to move out of the bladder;
squamous cell carcinoma of the pelvis of the kidney; can develop after years of irritation by a stone.

> **Urine**
>
> Specimens are examined for albumin, red blood cells, pus.
>
> **Renal function tests**
>
> Renal function tests are performed to detect any signs of renal failure.
>
> **Blood**
>
> Serum calcium and serum phosphate levels are estimated in order to detect metabolic disease which might cause a stone.
> Normal serum calcium: 2.1-2.6 mmol/l.
> Normal serum inorganic phosphate: 0.8-1.5 mmol/l.

Hydronephrosis

Hydronephrosis is a dilitation of the pelvis and calyces of the kidney due to a functional defect or to an obstruction of the ureter or urethra.

Primary (idiopathic) hydronephrosis is thought to be due to either (a) a congenital neuromuscular defect which prevents the passage of the normal contraction of the renal pelvis into the ureter so that urine builds up and stretches the pelvis; or (b) an incompetent ureteric orifice into the bladder which allows urine to pass backwards up the ureter when the bladder contracts. Primary hydronephrosis is the commonest form of hydronephrosis in young people.

Secondary hydronephrosis can be unilateral or bilateral. *Unilateral secondary hydronephrosis* can be caused by:
pressure on the upper end of the ureter by an abnormal renal artery;
obstruction of the ureter by a stone or neoplasm of the ureter;
stricture of the ureter after an operation or the passage of a stone;
pressure on the ureter by an external neoplasm.
Bilateral secondary hydronephrosis can be caused by:
enlarged prostate gland;
pelvic tumours, e.g. a fibroid tumour of the uterus;
pregnancy, possibly as a result of relaxation of the muscle in the ureters.

As the hydronephrosis enlarges renal tissue is thinned, the renal blood vessels are compressed, and there is degeneration of the nephrons and their replacement by fibrous tissue.

Complications

Renal failure	hypertension
pyelonephritis	pyonephrosis (the pelvis becoming a bag of pus)
cystitis	calculus formation

> **Urine**
>
> *Urine* may be normal. Pus cells and micro-organisms present if the hydronephrosis is infected.

Neoplasms of Kidney

Neoplasms of the kidney can be benign or malignant.

Benign neoplasms

Fibroma angioma leiomyoma lipoma
They are small and not clinically important.

Malignant neoplasms

(a) *Nephroblastoma* (Wilm's tumour, embryoma of kidney).

This is the commonest malignant neoplasm

of early childhood. It occurs usually before the age of 3 years. It arises from primitive mesodermal cells in the kidney and is composed partly of differentiated elements (glomeruli, tubules, etc.) and partly of undifferentiated oval cells. It grows rapidly, forming a mass at one pole of a kidney and breaking down into haemorrhages and necrotic areas, from which cysts are formed. It infiltrates local tissues and forms metastases in the lungs.

(b) *Hypernephroma* (renal carcinoma, adenocarcinoma of the kidney, Grawitz tumour).

This forms about 75 per cent of all renal malignant neoplasms and about 1 per cent of all malignant neoplasms in the body. It can arise anywhere in the kidney but most commonly in a pole, and forms a golden, brown or reddish mass with sharply defined edges. It is composed of large clear cells arranged in tubules, papillary or solid patterns, and contains lipoid which gives the growth its usually yellow colour. It can infiltrate the renal vein and thence the inferior vena cava, producing oedema of the legs, or on the left side the testicular vein (which opens into the left renal vein) producing a varicocele.

It forms metastases in:

lungs   lymph nodes   brain
bone   skin

Metastases in the lungs may be small or large, so-called 'cannon-ball' deposits.

Neoplasms of the Pelvis of the Kidney and Ureter

A *squamous cell carcinoma* of the pelvis of the kidney can occur as a complication of renal calculi. The epithelium develops an overgrowth of cells which eventually become malignant.

A *papilloma* starts as a benign neoplasm of the pelvis of the kidney and announces its presence by bleeding and causing haematuria. Some eventually become malignant.

A *papillary carcinoma* may arise in a papilloma or be malignant from the start. Several neoplasms may appear about the same time along the ureter and it is thought that they 'seed' themselves from cells from an original growth in the pelvis. Haematuria is common.

BLADDER

Cystitis

Cystitis is an inflammation of the mucous membrane of the bladder, which in the acute state becomes oedematous and inflamed. It can follow:

(a) in men: prostatic enlargement, urethral stricture,
(b) in women: stretching and deformation of the urethra during childbirth,
(c) in both sexes: pyelonephritis, catheterization, cystoscopy, operations on the urinary tract.

E. coli is the most common infecting microorganism.

In chronic cystitis fibrosis of the bladder wall develops and there may be a deposit of amorphous phosphates on the mucous membrane.

Urine

A mid-stream or supra-pubic stab specimen is examined for microorganism and cells.

Interstitial cystitis is a fibrosis of the bladder wall which can occur in middle-aged women and is of unknown origin; it is thought that it may be a form of collagen disease.

Diverticulum of the Bladder

A *diverticulum of the bladder* is a pouch of mucous membrane surrounded by fibrous tissue which projects through a hole in the muscle of the wall of the bladder. It can be:

(a) congenital: rare.
(b) acquired: it is forced out through a weak spot in the muscle during attempts to micturate against a bladder-neck obstruction, the likeliest cause of which is an enlarged prostate gland.

The diverticulum, having no muscle in its wall, cannot empty itself by contraction, but one that fills up during micturition may empty when the bladder relaxes.

Complications

Cystitis	hydronephrosis
pyelonephritis	stone in the diverticulum
carcinoma of the bladder	

Neoplasms of the Bladder

A *papilloma of the bladder* is a benign neoplasm which is often multiple. It is composed of a number of long or short vascular processes which project into the bladder and often bleed profusely.

A *carcinoma of the bladder* is a malignant neoplasm composed of squamous cells, of epithelial cells, or of glandular cells.

Factors in its production are:
aniline dyes used in industry and excreted in the urine
smoking possibly
schistosomiasis, which sets up a chronic inflammation of the bladder.

The carcinoma can ulcerate and become infected, with the production of cystitis and pyelonephritis. Hydronephrosis follows any obstruction of the ureteric opening into the bladder. The degree of malignancy of the tumour varies. It can spread through the bladder wall to invade:

lymph nodes	sacral plexus of nerves
rectum	vagina

Fistulae into the rectum and vagina can follow invasion.

Metastases form commonly in:

liver	lungs
bone	

Urine

A mid-stream specimen or a specimen obtained by suprapubic puncture is examined for red cells, pus, cancer cells and micro-organisms.

Chapter 17 The Skin

Developmental Abnormalities

This term is preferable to 'congenital abnormalities' as some of them are not apparent until some weeks after birth.

Haemangioma

A *haemangioma* is a tumour of blood vessels. The commonest in the skin is a 'port wine stain' on the face or neck. Some gradually disappear.

Sturge-Weber's disease is a combination of haemangioma of the face or scalp in the distribution of a branch of the trigeminal nerve with haemangioma of the meninges and degeneration or failure of development of the cerebrum beneath the intracranial lesion.

Cavernous naevus (strawberry mark)

This is a soft vascular tumour which enlarges up to about the age of nine months and then shrinks until it disappears completely or leaves behind fleshy swellings from which the enlarged blood vessels have disappeared.

Haemangiectatic hypertrophy

This is an association of a large naevus with hypertrophy of a limb. A lymphangioma (tumour of lymph vessels) may be present.

Cysts

Sebaceous cyst

A *sebaceous cyst* is formed by the blocking of the duct of a sebaceous gland. Such cysts are common in the scalp and anterior wall of the chest. They are lined with stratified cells and contain sebaceous material.

Epidermoid cyst (implantation dermoid)

An *epidermoid cyst* can arise by the implantation of epidermal cells into the dermis. They look like sebaceous cysts. They are lined with squamous cells and can become malignant.

Dermoid cyst

A *dermoid cyst* is a developmental abnormality, most commonly found at the angles of the eye or mouth.

Pilonidal cyst

A *pilonidal cyst* is due to blockage of a pilonidal sinus, a condition of uncertain origin, which occurs in early adult life in the sacro-coccygeal region. It can contain hair.

Warts

Verruca vulgaris (common wart) occurs usually in children due to a virus infection. Multiple warts are usual.

Molluscum contagiosum is a viral infection of the skin, producing umbilicated nodules a few millimetres in diameter.

Lupus Vulgaris

Lupus vulgaris is a form of tuberculosis of the skin. Both human and bovine bacilli can be responsible for it. Infection of the skin can be by:

(a) inoculation of the skin by dust infected with the bacilli,
(b) lymphatic spread,
(c) blood-borne invasion from a lesion elsewhere in the body,
(d) spread from infected lymph nodes or a tuberculous sinus.

The nodules of lupus vulgaris appear as flat, semi-clear patches, resembling apple-jelly in appearance, most commonly on the face. The usual tuberculous processes of inflammation and fibrosis go on in and around them. Cartilage can be invaded (but not bone), and in severe cases the cartilages of the nose are destroyed.

Fungal Infections

Fungi of various kinds can infect the skin. It is usual to describe them according to the part infected and not by the precise fungus which causes the infection.

Tinea capitis (ringworm of the scalp)

The fungus invades the horny layer of the skin, gets down the hair follicles and infects the hairs, which become brittle. Affected areas are circular and show hairs broken off about 3 mm from the skin. Scaling, papules and pustules appear in the scalp. The condition occurs only in childhood, for the skin at puberty acquires resistance, presumably by some hormonal action, to the fungus.

Tinea barbae (ringworm of the beard)

The fungus which causes this kind of ringworm spreads from cattle and horses to man, and the disease is usually seen in farm workers and grooms. The beard area develops papules and pustules, with swollen skin between them.

Tinea circinata

The fungus can spread from man to man or from animal to man. It forms circular lesions for it spreads peripherally and heals centrally.

Tinea axillaris et cruris (ringworm of the axilla and groin)

Erythematous patches develop in the axillae and the crural folds and skin adjacent to them.

Tinea pedis (athlete's foot)

This fungus is spread by walking about with bare feet in swimming pools, changing rooms and bathrooms. Other parts of the skin can be infected. Vesicles, pustules and white sodden patches of skin can form.

Tinea unguium (ringworm of the nails)

Infected nails become grey or brown, rough, dull and thickened, and break easily.

Thrush (stomatitis), *angular cheilitis* (of the lips), *vulvo-vaginitis* (of the vulva and vagina) are fungal infections caused by *Candida albicans*.

Scrapings

Scrapings of the skin and nails and samples of hair are examined microscopically for the fungus. Specimens are placed in a drop of potassium hydroxide on a slide. Hyphae are seen, and spores can be seen on hair.

Culture

Candida can be cultured on Sabouraud's medium.

Vasomotor Disorders

Chilblains

Chilblains are due to the action of cold on exposed skin in susceptible people. The arterioles go into spasm, the blood stagnates in dilated venules, and affected parts thus have an inadequate supply of oxygen. Oedema and degeneration and fibrosis of connective tissue follow.

Rosacea

Rosacea is a condition in which in susceptible people excessive and prolonged blushing is produced by the ingestion of hot food and drink, exposure to heat and emotional crises. It most commonly appears at 30-50 years, but can be present in adolescence. Women are more commonly affected than men. The usual sites are the forehead, nose, cheeks and chin. The facial blood vessels can become permanently dilated. Papules can develop from the hair follicles and discharge a fluid which often contains large numbers of a microscopic parasite called *Demodex folliculorum*.

Rhinophyma is an overgrowth of the skin of the nose due to an overgrowth of hair follicles and sebaceous glands.

Psoriasis

Psoriasis is a disease of the skin characterized by the recurrent appearance and disappearance of raised patches of red skin with sharply defined edges and scaling of the surface. The condition is usually inherited and appears at 10-20 years. The cause is unknown, but attacks can be precipitated by infections, injury to the skin and emotional crises. It occurs in various forms. The basic lesion is an overproduction of epidermal cells.

Lichen Planus

Lichen planus is characterized by the appearance of reddish or violet flat-topped shiny papules in the skin or mucous membrane of the mouth. The cause is unknown: it has been thought to be due to a virus, so far unidentified.

Urticaria

Urticaria is (a) a redness of the skin with itchy papules and weals or (b) oedematous swellings below the skin or in the mucous membranes. It is the result of dilatation and increased permeability of the smaller arterioles and of the capillaries. The arteriolar dilatation is due to release of acetylcholine, and the capillary dilatation is due to the release of histamine. The cause can be:

(a) *external:* insect bites, nettle stings, friction, jelly fish stings, scabies, dental treatment

(b) *internal:* foods, infections, emotional factors, drugs, parasites

Exfoliative Dermatitis

Exfoliative dermatitis (erythrodermia) is a redness and peeling of the skin due to:
(a) some drugs, e.g. gold, arsenic
(b) over-treatment of eczema, psoriasis, infective dermatitis
(c) malabsorption syndrome, etc.

In severe cases the peeling is very severe and much fluid and heat are lost.

Complications

Bronchopneumonia   renal failure

Acne Vulgaris

Acne vulgaris is a condition in which occur:
(a) excessive secretion by the sebaceous glands, causing the skin to become excessively greasy
(b) blocking of the hair follicles and sebaceous glands, producing blackheads, papules and pustules
(c) hyperkeratosis of the skin.

The condition begins at puberty and usually disappears in adult life. It is more common in men than women. It is thought to be due to androgen-oestrogen imbalance or an excessive production of androgens.

Complications

Secondary infection by staphylococci; keloid formation: a keloid is an excessive production of scar tissue.

Premalignant and Malignant Conditions

1. *Solar keratotis* is produced by irradiation by prolonged sunshine. Abnormal cells develop in the epidermis and a carcinoma can develop.
2. *Leukoplakia* is a chronic inflammatory state of the skin due to physical or chemical irritation. Patches can develop in the mucous membrane of the mouth in lichen planus, lupus erythematous and other conditions. Squamous cell carcinoma can develop in the patches.
3. *Basal cell carcinoma* of the skin (rodent ulcer) is the commonest malignant neoplasm in man. It can be single or multiple, can arise in apparently healthy skin or in sun-damaged skin. It does not form metastases in other parts of the body, but can invade the subcutaneous tissue and bone by direct spread.
4. *Squamous cell carcinoma* can develop in sun-damaged skin or in a patch of leukoplakia, and can spread to lymph nodes draining the area.
5. *Malignant melanoma* can arise anywhere in the skin but is most common on parts exposed to trauma or friction. It can arise in apparently healthy skin or in a naevus. Pigmented and abnormal cells exist, and the growth can spread to lymph nodes or form metastases in the liver or lungs.

Juvenile melanoma occurs before puberty and can undergo spontaneous regression and disappear.

Eczema and Dermatitis

Eczema and *dermatitis* are two terms for the same skin condition, in which the skin becomes inflamed, oedematous and itching, develops papules and vesicles, and sometimes develops lichenification (thickening).

It is convenient to use both terms and to use each in a different context.

Eczema (eczematous eruptions)

Eczema is used to describe skin eruptions for which no external cause can be found. It is possible that the original cause was external; but lesions appear without any contact with an external irritant and in patches spread over different parts of the body.

The condition is characterized by outbreaks of vesicles which irritate and weep, and which recur sporadically.

Atopic eczema

Atopic eczema starts in infancy; the distribution of eruptions is over the face, scalp, flexures (knee, elbow) and trunk. It is often associated with hay fever and asthma, which may also start in infancy or develop later in life.

There is a strong hereditary influence and an association with the formation of IgE antibody.

N.B. *Atopy* is a term used to include eczema, asthma and hay fever occurring as an inherited predisposition.

Dermatitis

Dermatitis is a term conveniently used to describe a skin lesion acquired as the result of the action of a definite external agent.

Contact dermatitis

Contact dermatitis is a hypersensitivity reaction. The patient has become sensitized (i.e. developed antibodies) to an allergen, and develops a skin reaction at subsequent contact with the substance, at the site of contact.

Many substances can act as allergens, e.g. nickel, nylon, rubber, cosmetics, plants, especially primula and chrysanthemum.

Patch test

This consists of applying to an area of normal skin a little of the substance to which the patient is thought to be sensitive and covering it with an occlusive dressing. The test is positive if an area of dermatitis appears in 24-48 hours. Another piece of the dressing is used as a control. Some people are sensitive to the dressing.

Primary irritant dermatitis

This is not caused by a hypersensitivity reaction. Agents which damage the skin, or penetrate or destroy the natural defences, are called 'primary irritants' and are likely to cause a reaction in most people. Damaging substances include acids, alkalis, chemicals, solvents (e.g. petroleum, white spirit).

Chapter 18 Metabolic and Deficiency Diseases

Diabetes Mellitus

Diabetes mellitus is a disorder of metabolism characterized by a high blood sugar and glycosuria (sugar in the urine). The incidence of the condition depends upon what standards are used in studies of blood sugar level and at what point a condition is considered to be pathological. *Hyperglycaemia* means an excessive amount of glucose in the blood. *Hypoglycaemia* means an inadequate amount of glucose in the blood. Studies of blood sugar levels and glucose tolerance tests in various people show a gradual change from the normal to the abnormal. In general, it is thought that the incidence of diabetes mellitus in Europe and North America is about 13 per 1 000. About half of these cases occur over the age of 40 years, are mild, and present for medical examination only when one of the complications of diabetes arises. About ten times that number have a blood sugar of over 6.7 mmol/l two hours after taking glucose 50 g by mouth and are regarded as cases of 'subclinical diabetes'.

The cause or causes of diabetes mellitus are unknown. Three established factors are:
(a) a hereditary factor, possibly a recessive gene: identical twins are liable to develop diabetes about the same time, and there is greater incidence of diabetes in relatives of a diabetic than there is in relatives of a non-diabetic;
(b) an association with overweight in people whose diabetes begins over the age of 40 years;
(c) removal of the pancreas or chronic pancreatitis.

An association between diabetes and a Coxsackie virus infection has been suggested.

Diabetes mellitus is the consequence of a relative or absolute lack of insulin. Insulin is produced in the beta cells of the islets of Langerhans in the pancreas, and lack of it interferes with the metabolism of carbohydrate, fat and protein. In 50-75 per cent of cases the beta cells show various signs of degeneration. In the others no pathological changes can be detected histologically; it is thought that in these cases there is a relative lack of insulin due to excess of insulin antagonists, which can be (1) excess of glucocorticoids from the adrenal gland as in Cushing's syndrome, (2) excess of growth hormone (GH) produced by the anterior lobe of the pituitary gland as in acromegaly.

The rise of blood sugar that occurs is thought to be due to there not being enough insulin to:
(a) facilitate the transport of glucose across cell membranes,
(b) utilize glucose within cells,
(c) prevent over-production of glucose from glycogen in the liver.

The two large groups of diabetics are:
1. Juvenile onset diabetics: the diabetes begins in childhood, is severe, and is frequently complicated by ketosis.
2. Maturity onset diabetics: the diabetes begins over the age of 40, is associated with overweight, and is often mild.

The division is not absolute, and some maturity onset diabetics can have severe symptoms.

Complications

Ketonaemia: the incomplete metabolism of fat causes the appearance of ketone bodes in the blood.

Diabetic crisis: occurs as a result of ketosis; keto-acids produce metabolic acidosis; coma and death occur in untreated cases.
Infections: especially staphylococcal skin infections.
Arterial degeneration: obliterative arterial disease in the legs; gangrene of feet.
Cataract and retinal degeneration.
Renal disease: pyelonephritis, nephrotic syndrome due to glomerulosclerosis (a deposit of hyaline material in the glomeruli), renal arteriolosclerosis; renal failure.
Neuropathy: a degeneration of peripheral nerves.
Large babies: born to diabetic mothers.

Urine

Glucose: present in variable amounts. Clinistix test is used.
Ketone bodies: present in severe diabetes and diabetic crises. Ketostix test is used.

Blood sugar

A single blood sugar estimation of over 10 mmol/l taken 1-1½ hours after a meal containing liberal amounts of carbohydrate (at least 50 g) indicates that the patient has diabetes.

Glucose tolerance test

Glucose tolerance is the ability of a person to remove excess of glucose from the body after the administration of a large amount. The oral test is the one used clinically; there is an intravenous test but it is rarely used clinically.

After an overnight fast the patient takes 50 g glucose (children 1 g per kilo body-weight up to a maximum of 50 g) diluted in 300 ml of water. The same amount of glucose is also present in 65 g liquid glucose B.P. which is diluted to 300 ml. Blood specimens are taken at half hour intervals for 2 hours; in an 'extended test' specimens are taken for 5 hours. The patient should sit throughout the test and not smoke, as lying down and smoking each delay emptying of the stomach and so absorption of the glucose.

The upper limits of normal for blood sugar are taken as approximately:

	fasting	peak	after 2 hours
venous blood	5.6	8.8	6.1 mmol/l

In diabetes mellitus the fasting blood sugar is normal or raised and the blood sugar is raised at the peak and after 2 hours.

During the test the urine is examined for sugar and ketones at 1 and 2 hours after the administration of glucose.

Hyperinsulinism

Hyperinsulinism is an excessive secretion of insulin due to:
(a) usually an insulinoma of the pancreas: an insulinoma is an adenoma formed of beta cells of the islets of Langerhans, can develop anywhere in the pancreas, and grows to a diameter of about 2 cm;
(b) occasionally a generalized overgrowth of islet cell tissue in the pancreas;
(c) occasionally a carcinoma of islet cell tissue.

An excessive amount of insulin is produced intermittently and causes the blood sugar to fall below 2.2 mmol/l at which level signs of hypoglycaemia (low blood sugar) appear – sweating, rapid pulse, tremor, confusion, abnormal behaviour of various kinds, coma.

> **Blood**
>
> *Blood glucose:* abnormally low (below 2.2 mmol/l) during attacks.
> *Prolonged fast test:* the patient is admitted to hospital and given only unsweetened drinks for 48 hours. The blood sugar will fall below 2.2 m mol/l if the patient has hyperinsulinism, and symptoms will be relieved by the injection of 50 ml of 50 per cent glucose (glucose 25 g).
> *Glucagon test.* 1 mg of glucagon is given intramuscularly. If the patient has hyperinsulinism the blood glucose rises sharply within 30 minutes and then falls to below 2.2 mmol/l. The rise, but not the fall, will occur in normal people.
> *Tolbutamide test.* A fasting patient is given sodium tolbutamide 1000 mg in 20 ml distilled water. The blood glucose is measured every 30 minutes for 3 hours. All people show a fall in blood glucose for 1-2 hours. After 120-180 minutes the blood glucose has returned to 70 per cent of its original level in normal people. In patients with hyperinsulinism there is either no rise or a much lower one than 70 per cent.

Gout

Gout is a condition in which there is an excess of uric acid in the blood and tissue-fluids with a deposit of urate crystals in some joints and elsewhere.

Uric acid is the end product of purine metabolism. Purines or purine bodies are nucleoproteins. Uric acid is excreted into the urine by the distal part of the renal tubules.

Gout can be primary or secondary.

(a) *Primary gout* is gout for which no cause can be found. There may be a familial tendency to overproduce uric acid. It occurs in:

men after puberty,
women after the menopause,
teetotallers as often as in alcoholics,
upper social classes more than in lower social classes.

(b) *Secondary gout* is the result of an excessive purine intake or breakdown, or of a failure of excretion, and occurs in:

leukaemia	impaired renal tubular function
psoriasis	
ketosis	excess alcohol consumption
thyroid deficiency	
polycythaemia	hyperparathyroidism

actions of certain drugs (e.g. salicylates) on kidney function.

Pathological changes are the same in primary and secondary gout. The uric acid level in the serum is raised, and sharp rises or falls in its levels appear to precipitate attacks of gout. Crystals of uric acid are deposited in the joint fluid and joint structures. The joint fluid is invaded by leucocytes, some of which are able to absorb some of the crystals. An acute synovitis of the joint is followed by acute arthritis of the whole joint. Any joint in a limb can be affected, but classically the one most likely to be affected is the metatarso-phalangeal joint of a big toe. With repeated attacks of arthritis, urates are deposited in the joint cartilage and underlying bone.

Tophi are deposits of urates which can develop in bone, the pinna of the ear or the renal tract.

Complications

Ankylosis of joint
Uric acid stone in renal tract.

> **Blood**
>
> Serum uric acid: raised. Normal: men 210-450 μmol/l; women 120-380 μmol/l.

> Erythrocyte sedimentation rate (ESR): raised during an attack. Normal: males 0-20 mm, females 0-30 mm, in 1 hour.

Phenylketonuria

Phenylketonuria is an uncommon error of metabolism transmitted by a recessive gene. It occurs in about 1 in 15,000 children and is equally common in boys and girls.

Due to the lack of a particular enzyme the normal breakdown of the aminoacid phenylalanine into tyrosine is blocked, with phenylalanine building up in the blood and cerebrospinal fluid and appearing in the urine. Most patients are severely mentally retarded, presumably because an excess of phenylalanine prevents proper cerebral development, but occasionally phenylketonuria is found in a person of normal intelligence. The brain is small, and demyelination of nerve tracts in it can sometimes occur. Lack of tyrosine inhibits the development of melanin (which forms pigment in the skin and elsewhere) and in people of the white race the skin is fair and the eyes blue. Eczema, fits and hypertonia often occur.

> **Guthrie test**
>
> A spot of blood is collected on to filter paper from a baby's foot between 6th and 14th day of life. The test is a microbiological one in which the excess of phenylalanine allows the growth of *B. subtilis* in cultures in which the growth would be inhibited.
>
> **Blood**
>
> The phenylalanine level in the blood is estimated in babies with a positive Guthrie test.

VITAMIN DEFICIENCIES

Pathological changes due to vitamin deficiencies appear if the diet (which is the principal source of vitamins) contains less than the minimum amount of vitamins necessary to maintain the health of the tissues, or a malabsorption syndrome prevents their absorption in adequate amounts. As there is likely to be a deficiency of more than one vitamin at a time, pathological changes due to the absence of one particular vitamin are uncommon clinically and the changes that occur are likely to be due to lack of several vitamins and to other dietary deficiencies such as protein deficiency.

Vitamin A Deficiency

The main sources of vitamin A are:
liver   fish-liver oil   eggs
butter   cheese.

It can be formed in the body from carotenes, chemical substances present in green vegetables, apricots and red palm oil, but this is not as important a source as that of the other foods. As it is a fat-soluble vitamin lack it is likely to occur when the diet is inadequate in fat. It is more common in the Far East and Africa than in the West.

Lack causes:
(a) poor night vision: vitamin A forms part of the molecule of visual purple (rhodopsin), the light sensitive substance in the rods of the retina,
(b) degeneration of the epithelium of the respiratory and urinary tracts,
(c) xerophthalmia: a degeneration of the conjunctiva and cornea.

Vitamin B Deficiency

(a) **Vitamin B_1 (aneurine, thiamine)**

Vitamin B_1 occurs in:
the germ and outer layers of cereals
nuts   beans   peas
liver   kidney   eggs   pork.

Deficiency is most likely to occur in the parts of the Far East where polished rice (i.e. without the outer layers) is the staple diet. In Western countries it can occur as a complication of chronic alcoholism, in which a low vitamin B intake is likely.

Beri-beri is the condition produced by lack of vitamin B_1.
(a) In the 'wet' form the heart hypertrophies and then dilates with the production of congestive heart failure, oedema and effusions into the peritoneal, pleural and pericardial cavities.
(b) In the 'dry' form there is degeneration of nervous tissue: demyelination and degeneration of peripheral nerves and patches of degeneration in the pons, medulla oblongata and the posterior columns of the spinal cord.

(b) Riboflavin

Riboflavin is a vitamin of the B group found in many foodstuffs, especially:
milk cheese eggs
yeast liver green vegetables.
It is destroyed by light, and milk exposed in bottles to sunlight quickly loses what it has. Lack of it is most likely to occur in people living in Africa, India and the Far East.

Lack causes:
(a) a seborrheic dermatitis on the face, scrotum or vulva,
(b) superficial glossitis: the surface of the tongue loses its papillae and becomes smooth or fissured,
(c) sometimes invasion of the cornea (which is normally avascular) by blood vessels, with degeneration of the corneal epithelium.

(c) Vitamin B_6 (pyridoxine)

Vitamin B_6 is present in many foodstuffs, especially:
wheat germ liver yeast
cereals peas beans
  Lack causes:
(a) seborrheic dermatitis on the face,
(b) glossitis,
(c) hypochromic anaemia, apparently due to a failure of the red blood cells to absorb iron in the bone marrow,
(d) granulopenia, a reduction in the number of granulocytes in the blood.

(d) Vitamin B_7 (nicotinamide, nicotinic acid)

Vitamin B_7 is present in:
cereals yeast
meat liver
In maize it is present in a bound form, from which it cannot be released for nutritional purposes. Shortage occurs mainly in people who live largely on maize, in chronic alcoholics and in patients with a malabsorption syndrome.

Pellagra is due to lack of vitamin B_7. It is characterized by:
(a) dermatitis on the parts of the skin exposed to light,
(b) glossitis: inflammation of the tongue with loss of papillae, fissures and ulceration,
(c) inflammation of the mucous membrane of the mouth and fissures at its corners,
(d) neuropathy: degeneration of peripheral nerves,
(e) dementia: due to degeneration of cells in the cerebral cortex,
(f) diarrhoea.

(e) Vitamin B_{12} deficiency

See p. 94

(f) Folic acid deficiency

See p. 96

(g) Vitamin C (ascorbic acid)

Vitamin C is found in:
green vegetables oranges lemons
black currants potatoes rose hips, etc.
It is rapidly destroyed by cooking and in food kept warm. Daily human requirements are about 50 mg. Larger amounts (up to 75 mg) are required during infections or stress.

It is essential for the formation of collagen and bone. Lack of it causes degeneration of capillary wall, inadequate calcification of bone, etc.

Scurvy is due to lack of vitamin C. It is characterized by:
(a) bleeding into the gums, skin and subcutaneous tissue, and under the periosteum,
(b) imperfect development and calcification of bone,
(c) slow healing of wounds,
(d) anaemia.

Saturation test

Ascorbic acid is given in a large dose (5 mg per lb body weight) every morning for several days and the amount excreted in the urine is measured 4-7 hours later. If there is a vitamin C deficiency the vitamin is absorbed and not excreted.

Ascorbic acid content

The ascorbic acid content of plasma, leucocytes and platelets is measured. Plasma: normal 6-12 mg/l.

Chapter 19   The Nervous System

The essential features of pathological changes in the nervous system are:

1. The number of nerve cells is never increased. Damaged nerve cells may recover, but if a cell **is destroyed by disease** or injury it is not replaced.

2. Degeneration of the nerve fibres of a tract follows injury or disease of the fibre or its cell, and produces an interruption and often complete stoppage of the functions performed by that tract. Degeneration of a sensory fibre interferes with the transmission of sensation, degeneration of a motor fibre interferes with motor functions, and so on.

3. Provided that the nerve cell is not damaged beyond repair, a nerve fibre will make an attempt to regenerate itself by growing along its former myelin sheath down to its former ending, but sometimes a fibre gets into the wrong myelin sheath, a sensory fibre, for example, going down the sheath of a severed motor fibre and so failing to become functional.

4. Demyelination is a common pathological process. In demyelination, the myelin sheath round a nerve fibre degenerates and its degenerated remains are phagocytosed, i.e. absorbed by phagocytic scavenger cells. Demyelination interferes with the conduction of impulses along a nerve fibre and is followed by degeneration of the fibre.

5. Gliosis is an increase in the number of glial cells in an area. Gliosis commonly follows degeneration and death of nerve cells and fibres. Glial cells form a kind of fibrous scar; they cannot take over the function of nerve cells.

6. A space-occupying lesion of the central nervous system (CNS) can be:
a tumour
a haematoma
an abscess
a foreign body.

As, after early childhood, the brain and spinal cord are enclosed within a rigid, unyielding box formed by the skull and vertebral column, the presence of a space-occupying lesion increases the pressure within the box. This increase is reflected in the CSF pressure.

Such a lesion produces two kinds of change:
(a) the increased pressure within the skull compresses the brain, flattening it against the skull and tending to push the brain-stem down the foramen magnum;
(b) the position of the lesion will cause localizing symptoms and signs according to its precise position, e.g. a tumour of the visual cortex in an occipital lobe will cause a disturbance of vision.

7. Many changes in the CNS have an effect upon the CSF, and examination of a specimen of CSF obtained by lumbar puncture is an essential part of any examination where disease of the CNS is suspected.

Cerebrospinal fluid (CSF)

5-6 ml. are required. The specimen should be collected in a dry, sterile, screw-capped bottle. Two bottles should be available: the first is used for CSF that has accidentally become contaminated with blood, the second for CSF when it has become clear. If meningitis is suspected, the specimen should be kept warm and sent as quickly as possible to the laboratory as the meningococcus soon dies in the cold. If microbiological examination is not required, the specimen need not be kept warm.

Test	Normal	Abnormal
Appearance	clear, colourless	(a) turbid in suppurative meningitis (b) clear or slightly turbid in tubercular meningitis (c) blood-stained in subarachnoid haemorrhage and when a blood vessel is pricked during lumbar puncture.
Pressure	60-150 mm of fluid with body in lateral horizontal position.	Raised in space-occupying lesions, haemorrhage, meningitis
Protein	0.15-0.40 g/l	Raised in infections, haemorrhage, old age. Less in childhood.
Globulin (Pandy test)	Negative	Positive in meningitis, subarachnoid haemorrhage. Strongly positive in syphilis of CNS.
Lange gold curve	0—0	P=paretic, e.g. 5555543100 L=luetic, e.g. 0123332100 M=meningitic, e.g. 0011233221
Chloride	120-130 mmol/l	Reduced in tubercular meningitis
Glucose	2.5-3.9 mmol/l	Reduced in suppurative and tubercular meningitis.
Cells	0-5 lymphocytes/cu.mm.	(a) lymphocytes increased in tubercular meningitis, viral meningitis, syphilis of CNS; (b) polymorphs present in suppurative and tubercular meningitis; (c) red cells present in subarachnoid haemorrhage and when vessel has been pricked in puncture.
WR reaction	Negative	Always positive in GPI; usually positive in other forms of CNS syphilis.
Organisms	Sterile	Organisms isolated in suppurative and tubercular meningitis.

CONGENITAL DEFORMITIES

Anencephaly

Anencephaly is failure of development of the cerebral hemispheres and is incompatible with life after birth.

Hydrocephalus

In hydrocephalus the ventricles of the brain are dilated and filled with an excessive amount of CSF.

The causes are:
(a) any malformation which prevents the

passage of CSF down the aqueduct of Sylvius, which runs between the 3rd and 4th ventricles, or prevents it escaping from the 4th ventricle into the subarachnoid space;
(b) rarely an excessive secretion of CSF or a failure of absorption into the intracranial venous sinuses;
(c) acquired: in later life meningitis or a tumour of the brain may block the passage of CSF.

The ventricles become more and more dilated, brain tissue is compressed, and the cortex can become little more than a thin sheet. Spontaneous arrest of a congenital hydrocephalus can occur. The increasing pressure on the brain and its damage causes mental retardation, spasticity, epilepsy and blindness.

The congenital form is sometimes associated with spina bifida.

Spina Bifida

Spina bifida is a congenital abnormality involving the vertebral column and the spinal cord. The defect is usually in the lumbar region. It is a result of a failure to close of the vertebral arch, with or without a failure to close of the neural canal. Various degrees can occur:
(a) *spina bifida occulta:* the vertebral column is defective posteriorly, but the spinal cord and meninges are not affected.
(b) *meningocele:* the meninges protrude through the opening in the vertebral column; the spinal cord is not affected.
(c) *myelomeningocele:* the meninges, spinal cord and spinal nerves protrude through an opening in the vertebral column.
(d) *myelocele:* neither the vertebral arch nor the neural tube have closed, and nervous tissue is present on the surface of the body, with CSF leaking from a red granular surface; it is not compatible with life.

Spina bifida is sometimes associated with hydrocephalus.

Cerebral Palsy

Cerebral palsy is any condition in which there is an association, in varying degree, of muscular spasticity, involuntary movements and other conditions (mental retardation, epilepsy, blindness) as a result of a failure of normal development of the brain.

The causes are:
(a) a failure of the brain to develop normally, possibly as a result of a gene abnormality,
(b) infections of the mother and fetus during early pregnancy,
(c) irradiation of the maternal pelvis during pregnancy,
(d) kernicterus due to blood group incompatibility,
(e) anoxia before or at birth,
(f) birth injuries,
(g) meningitis or brain injury after birth.

Pathological changes include:
cerebral agenesis: the convolutions and other parts of the brain are small and ill-developed with scanty or abnormal cells and fibres;
areas of gliosis and cyst formation;
thickened membranes.

VASCULAR DISEASE OF THE BRAIN

1. Atheromatous degeneration of arterial wall

This is part of a general degeneration of the endothelium of arteries. Extensive disease of the carotid and vertebral arteries can occur. The blood supply to the brain is diminished, causing interference with cell activities and functioning of the part of the brain involved.

2. Thrombosis

Blood clots on the diseased endothelium of an atheromatous artery and causes a sudden interruption in the supply of blood through that particular artery with the production of a cerebral infarction. Brain cells die in the infarcted area, which becomes gliotic and cystic. Some recovery may take place at the fringe of the infarction.

3. Embolism

This is the blocking of an artery by an embolus, a piece of tissue detached from another site in the body, usually:
a piece of vegetation from a heart valve in rheumatic fever;
a piece of a thrombus from the inner wall of the left ventricle in a fibrillating heart;
a piece of degenerated tissue from the endothelium of an atheromatous carotid or vertebral artery.

Interference with cerebral function is sudden and produces an infarct.

4. Haemorrhage

Haemorrhage into the substance of a cerebral hemisphere occurs as the result of the rupture of an artery, usually one of the perforating arteries supplying the interior of the hemisphere. The cause of the bleeding can be:
an atheromatous cerebral artery
hypertension
purpura
a malignant tumour of the brain
anti-coagulant treatment.

The blood forces the nervous tissue apart and may rupture into a ventricle or on to the surface of the brain. The haemorrhage is a common cause of death.

5. Aneurysm

A so-called 'berry' aneurysm occurs in a cerebral artery as the bulging of the endothelium through a defect in the muscle and fibrous wall of an artery. Aneurysms usually occur on the circle of Willis or one of its branches, and usually at the bifurcation of an artery. There may be more than one. The cause of these aneurysms is uncertain. Some may be congenital, but they are not usually large enough to cause any symptoms or signs unless they rupture. The average age for rupture is 50 years. When they rupture they bleed into the subarachnoid space at the base of the brain. If the patient survives the first rupture, he is likely to die of another.

6. Angioma

An angioma is a mass of tangled, dilated, intercommunicating arteries and veins, formed in the meninges, usually as a congenital deformity. They produce symptoms by pressing on the underlying brain or by rupturing.

7. Venous thrombosis

Clotting of blood in one of the intracranial sinuses draining the brain can be due to:
(a) increased coagulability of the blood, e.g. in dehydrated infants or old people,
(b) the spread of infection from the middle ear, which is closely related to the sigmoid sinus running in a bony groove on the inside of the skull, or from a septic area on the face through the veins through which blood passes from the face into the orbit and thence backwards into the cavernous sinus immediately behind the orbit.

INJURIES OF THE BRAIN

The brain may be injured by a blow to the head, whether or not a fracture of the skull is produced.

1. Bruising and tearing

Bruising and tearing of the surface of the brain can occur. The inferior aspects of the frontal and temporal lobes are the parts usually affected. A *contre-coup* injury is one to the part of the brain opposite to the point of impact and is the result of the jolt of the brain against the skull. Bleeding from torn blood vessels can compress the brain and cause further damage. Compression is increased by an oedema that develops in the damaged tissue or around it.

2. Subarachnoid haemorrhage

Subarachnoid haemorrhage is bleeding into the subarchnoid space between the arachnoid membrane and the pia covering the brain. Compression of the brain beneath the haemorrhage is likely.

3. Extradural haemorrhage

Bleeding into the extradural space between the dura mater and the skull is known as extradural haemorrhage. The middle meningeal vessels, which run through the temporal bone and groove the inner surface of the temporal and parietal bones, are particularly liable to be torn. Compression of the brain occurs. A *chronic subdural haematoma* may follow a slight injury to the head, a small vein being torn where it passes across the subdural space. A haematoma forms, becomes surrounded by a capsule of fibrous tissue, and gradually enlarges; the fluid within the capsule may be liquid blood, a clot, or clear yellow fluid. The brain is compressed.

INFECTIONS OF THE BRAIN

Encephalitis and meningitis are the result of infection of the brain and meninges (the arachnoid membrane and pia mater) by various organisms.

1. Viral encephalitis and meningitis

Among the viruses which can cause encephalitis and meningitis are:

arboviruses   Coxsackie viruses
ECHO viruses   herpes viruses
measles virus   mumps virus

In these infections the brain and spinal cord may look normal, although sometimes parts of them are swollen or soft. On microscopic examination the nervous system is seen to be inflamed and invaded at first by polymorphs and later by lymphocytes. The lesions are not suppurative, i.e. no pus is formed. The neurones show evidence of degeneration and the damaged tissue is invaded by glial cells. The various kinds of virus infection produce generally similar changes, but they differ in the part of the nervous system affected.

CSF

Protein   *Glucose*   *Chloride*
Normal or   Normal   Normal
increased
Cells
Polymorphs and lymphocytes in early stages, then lymphocytes 50-200 per mm.³
Brain biopsy
May be necessary for exact diagnosis.

---

2. Meningococcal meningitis

Meningococcal meningitis is the result of infection by the meningococcus.

The *meningococcus (Neisseria meningitidis)* is oval or bean-shaped. Meningococci live in pairs, side by side. Four groups are known:

group A: responsible for most epidemics;
group B: responsible for some sporadic cases; usual organism found in healthy carriers;
group C: responsible for some sporadic cases;
group D: rarely causes disease.

The meningococcus is present in the throat of about 5 per cent of healthy people. During an epidemic the percentage of carriers is much increased and can be as high as 90 per cent of people in the epidemic area.

Infection occurs in 3 stages:
1. The meningococcus multiplies in the nasopharynx. Slight inflammation can occur. Most cases proceed no further.
2. The blood is invaded by the organisms, with the production of a meningococcal bacteriaemia. Petechiae (small spots) can occur in the skin. The meninges may be invaded without the occurrence of a meningitis, the organisms sometimes residing there for months or years. Rarely a haemorrhage into the adrenal glands produces adrenal cortical damage and death within 24 hours.
3. An acute meningococcal meningitis begins.

Sporadic attacks can occur; and epidemics break out, especially where people are living in overcrowded conditions, e.g. refugee camps.

The meninges become acutely inflamed. Polymorphs and an exudate rich in fibrin occur around the blood vessels and in the sulci of the brain. This is a suppurative meningitis, i.e. pus forms.

Other organisms causing a similar kind of meningitis:
pneumococcus
haemophilus influenzae
staphylococcus
E. coli

3. Tubercular meningitis

Tubercular meningitis is part of a generalized infection of the body (miliary tuberculosis), arising usually from a tubercular focus in a lung.

The meninges become thick and opaque, and multiple tubercles are visible as little white spots. A sticky exudate covers the surface of the brain and spinal cord. Hydrocephalus occurs if the exudate prevents the passage of CSF from the 4th ventricle into the subarachnoid space. Occasionally a *tuberculoma* (a localized collection of tubercular material) forms within the brain; recurrence of infection can arise from one.

Adhesions can form in the meninges, especially at the base of the brain. Degenerative changes in the walls of the small cerebral arteries cause degeneration of nerve cells and fibres.

CSF

Protein	*Lange gold curve*	*Glucose*
increased	M	decreased
Chloride decreased	*Cells* polymorphs 200-300/mm.^{3}	

Organisms
meningococci found on staining or culture

CSF

Protein	*Lange gold curve*	*Glucose*
increased	Weak M	decreased
Chloride decreased to 80-120 mmol/l.	*Cells* lymphocytes and some polymorphs 50-500/mm.^{3}	

Organisms
Myco. tuberculosis found on staining with Ziehl-Neelsen stain

4. Brain abscess

An abscess in the brain can be due to:
(a) spread of infection from the middle ear, mastoid process, nasal sinus, venous sinus;
(b) spread of infection from osteomyelitis of the skull;
(c) a penetrating wound of the brain;
(d) blood-borne infection from a lung abscess, bronchiectasis or empyema;
(e) acute endocarditis.

An abscess is usually single. It can occur in any part of the brain, but infection of the ear is likely to produce an abscess in the temporal lobe or cerebellum, and infection of a frontal sinus is likely to produce one in the frontal lobe.

An abscess is surrounded by oedematous brain tissue, and if it persists it becomes surrounded by glial tissue, which forms a capsule around it. It gradually enlarges and increases the intracranial pressure. It can rupture into a ventricle or on the surface of the brain.

5. Syphilis

The brain can become infected during the generalized spread of syphilis in the primary and secondary stages of the disease.

Meningo-vascular syphilis can occur about 3-5 years after the primary infection. The endothelium of the cerebral arteries becomes inflamed and they are surrounded by a cuff of lymphocytes and plasma cells.

CSF		
Protein	*Lange gold curve*	*Glucose*
increased	L or P	usually normal
Chloride usually normal	*Cells* lymphocytes 10-500/mm^3	*WR* usually positive

General paralysis of the insane (GPI) occurs 5-15 years after the primary infection. Spirochetes in the cerebral cortex multiply, producing degeneration and death of brain cells. The convolutions shrink and the sulci widen.

CSF		
Protein	*Lange gold curve*	*Glucose*
normal or increased	P	usually normal
Chloride usually normal	*Cells* lymphocytes 40-100/mm^3.	*WR* positive

DEMYELINATING DISEASES

The demyelinating diseases are diseases in which the myelin sheath surrounding the nerve fibres degenerates and disappears. The commonest of these is disseminated sclerosis.

Disseminated sclerosis

Disseminated or multiple sclerosis is a disease of unknown causation. It has been attributed to a slow acting virus and has been thought to be an auto-immune disease.

It begins in adolescence or early adult life and is characterized by attacks separated by intervals of months or years. In the acute phase patches of nervous tissue in the brain and spinal cord become swollen and pink. As the acute phase settles down the patch becomes grey, smaller and firm. Demyelination of involved fibres follows; eventually the nerve fibres die and the damaged tissue is replaced by glial tissue. In severe cases extensive damage is done to the nervous system, but in many cases only slight damage is done.

CSF		
Protein	Lange gold curve	Glucose
normal or slightly increased	normal or weak P	normal
Chloride	Cells	WR
normal	moderate increase in lympho-cytes 10-50/mm.^{3}	negative

Acute disseminated encephalomyelitis

In this condition demyelination of nerve fibres in the brain occurs as a sequel to (a) an acute viral infection – measles, German measles, chickenpox, viral infection of the lung; (b) vaccination against smallpox or rabies. The demyelination is thought to be an immune reaction.

DEGENERATIONS

Various degenerative diseases of the brain occur. Their causes are usually unknown.

Paralysis agitans (Parkinson's disease)

This is a disease of late adult life. The basal ganglia of the brain (the lenticular and caudate nuclei) are affected. The nerve cells in them degenerate and disappear, and the ganglia shrink. Interference with their function produces rigidity, poverty of movement, and tremor. Degeneration of the cerebral cortex produces dementia in prolonged cases.

Similar effects can be produced by carbon monoxide poisoning, degeneration of the arteries supplying the ganglia, and as a side-effect of some tranquillisers..

Huntington's chorea

This disease is transmitted by a dominant gene, being inherited by about half the children of an affected person. The brain shows degeneration of the cortex and basal ganglia. Nerve cells in them die and are replaced by glial tissue.

Dementia

Senile dementia occurs in old people. Cells of the cerebral cortex degenerate and eventually disappear. The convolutions shrink and the sulci widen. The frontal poles are commonly more affected than the rest of the cerebral hemispheres. Senile plaques are round or irregular granules of uncertain origin that occur in the cortex in some cases.

Presenile dementias (Pick's disease, Alzheimer's disease, etc.) are similar degenerations, with individually characteristic features, which produce dementia before the senile period, usually in middle life.

Dementia can also be due to:
arteriosclerotic disease of cerebral vessels,
Huntington's chorea,
paralysis agitans,
disseminated sclerosis.

NEOPLASMS OF THE NERVOUS SYSTEM

Neoplasms of the nervous system can be primary or secondary.

1. Primary Neoplasms

Primary neoplasms of the nervous system can be benign or malignant.

Meningioma

This neoplasm arises from cells of the meninges and is composed of fibroblasts usually arranged in a whorled pattern. It forms a firm, spherical, 'golf ball' mass. Most are benign, although they can cause symptoms by pressing on underlying areas of brain. About 10 per cent become locally malignant, i.e. they grow into the brain-tissue or skull but do not form metastases.

Neurofibroma

This neoplasm arises from cells in the sheath of a nerve and grows to form a cylindrical mass composed of fibroblastic cells. More than one may be present. Neurofibromatosis (von Recklinghausen's disease) is the name given to the condition in which multiple neurofibromas are present. A neurofibroma is usually benign, but occasionally a single one becomes malignant. Pressure symptoms are likely when one grows in a confined space, such as on a spinal nerve within the spinal canal or on the eighth cranial nerve in the internal auditory canal in the temporal bone.

Gliomas

These are malignant neoplasms derived from glial cells and are composed of various kinds of cells with different degrees of malignancy. The common types are:
astrocytoma   ependymoma
medulloblastoma   oligodendroglioma

(a) ASTROCYTOMA

This, the commonest of the gliomas, occurs at any age – in the cerebral hemisphere of an adult or in the cerebellum of a child. It forms a soft, infiltrating mass with cystic and haemorrhagic areas in it. Astrocytomas are sub-classified as Grade I-IV according to the type of cell and degree of malignancy, Grade IV being the most abnormal and the most malignant.

(b) EPENDYMOMA

This arises in the cells lining the cerebral ventricles or the central canal of the spinal cord or in those covering the choroid processes in the ventricles. They are composed of cells of varying appearance and different degrees of malignancy, being classified, like astrocytomas, into Grades I-IV, Grade IV being the most abnormal and the most malignant.

(c) MEDULLOBLASTOMA

This is a malignant growth which occurs in the cerebellum of children and is thought to arise from fetal cells trapped in it in the course of development. If forms a soft, grey mass composed of small, oval and 'carrot-shaped' cells, often arranged in rosettes. Metastases can develop on the spinal cord, being 'seeded' in the CSF from the original growth.

(d) OLIGODENDROGLIOMA

This is an uncommon glioma. It occurs as a soft mass in the cerebral hemisphere of an adult and is composed of small cells. It is only locally malignant.

Other primary neoplasms

Other primary neoplasms can arise within the skull from:
the pituitary gland,
the pineal gland,
blood-vessels.
  Other primary intracranial tumors can be:
(a) *pituitary tumours*
(b) *pineal tumours:* arise in the pineal gland and sometimes cause precocious puberty by pressing on the cells around the gland whose function is to inhibit the onset of puberty.

2. Secondary Neoplasms

About 20 per cent of neoplasms which occur in the brain are carcinomas secondary to a primary carcinoma elsewhere in the body. Commonly the source of origin is:

lung   breast
stomach   kidney
malignant melanoma of the skin.

More than one may be present. The neoplasm is composed of the same type of cell as the primary growth.

DISEASES OF THE SPINAL CORD

Poliomyelitis

Poliomyelitis is an infection of the CNS by the poliovirus.

Poliovirus is one of a large group of viruses with a roughly cuboid shape. Three types known:
1. responsible for most epidemics
2. responsible for some small attacks
3. occasionally causes epidemics.

Infection with one type does not confer immunity against one of the others.

The virus is present in the pharynx and faeces for a few days before infection is apparent. It is spread by faeces and faecal contamination. The virus multiplies in the pharynx and intestinal tract and enters the CNS either along nerves or via the blood.

The virus attacks specifically the anterior horn motor cells in the spinal cord. The cells are damaged and may die. Transmission of impulses along the motor nerves is impaired temporarily or completely interrupted with the production of paralysis, muscular wasting and loss of tendon reflexes.

Tabes dorsalis

This is a syphilitic disease of the spinal cord which begins 5-15 years after the primary infection. The nerve-fibres of the posterior column degenerate and are replaced by fibrous tissue. This causes sensory loss and degenerative changes in joints and skin.

CSF		
Protein	*Lange gold curve*	*Glucose*
normal or increased	normal or weak. P or weak L	normal
Chloride normal	*Cells* lymphocytes increased 10-50/mm.³	*WR* usually positive

Syringomyelia

This is a disease of unknown origin. A cyst enclosed within glial tissue develops in the region of the posterior horns of the spinal cord, usually in the cervical region. The spinal cord in the area becomes swollen and the meninges over it thickened. The nerve fibres conveying sensations of pain and temperature cross in this region from one side to the other, and their compression produces the characteristic clinical feature of the disease: the patient develops anaesthesia for pain and temperature in affected parts while retaining other sensations unimpaired.

Enlargement of the cyst compresses in time other tracts in the spinal cord, causing paralysis and loss of reflexes.

Syringobulbia is an extension of the cyst upwards into the medulla oblongata.

Subacute combined degeneration of the cord

This is a degeneration of fibres in the posterior and lateral columns of the spinal cord. It is due to lack of vitamin B_{12} and usually occurs in association with a megaloblastic anaemia.

The sensory fibres in the posterior column of the cord and the pyramidal tract are affected. Their myelin sheaths degenerate and are absorbed, and the fibres then degenerate.

DISEASES OF PERIPHERAL NERVES

Peripheral neuropathy

The term *neuropathy* is preferred to *neuritis* or *polyneuritis* for the condition is usually a degeneration and only rarely an inflammation. It can be due to:
1. lack of part of the vitamin B complex: alcoholism, beri-beri, malabsorption syndrome, starvation;
2. metabolic disease: diabetes mellitus, myxoedema, amyloid disease;
3. connective tissue disease: rheumatoid arthritis, polyarteritis nodosa;
4. carcinoma: most commonly carcinoma of the bronchus (lung);
5. poison: arsenic, bismuth, copper, lead;
6. infection: leprosy.

Whatever the cause the type of degeneration is the same. Peripheral nerves are affected; their myelin sheaths degenerate and the degenerated material is absorbed by phagocytic cells. In leprosy the nerves become thickened by inflammatory changes.

Chapter 20 The Pituitary, Thyroid and Adrenal Glands

PITUITARY GLAND

The common conditions to affect the pituitary gland are:
neoplasms of the gland or of neighbouring structures,
interference with the blood supply,
trauma,
dysfunction of the hypothalamic-pituitary complex.

The *hypothalamic-pituitary complex* consists of the hypothalamus of the brain, the pituitary gland and the stalk which connects them. Several hormones are secreted in this complex and released from the gland to act upon other endocrine glands and tissues. Diseases of the complex are likely to produce either an undersecretion or an oversecretion of its hormones, with the production of changes in the glands and tissues they act upon.

The *pituitary gland* is composed of an anterior lobe and a posterior lobe, which are different in origin, structure and function.

The *anterior lobe* is composed of chromophobe (non-staining) cells: 50 per cent; acidophil (acid-staining) cells: 40 per cent; basophil (base-staining) cells: 10 per cent. It produces:

ACTH: adreno-cortico-trophic hormone, which stimulates the cortex of the adrenal gland to produce cortisol and androgens.
GH: growth hormone, which controls growth and helps to maintain blood-glucose levels.
TSH: thyroid-stimulating hormone, which stimulates the thyroid gland to produce its hormones.
FSH: follicle-stimulating hormone, which in females ripens the ovarian follicle and in males stimulates spermatogenesis in the testis.
LH: luteinizing hormone, which aids the maturation of the ovarian follicle, and the release of the ovum; it luteinises the follicle, i.e. it converts it into the corpus luteum.
ICSH: interstitial-cell-stimulating hormone, which is the same as LH of female but in the male is not called LH because it has no luteinizing function; it stimulates the interstitial cells of the testis to produce testosterone.
Luteotrophic hormone (prolactin, lactogenic hormone): stimulates the breasts, already prepared by oestrogen, to secrete milk.
Releasing factors: hormones of the hypothalamus which stimulate the release of some hormones of the pituitary. CRF (corticotrophin releasing factor) regulates the release of ACTH. TRF (thyrotrophin releasing factor) regulates the release of TSH.

The *posterior lobe* is composed of neuroglial cells and fibres. It produces:
ADH: anti-diuretic hormone, which acts on the distal renal tubules and makes them absorb water from the fluid passing down them.
oxytocin: which (1) causes the pregnant uterus to contract, so being one of the factors contributing to the onset of labour; (2) causes contraction of the

myo-epithelial tissue of the breast so that milk is ejected in lactation.

Tests of Hypothalmic-Pituitary Function

The functions of the hypothalamic-pituitary complex are assessed by:
(i) measuring the amounts of its hormones in the plasma
(ii) measuring the output of the other endocrine glands it controls.

1. ACTH assessment

The amount of ACTH in the plasma is measured by direct radio-immunoassay. An excess of ACTH is a reliable result, but the value of a reduction of ACTH is not so easily assessed as there is only a small difference between normal and subnormal values.

2. Lysine vasopressin test

Lysine vasopressin is a synthetic corticotrophin (i.e. it acts like corticotrophin-releasing factor of the hypothalamus). It stimulates the anterior pituitary to release ACTH. Blood is taken before injection of lysine vasopressin and 30 and 60 minutes afterwards. Cortisol levels in the specimens are measured.

Normal response

Cortisol levels in the plasma should rise to at least 168 nmol/l above the control level (because ACTH stimulates the adrenal cortex to secrete cortisol).

Subnormal response

A failure of the plasma cortisol to rise indicates inability of the anterior pituitary to secrete ACTH. This conclusion assumes that the adrenal cortex is capable of responding to ACTH, i.e. that primary adrenal failure has been excluded.

3. Insulin stress test

This test is used to measure the response of the cerebro-hypothalamic-pituitary-adrenal complex to hypoglycaemia. In normal people hypoglycaemia stimulates the secretion of both growth hormone (GH) and cortisol. After samples of blood have been taken as controls, insulin is injected intravenously to reduce the blood glucose below 2.2 mmol/l. Samples of blood are taken and examined for GH and plasma cortisol.

Normal response

(i) Rise of plasma GH level to 50-70 µg/l half to one hour after hypoglycaemia is achieved.
(ii) Rise of plasma cortisol level above control level of at least 190 nmol/l.

Hypopituitary response

(i) Subnormal or absent rise in plasma GH levels.
(ii) Subnormal rise in plasma cortisol due to failure of anterior pituitary to secrete ACTH. The latter conclusion assumes that the adrenal cortex is capable of responding to ACTH, i.e. that primary adrenal failure has been excluded.

4. Metyrapone (metopirone) test

Metyrapone blocks the action of the enzyme responsible for the final stage of cortisol synthesis in the adrenal cortex. The gland therefore secretes a cortisol precursor which does not suppress the secretion of ACTH and which can be estimated as 17-oxogenic steroids in the urine.
(i) A 24-hour collection of urine is made for control estimation of 17-oxogenic steroids.
(ii) Metyrapone is given orally in 4 doses of 750 mg at 6-hourly intervals.
(iii) 24-hour urine collections are made on the day of dosage and the day after.

Normal response

ACTH secretion increases because the negative feedback mechanism is not working; this causes an increase in secretion of the cortisol precursors, and urinary excretion of 17-oxogenic steroids should increase considerably over the control level.

Subnormal response

Suggests a failure of the hypothalamus to secrete the corticotrophin-releasing factor or a failure of the anterior pituitary to secrete ACTH. This conclusion assumes that the adrenal cortex is capable of responding to ACTH, i.e. that primary adrenal failure has been excluded.

Neoplasms of the Pituitary Gland

Neoplasms of the pituitary gland can be:
primary
secondary.

Primary neoplasms

Primary tumours are likely to produce:
(a) an excess of the hormone produced by the particular cell from which the neoplasm arises
(b) a diminution in the secretion of other hormones because of pressure on secreting tissues of the tumour growing within the pituitary fossa. In consequence the pathological and clinical features are likely to be complex.

CHROMOPHOBE TUMOUR

A *chromophobe tumour* arises from chromophobe cells in the anterior lobe. It is the commonest of the pituitary tumours and is composed of clear cells; degenerative areas and cysts can appear in it. It compresses the rest of the gland, causes the pituitary fossa to enlarge, and can press on the optic nerves or chiasma, on the clinoid processes of the sphenoid bone (which become eroded), and on the hypothalamus and midbrain (sometimes causing hydrocephalus), and can invade neighbouring structures, such as the sphenoid and nasal sinuses. It produces hypopituitarism by compressing the rest of the gland.

ACIDOPHIL TUMOUR

An *acidophil tumour* arises from acidophil cells in the anterior lobe. It is less common than a chromophobe tumour. It produces gigantism in childhood and adolescence and acromegaly in adult life (see below).

BASOPHIL TUMOUR

A *basophil tumour* arises from basophil cells in the anterior lobe. It is rare, always very small, and does not enlarge the pituitary fossa nor press on neighbouring structures. It is associated with Cushing's syndrome.

CRANIOPHARYNGIOMA

A *craniopharyngioma* is a tumour arising from embryological remnants either in or just above the gland. The tumour can grow to the size of a golfball and is solid or cystic or sometimes shows calcification.

Secondary neoplasms

A secondary tumour can arise in the pituitary gland, being usually from a primary carcinoma in the breast or bronchus. A nasopharyngeal carcinoma can invade the pituitary fossa directly.

Hyperpituitarism

1. Excess of GH

A neoplasm of acidophil cells of the anterior lobe produces an excessive amount of GH (growth hormone). This causes: gigantism or acromegaly.
  (a) *Gigantism* is the result of an excess of GH in childhood or adolescence before the epiphyses of bones have fused with the shafts and while growth is still possible. The patient becomes excessively tall. Muscular development is increased and sexual precocity may be present. Features of acromegaly can develop in later life.
  (b) *Acromegaly* is the result of an excess of GH after the epiphyses have fused. Bones become larger; the face is elongated and coarsened, the mandible sticks out, the frontal sinuses enlarge, the hands and feet enlarge. The larynx hypertrophies, the thyroid gland may enlarge. Secondary effects are:
  (i) muscular wasting, hypogonadism and myxoedema due to the destruction of other pituitary cells by pressure from the tumour,
  (ii) diabetes mellitus, because GH has anti-insulin properties,
  (iii) acromegalic cardiac myopathy.

2. Excess of ACTH

A neoplasm of basophil cells of the anterior lobe produces an excess of ACTH. This causes: Cushing's syndrome (see p. 172).

Tests for Gigantism and Acromegaly

Radio-immunoassay of plasma GH

Always above 10 µg/l and usually above 20 µg/l.

Serum calcium

High normal or raised in about 20 per cent of cases. Normal: 2.1-2.6 mmol/l.

Serum inorganic phosphate

Raised in about 20 per cent of cases. Normal: 0.8-1.5 mmol/l.

Glucose tolerance test

The feed-back mechanism normally controlled by the blood glucose level becomes abnormal in gigantism and acromegaly. The plasma HG level remains high and unchanged when the blood glucose level rises (normally the plasma HG level falls).

Hypopituitarism

Hypopituitarism is the condition due to failure of anterior lobe function and varies in degree according to the cause. Usually more than one hormonal output is affected, and rarely is the reduction limited to one particular hormone. Panhypopituitarism is failure of all pituitary hormones. The pathological and clinical features differ according to whether it occurs before or after puberty.

Prepubertal panhypopituitarism

Prepubertal panhypopituitarism is the result of destruction of the pituitary gland or a failure of hypothalamic-pituitary function in childhood. It can be due to:
brain trauma at birth;
tubercular or other meningitis;
craniopharyngioma.
No cause for a hypothalamic-pituitary dysfunction is usually found.

The effects are:
(a) a shortage of GH (growth hormone) produces dwarfism and attacks of hypoglycaemia,
(b) a shortage of ACTH (adreno-corticotrophic hormone) causes a reduction of cortisol secretion by the cortex of the adrenal gland.

Fröhlich's syndrome (dystrophia adiposogenitalis) is a very rare form of hypopituitarism characterized by:
obesity
dwarfism (in most cases; in some there is an adequate secretion of GH and dwarfism is not present)
genital infantilism
diabetes insipidus

Adult hypopituitarism

Adult hypopituitarism is a failure of pituitary function in adult life due to:
(a) infarction, the result of severe haemorrhage and shock during childbirth (Sheehan's syndrome)
(b) a neoplasm of the pituitary gland, especially chromophobe adenoma and craniopharyngioma
(c) a neoplasm pressing on the pituitary gland
(d) a chronic granulomatous lesion (tuberculosis, syphilis)
(e) destruction of the pituitary gland by radiotherapy for acromegaly or Cushing's disease
(f) surgical removal of the gland.

According to the precise hormone missing the results are:
1. Gonadal failure (hypogonadism), amenorrhoea, infertility, impotence, sterility, genital hypoplasia, sparse pubic and axillary hair due to lack of FSH and LH (ICSH).
2. Secondary hypothyroidism: due to lack of TSH.
3. Hypoglycaemia: due to lack of ACTH and GH.
4. Liability to infection: due to lack of ACTH.

Insulin stress test

In patients with lowered GH secretion there is usually a subnormal rise in plasma GH ½-1 hour after hypoglycaemia has been induced.

Glucose tolerance test

There may be a failure of the normal rise in GH level in the plasma when the blood of glucose level falls 3-4 hours after the administration of glucose.

Diabetes insipidus

Diabetes insipidus is a result of a failure of the hypothalamic-pituitary complex to produce and release ADH (antidiuretic hormone). ADH stimulates the distal tubules of the kidney to reabsorb water from the fluid passing through them.

Diabetes insipidus is due to damage to the hypothalamic-pituitary complex by:
(a) neoplasm of the pituitary gland or neighbouring structures,
(b) chronic granulomatous lesions at the base of the brain (sarcoidosis, tuberculosis, syphilis),
(c) meningitis,
(d) head injury,
(e) intracranial operations.
The patient excretes large amounts of dilute urine.
Other signs of pituitary malfunctioning may be present.

> **Urine**
>
> *Specific gravity* (SG): if the patient is deprived of fluid for several hours so that his body-weight falls by 5 per cent, SG of urine does not rise above 1 010.

ADRENAL GLANDS

The adrenal glands are composed of two separate glands:
the cortex
the medulla.

Cortex of the Adrenal Gland

Disease of the cortex produces either increased cortical activity or decreased cortical activity.
The hormones of the adrenal cortex are:

1. *Glucocorticoids*

Mainly cortisol, and small amounts of corticosterone. Glucocorticoids act in opposition to insulin, i.e. they raise the blood sugar. Secretion of glucocorticoids is stimulated by ACTH from the pituitary gland. When there is a high level of circulating glucocorticoids in the blood the secretion of ACTH by the pituitary gland is suppressed (negative feedback mechanism).

2. *Mineralocorticoids*

Aldosterone is the most important. Aldosterone causes the retention of sodium and the excretion of potassium in the urine. Mineralocorticoids are not ultimately under the control of ACTH.

3. *Sex hormones*

Mainly androgens and a little oestrogen. They have little sex hormone activity normally compared with the same hormones produced by the gonads. Their secretion is stimulated by ACTH.

Increased cortical activity

Increased cortical activity can be a result of:
1. Generalized bilateral overgrowth (hyperplasia of cortex).
2. Hyperfunction without an increase in the size of the glands.
3. Adenoma or carcinoma of the cortex.
4. Excess ACTH production.
The syndromes due to various kinds of increased cortical activity are:
Cushing's syndrome,
Conn's syndrome,
adrenogenital syndromes.

CUSHING'S SYNDROME

Cushing's syndrome is a syndrome produced by an excessive secretion of glucocorticoids by the adrenal cortex. It occurs at 30-40 years of age and more commonly in women than men.

Causes

1. Bilateral cortical overgrowth due to overstimulation by excessive amounts of ACTH produced by the anterior lobe of the pituitary gland.
2. Occasionally a small basophil or chromophobe adenoma of the pituitary gland is present and the cause of the over-secretion. In other cases the pituitary gland appears to be overstimulated by the hypothalamus or a higher centre in the brain.
3. An adenoma or carcinoma of the cortex of the adrenal gland.
4. An ectopic ACTH-secreting 'non-endocrine' neoplasm.
5. Prolonged administration of cortisone, cortisol, etc.

Clinical features

The clinical features and biochemical findings are directly due to the excessive amount of glucocorticoids. The patient is likely to develop obesity, hypertension, a plethoric facies, striae of the skin, muscular wasting, diabetes mellitus, and osteoporosis (with pathological fractures and compression of the vertebral bodies).

Plasma cortisol

The normal plasma cortisol is 84-700 nmol/l. There is a normal diurnal rhythm:
minimum at midnight-4.00 hours: 84-196 nmol/l.
maximum at 8.00-9.00 hours: 196-700 nmol/l.
Patients with Cushing's syndrome lose this diurnal variation and have raised levels at all times of the day, e.g. 300-2 000 nmol/l.

Urinary 17-hydroxycorticosteroids

Raised in some patients with Cushing's syndrome, but not in all.

Dexamethasone suppression test

(1) On the lower dose patients with Cushing's syndrome show no suppression of plasma cortisol or urinary 17-hydroxycorticosteroid levels.
(2) On the high dose: (a) patients with adrenal hyperplasia show suppression; (b) most patients with carcinomas and some with adenomas show no suppression.

Glucose tolerance test

A diabetic curve is likely.

CONN'S SYNDROME

Conn's syndrome (primary aldosteronism, hyperaldosteronism) is a syndrome due to the presence of an adenoma of the zona glomerulosa of the adrenal cortex or less commonly to a generalized overgrowth of the zone. The cells in this zone are yellow, and an adenoma is yellow or orange and can grow up to 4 cm diameter. More than one adenoma may be present.

There is an excessive production of aldosterone from the abnormal tissues. This causes a loss of potassium in the urine and the consequent reduction of potassium in the blood causes muscular weakness and occasionally temporary paralysis. Sodium retention occurs, but oedema does not occur. There is a metabolic alkalosis. A moderate degree of hypertension is usually present.

Blood

Serum potassium: reduced. Normal: 3.5-5.0 mmol/l.
Serum sodium: normal or raised. Normal: 135-148 mmol/l.

Urine:

A 24-hour specimen is examined for potassium. The amount is likely to be high.

ADRENOGENITAL SYNDROMES

Congenital adrenal hyperplasia

This is a rare condition in which enzyme deficiencies interfere with the production of cortisol. The lack of cortisol stimulates excessive ACTH production, and this causes adrenal hyperplasia and an excess of adrenal androgens. The clinical features depend on the sex of the patient and the age at which the patient is noticeably affected.

Females. At birth: pseudohermaphroditism (i.e. genitalia have a male appearance). Older girls: virilization.

Males. Infants: precocious development of the genitalia

Boys and adolescents: precocious development of secondary male sexual characteristics, but testicular atrophy

Other adrenogenital syndromes may be due to adenoma, carcinoma or hyperplasia of the adrenal cortex.

Urine

Excretion of 17-oxosteroids is raised (because excess ACTH stimulates the production of androgens). 17-hydroxycorticosteroids are raised due to excretion of cortisol precursors.

Barr body

If the sex of a person is in doubt, the genetic sex is decided by examining cells obtained by a buccal smear from the epithelium of the inside of the mouth. A Barr body is present in many cells if the person is genetically a female. A Barr body is a small stainable spot found in the cells close to the membrane of the nucleus and is formed by two X chromosomes (i.e. the female sex chromosomes).

CARCINOMA OF THE ADRENAL CORTEX

Carcinoma of the adrenal cortex is rare. It can develop at any age, and quickly spreads into surrounding tissues and forms metastases in the liver. The results may be:
(a) no endocrine abnormalities,
(b) Cushing's syndrome,
(c) an adrenogenital syndrome,
(d) a mixed syndrome with features of Cushing's syndrome and adrenogenital syndrome.

Decreased cortical activity

Insufficiency of the cortex can be acute or chronic.

(a) ACUTE ADRENAL INSUFFICIENCY

Acute adrenal insufficiency (adrenal crisis) is due to a severe failure of adrenocortical hormonal secretion, which can occur in:
(a) infants with an adreno-genital syndrome who lack a particular enzyme necessary for the formation of cortisol,
(b) virulent infections producing a haemorrhagic necrosis of the gland, e.g. meningococcal septicaemia in infancy,
(c) patients with Addison's disease,
(d) patients who have had their adrenal glands removed and whose maintenance dose of cortisone or fludrocortisone has not been increased in any condition producing vomiting or diarrhoea,
(e) patients who have been taking glucocorticoids to suppress the hypothalamic-pituitary-adrenal axis and have not been given a larger dose to cover childbirth, a surgical operation or other stressful condition.

Deficiency of glucocorticosteroid causes hypoglycaemia, weakness and stupor. Deficiency of aldosterone causes an excessive excretion of sodium and water in the urine, hypotension and circulatory collapse.

(b) CHRONIC ADRENAL INSUFFICIENCY

Primary insufficiency

Primary insufficiency of the adrenal cortex, or Addison's disease, is due to failure of the adrenal cortex itself. The causes are:
(a) atrophy of the adrenal glands, for a reason which is not definitely known but is probably an auto-immune reaction (it is often found in association with other auto-immune conditions),
(b) tuberculosis of the adrenal glands, secondary to tuberculosis of the lungs, peritoneum, urinary tract or endometrium,

(c) secondary carcinoma of the adrenal glands; the primary growth is usually in the bronchus (lung),
(d) chronic granulomatous disease involving the glands.

According to the cause, the glands show atrophy, fibrosis, calcification, tuberculous degeneration, neoplastic changes, etc.

The changes produced are similar to those produced by acute adrenal insufficiency, but are more prolonged and not so acute.

Features of the diseases are attributable to lack of hormones:

Lack of cortisol causes hypoglycaemia. It also stimulates ACTH secretion, causing pigmentation. (ACTH has a chemical composition similar in part to MSH, melanophore-stimulating hormone, a pituitary gland hormone which produces pigmentation.)

Lack of mineralocorticoids (aldosterone): loss of sodium leads to dehydration; retention of potassium; metabolic acidosis.

Lack of sex hormones: there may be retarded growth in children and loss of hair in women.

Secondary insufficiency

This is due to lack of ACTH in pituitary hypofunction.

The features are mainly those of glucocorticoid insufficiency. There is *no pigmentation* because there is a lack of ACTH. There is no loss of aldosterone because mineralocorticoids are not under the ultimate control of ACTH, so there are no features of mineralocorticoid loss.

Tests for Adrenal Insufficiency

Plasma cortisol: low or undetectable levels.
Urine:
17-hydroxycorticosteroids   low or absent
17-oxogenic steroids low or absent
Glucose tolerance test: flat curve.
Response to stimulation by ACTH.

If plasma cortisol level does not rise during the test, there is a primary lesion of the adrenal cortex. If there is a subnormal rise or a delayed rise, adrenal insufficiency is probably secondary to pituitary hypofunction.
Metyrapone (Metopirone) test: a subnormal response indicates a deficiency of hypothalamic or pituitary secretion, if the adrenal cortex is responding normally to ACTH.

Medulla of the Adrenal Gland

Primary and secondary neoplasms of the medulla can occur. The primary tumours are: phaeochromocytoma, neuroblastoma, ganglioneuroma.

Phaeochromocytoma

A *phaeochromocytoma* is usually benign but can be malignant, occurs most commonly at the age of 20-50 years, and grows into a spherical or oval mass with a reddish-yellow appearance on section. In about 10 per cent of cases it occurs elsewhere than in the adrenal gland. Its cells produce an excessive amount of adrenaline and noradrenaline, and patients suffer episodes of hypertension, sweating, irregularity of the heart's action, pounding in the head, abdominal pain, etc.

Necrosis of the neoplasm or haemorrhage into it produces attacks of circulatory collapse and hypotension.

Urine

The 24 hour urinary excretion of VMA is raised. VMA (vanillylmandelic acid) is an end product of the metabolism of adrenaline and noradrenaline.

Neuroblastoma

A *neuroblastoma* is a malignant neoplasm arising in nerve-cells of the sympathetic system in infancy or early childhood. The adrenal medulla is the commonest site. It is formed of small round cells, often arranged in rosettes, and can become necrotic and haemorrhagic. It grows quickly into a large mass and forms metastases, especially in bone.

Ganglioneuroma

A *ganglioneuroma* is a small tumour of nervous and fibrous tissue which develops in the sympathetic chain or in the adrenal medulla to form a small, encapsulated, firm and often lobulated tumour. It is usually benign, but can become malignant.

Secondary neoplasms

Secondary carcinomas can develop in the adrenal medulla.
The commonest source of origin is: carcinoma of the bronchus (lung).

Tests of Adreno-Cortical Function

Tests measure the amounts of steroids present in plasma and urine. The amounts are increased in excessive adreno-cortical activity and decreased in reduced adreno-cortical activity.

Plasma

Plasma cortisol

The amount of 11-hydroxycorticosteroids in the plasma is measured. This is called the 'cortisol' level, but it includes corticosterone as well as cortisol. The amount produced is normally subject to diurnal variation, being highest at 8.00-9.00 hours and diminishing to its lowest level at midnight-4.00 hours.
Normal range: 84-700 nmol/l.
Midnight-4.00 hours: 84-196 nmol/l.
8.00-9.00 hours: 196-700 nmol/l.
Levels are increased in obesity and in pregnancy and when the patient is taking oestrogens (including contraceptive pill).

Urine

1. *17-oxogenic steroids and 17-hydroxycorticosteroids in urine*

The excretion of these substances, which are products of metabolism, gives a measure of urinary cortisol excretion. Normal excretion rate in adults of 17-oxogenic steroids is:
Males 11-63 µmol/24 hours
Females 5-55 µmol/24 hours.
Normal excretion varies with age, being lower in children and older people.
These steroids are measured during tests of stimulation and of suppression of the pituitary gland and adrenal cortex. They are decreased in Addison's disease, panhypopituitarism and myxoedema.

2. *17-oxosteroids in urine*

These give a measure of androgen excretion. Normal excretion:
Male adults 14-65 µmol/24 hours
Female adults 10-40 µmol/24 hours.
Levels depend on the age of the patient. Excessive amounts occur in adreno-genital syndromes and adrenal tumours, especially virilizing tumours.

Response to stimulation by ACTH

These tests measure the response of the adrenal cortex to stimulation by ACTH or synacthen, a synthetic ACTH. The normal response is an increase in plasma cortisol and urinary 17-hydroxycorticosteroids.

1. *Quick test for adrenal insufficiency*

At 9.00 hours blood is taken for cortisol estimation. Tetracosactrim (Synacthen) 250 µg in normal saline is given intramuscularly. Two specimens of blood are taken at half-hourly intervals.
Normal: control level at least 140 nmol/l. After tetracosactrim one sample should rise by about 280 nmol/l. Lower response indicates an impairment of adrenal cortical function.

2. *Prolonged test: response to stimulation by ACTH*

This test measures the response of the adrenal cortex to stimulation by ACTH. In it:
(a) a sample of plasma is examined at 9.00-10.00 hours for cortisol; and the amount of 17-oxogenic steroids in a 24 hour urine specimen is measured,
(b) then ACTH-gel 40 mg is injected intramuscularly twice a day for 3 days,
(c) on the morning of the 3rd day a sample of plasma is examined and the urinary steroids measured for 24 hours.
Normal response:
(a) plasma cortisol level on 3rd day: over 1 600 nmol/l
(b) 17-oxogenic steroids in urine: over 140 µmol/24 hours.

Addison's disease: no increase in cortisol level or in amount of urinary steroids excreted.
Adrenal atrophy due to pituitary failure; a step-wise increase in both but rarely to same level as normal.

Response to dexamethasone

Normally the administration of dexamethasone (a synthetic glucocorticoid) suppresses the secretion of ACTH, and therefore the secretion of cortisol by the adrenal cortex is suppressed.
1. 24 hour samples of urine are collected for two days, and blood samples are taken at 9.00 hours on both days.
2. Dexamethasone 0.5 mg is given orally every 6 hours for two days.
3. Dexamethasone 2.0 mg is given orally every 6 hours for a further two days.
   Blood is collected daily before the first dexamethasone dose, and 24 hour urine collections are made during the test.
Normal response. Plasma cortisol and urinary excretion of 17-hydroxycorticosteroids fall to below half the control values.
Cushing's syndrome. While the patient is receiving the lower dose of dexamethasone there is no suppression. While he is receiving the higher dose the result depends on the cause of the disease:
(a) A patient with hyperplasia of the adrenal cortex shows suppression;
(b) a patient with a carcinoma usually does not show suppression; some patients with adenoma do not show suppression;

> (c) a patient with ACTH-secreting carcinoma outside the adrenal gland does not show suppression.

THYROID GLAND

Goitre

A *goitre* is an enlarged thyroid gland. It may be simple or colloid.

Simple goitre

A simple goitre is a generalized enlargement of the gland. It can occur:
(1) when there is a shortage of iodine in drinking water and food, as in some mountainous parts of the world;
(2) when there has been interference with the production of thyroid hormones by drugs, e.g. PAS (para amino salicylic acid), thiocyanate;
(3) when there is a demand for extra thyroxine as at puberty and in pregnancy.

In these cases the amount of thyroxine in the blood is reduced, and this reduction stimulates the anterior lobe of the pituitary gland to produce more TSH (thyroid-stimulating hormone) and the TSH tries to stimulate the thyroid gland to produce more thyroxine, which it cannot do. The gland is enlarged and there is an increase in the number of its cells.

The gland may return to normal. However if the abnormal conditions persist for too long, a colloid goitre develops.

Colloid goitre

The vesicles of the gland are distended with colloid. The goitre may be:
(1) *diffuse,* usually at first, and then
(2) *nodular.* The gland is then enlarged by nodules (usually more than one) which differ in size and are scattered irregularly through the gland. Each nodule is enclosed in a thin or ill-developed capsule. These nodules are mostly areas which have atrophied after cessation of stimulation by TSH, which caused the original hypertrophy. Some contain areas of hyperplastic tissue. Cysts, haemorrhages and areas of calcification can occur.

Complications

Pressure: on trachea, oesophagus and great veins.
Haemorrhages: sudden haemorrhages into the gland can enlarge it and cause acute pressure symptoms.
Hyperthyroidism: sometimes called a toxic nodular goitre.
Carcinoma: in about 5 per cent of cases.

Hyperthyroidism

Hyperthyroidism (thyrotoxicosis) is the condition due to an oversecretion of thyroid hormones. It occurs as:
Graves' disease
toxic nodular goitre.

Graves' disease

Graves' disease (exophthalmic goitre) occurs more commonly in women than men and usually between 15 and 45 years of age.

It is thought to be an autoimmune disease. LATS (long-acting thyroid stimulator) is present in the blood; it is a gamma-globulin with the characteristics of an IgG antibody produced by lymphocytes and has effects on the thyroid gland similar to those of TSH (thyroid-stimulating hormone of the anterior lobe of the pituitary gland) but has a much more prolonged action.

The thyroid gland is firm and vascular. The follicles are enlarged, lined with cubical or columnar epithelial cells, and contain only a little colloid, staining palely. The tissue between the vesicles is invaded by lymphocytes and plasma cells. Areas of fibrosis appear.

Complications

Cardiac arrthymias and myopathy.
Muscle wasting, especially of the shoulder and pelvic girdle.
Myxoedema of skin in front of the tibia, due to a deposit of mucopolysaccharides in the skin.
Exophthalmos: the eyes project because the orbital tissues are infiltrated by lymphocytes, plasma cells and other cells, and there is a deposit of mucopolysaccharides.

Toxic nodular goitre

A *toxic nodular goitre* is a nodular goitre in which the nodules start to produce an excess of thyroid hormones. Why they should do this is unknown. The condition occurs usually over the age of 50 years and is a little more common in women than men. There is no excess of LATS (long-acting thyroid stimulator) in the blood.

Tests in Hyperthyroidism

TSH stimulation test: no rise in TSH after injection of TRH (thyrotrophin releasing factor) because the thyroid gland is producing high levels of thyroxine independently of pituitary stimulation (negative feedback is operating).
Protein bound iodine: high
Serum thyroxine: high
T_3 *uptake test:* high resin uptake.
Radio-active iodine tests: uptake by the thyroid gland is high; urinary excretion is low.

Hypothyroidism

Hypothyroidism is the condition due to an underproduction of thyroid hormones. It can occur as:
cretinism
myxoedema

Cretinism

Cretinism is hypothyroidism in infancy. It can be due to:
(a) congenital absence of the thyroid gland
(b) congenital absence of one of the enzymes necessary for the production of thyroxine
(c) shortage of iodine during intra-uterine life (in places where simple goitres occur, for the same reason)
(d) treatment of a hyperthyroid mother during pregnancy with large doses of a thyroid-depressing drug.

In congenital abnormalities no thyroid tissue or only a small nodule is present. With an enzyme defect the gland is large but functionless as thyroxine cannot be produced. With iodine deficiency, the gland is usually small and fibrosed, but there may be a goitre.

Myxoedema

Myxoedema is hypothyroidism in adult life. The term 'myxoedema' is taken from one feature of the disease — the swelling of some tissues due to infiltration by a mucinous substance. It is more common in women than men, and usually occurs at 30-50 years of age.

Causes of myxoedema.

1. In many cases it is idiopathic, i.e. the cause is unknown.
2. Hashimoto's disease.
3. Many patients have circulating antibodies to thyroglobin or other thyroid antigens, but may not have a history of Hashimoto's disease.
4. Thyroiditis: e.g. Riedel's thyroiditis, viral thyroiditis.
5. Iodine deficiency.
6. Following treatment for hyperthyroidism:
(a) irradiation
(b) too extensive a thyroidectomy
(c) anti-thyroid drugs.
7. Lack of TSH due to hypopituitarism.

In idiopathic myxoedema and when myxoedema is due to lack of stimulation by the pituitary gland, the thyroid gland is small and fibrosed. When myxoedema is due to Hashimoto's disease the thyroid gland is enlarged.

Features of myxoedema

1. Myxoedema: a mucinous material infiltrates subcutaneous tissues, especially in the pretibial region, and the larynx, producing a croaky voice and hoarseness.
2. Slowing of body processes; sensitivity to cold; hair falls out.
3. Bradycardia; hypertension due to increased peripheral resistance.
4. Anaemia.
5. Mental slowing.

Tests for Hypothyroidism

Protein bound iodine: low
Serum thyroxine: low
T_3 uptake: low resin uptake
Radioactive iodine tests: thyroid uptake low; urinary excretion high.

Thyroiditis

Thyroiditis is inflammation of the thyroid gland.
1. *Acute suppurative thyroiditis.* Infection by a pyogenic organism is rare.
2. *Viral thyroiditis.* An acute inflammation can be caused by several viruses – Coxsackie, adenoviruses, ECHO, mumps. The gland becomes swollen and infiltrated by lymphocytes. Thyroid hormones, liberated suddenly from the gland, can produce a short attack of hyperthyroidism.
3. *Hashimoto's disease.* This is an autoimmune disease. It occurs more commonly in women than men and usually at the age of 30-50 years. The gland becomes enlarged, hard, infiltrated by lymphocytes and eventually fibrosed. Myxoedema develops as thyroid function fails.

Blood

Erythrocyte sedimentation rate (ESR): raised.
Serum gamma globulins: raised
Serological tests: 3 antibodies may be found, one is an antibody to thyroglobulin and the other two to parts of the cells of the thyroid gland. A high titre of one or more of these antibodies is found.

---

4. *Riedel's thyroiditis.* This is a rare disease of unknown origin in which the gland is converted into dense avascular fibrous tissue and becomes adherent to the skin and other structures. Myxoedema develops in about a quarter of the patients.

Carcinoma of the Thyroid Gland

Carcinoma of the thyroid gland can appear as:
(a) *Papillary type.* This occurs in childhood or early adult life. The growth is composed of papillae of thyroid cells projecting into a cyst. Spread occurs into cervical lymph nodes and less commonly by the blood stream into bones and lungs.
(b) *Follicular type.* This occurs usually in middle age. A large grey mass of malignant thyroid cells is formed. Spread occurs by the blood stream to bones and lungs and less commonly by lymph vessels to lymph nodes.
(c) *Anaplastic type.* This occurs usually in old age, is composed of very malignant undifferentiated cells, large and small, rapidly spreads via blood and lymph, and is fatal within a few months.

Tests of Thyroid Function

Tests of thyroid function fall into three groups:
I.   Measurements of circulating pituitary hormones

II. Measurements of circulating thyroid hormones
III. Radio-active iodine tests

I. Measurements of circulating pituitary hormones

1. *TSH levels* (thyroid-stimulating hormone)

TSH in the plasma is measured by radioimmunoassay. The results are useful in determining the cause of hypothyroidism. TSH levels are high when hypothyroidism is due to failure of the thyroid gland itself, because the negative feedback is not operating. TSH levels are low when hypothyroidism is due to failure of the pituitary gland.

2. *TSH stimulation test*

Thyrotrophin - releasing factor (TRF) is injected and plasma TSH levels are measured at intervals. Peak levels occur about 20 minutes later.

In *primary hypothyroidism* (i.e. due to failure of the thyroid gland) very high levels of TSH occur because the negative feedback is not operating. In *thyrotoxicosis* there is no rise of TSH because high circulating levels of thyroid hormones are operating the negative feedback mechanism, preventing the release of TSH from the pituitary gland.

II. Measurements of circulating thyroid hormone

1. *Protein-bound iodine*

Protein-bound iodine (PBI) is composed mainly of thyroxine (T_4) with a small amount of the more active triiodothyronine (T_3), and the amount of it is an indication of the amounts of the hormones which are being secreted by the thyroid gland.

Normal range: 300-600 nmol/l plasma.

The amount is increased in: hyperthyroidism, pregnancy, women taking contraceptive pills containing oestrogens.

The amount is decreased in: hypothyroidism and in the nephrotic syndrome, because the amount of thyroid-binding globulin (TBG) is reduced.

The test is invalidated if the patient has:
(a) recently taken any drug containing iodine (N.B. iodine is often present in cough and asthma preparations),
(b) has been administered an iodine-contrast medium for an X-ray (which can remain in the body for a long time),
(c) has recently taken any mercurial compound.

2. *Serum thyroxine*

Thyroxine (T^4) is bound mainly by a protein called thyroxine-binding globulin (TBG). By radio-active techniques involving TBG the amount of T^4 in the blood is measured.

Normal range (varies with method used): 60-138 nmol/l.

The amount is increased in hyperthyroidism and decreased in hypothyroidism. The test is not invalidated by any iodine that has been taken.

3. *Triiodothyronine uptake test*

This test is an indirect measure of 'free' or available binding sites for T_3 on thyroxine-binding globulin

((TBG). Radioactive T_3 ($^{125}IT_3$) and a resin are added to serum. The amount of T_3 taken up by the resin is measured. TBG has a greater affinity for T_4 (thyroxine) than for T_3, and any T_3 which is not taken up by TBG will be absorbed by the resin.

In *thyrotoxicosis* the uptake of T_3 by resin is high because available binding sites on TBG are already occupied by excess T_4 (thyroxine). In *hypothyroidism* T_3 uptake by resin is low because less thyroxine is circulating and more binding sites are available for T_3 on TBG. The T_3 is taken up by TBG and not by the resin.

The test is not invalidated by any iodine taken previously, but the results are influenced by alterations in the amount of TBG circulating (e.g. in the nephrotic syndrome it is diminished).

4. *Free thyroxine*

Free thyroxine is the amount of thyroxine not bound to protein in the blood. It is thought to be the active principle, the PBI being thought to be inert and used as a reservoir from which free thyroxine is withdrawn. The amount can be measured, but the test is not usually done as a routine test.

A 'free thyroxine index' is derived mathematically by combining results of PBI and T_3 uptake tests. The 'index' is proportional to the amount of free thyroxine present.

III. Radio-active iodine tests

These tests measure either:
(a) the rate at which the thyroid gland accumulates radio-iodine; or
(b) the rate at which the thyroid gland discharges radio-labelled hormone into the blood.

Most of these tests are better at detecting hyperthyroidism than hypothyroidism.

1. *Thyroid uptake tests*

A test dose of radio-iodine is administered and the amount taken up by the gland is measured over the front of the neck at some specific time later (usually some hours, but can be between 10 minutes and 24 hours). The radio-isotopes ^{132}I and ^{131}I are used. ^{99m}Tc (technetium) is a non-iodine radio-isotope which can be used; it is concentrated in the same way as iodide in the gland, and the radiation dose to the gland from it is smaller than that from iodine-radioisotopes.

The uptake is high in hyperthyroidism and low in hypothroidism.

2. *Urinary excretion test*

The amount of radio-iodine excreted in the urine after a test dose of radio-iodine is measured at intervals. This test is particularly useful in the diagnosis of hypothyroidism. The excretion of the radio-iodine depends on the amount taken up by the thyroid gland (assuming that renal function is normal). The amounts excreted are high in hypothyroidism because iodine is not being taken up by the thyroid gland, and they are low or absent in hyperthyroidism.

3. *Organic radio-iodine test*

When the isotope ^{131}I is synthesized into thyroid hormone it appears in the circulating blood bound to protein. The amount of protein-bound ^{131}I in the plasma is an indication of the rate at which the thyroid gland is using iodine. The test is useful in the diagnosis of hyperthyroidism.

4. *T$_3$ suppression test*
In normal people the administration of thyroid hormone by mouth suppresses thyroid function for a time. In hyperthyroidism (and sometimes in patients with a non-toxic nodular goitre) this suppression does not occur. T$_3$ is given by mouth in dose of 80-120 μg daily for 7 days. The uptake of the gland after the test is compared with that before the test.

Chapter 21 Muscles, Joints, Bones, Parathyroid Glands

MUSCLES

Infections

Muscles may be infected:
(a) in certain virus diseases, especially viruses of the Coxsackie group, as in Bornholm disease (epidemic myalgia), in which small areas of inflammation and degeneration appear in voluntary muscle.
(b) by the spread of infection from adjoining tissues – bone, connective tissue, skin.
(c) in gas gangrene.
(d) in trichiniasis due to eating pork infected with *Trichinella spiralis*, the pork tapeworm.

Polymyositis

Polymyositis is a term used to describe a group of conditions in which inflammatory and degenerative changes take place in voluntary muscle and are associated usually with collagen disease, connective tissue disease or malignant neoplasms. The nature of the condition is not clearly understood. It can appear as:
(a) an inflammatory and degenerative state of muscles only, thought to be a specific auto-immune disease;
(b) an inflammatory and degenerative state of muscle associated with some evidence of collagen disease;
(c) an inflammatory and degenerative state of muscle associated with severe collagen disease, especially rheumatoid arthritis, and with skin and connective tissue lesions – erythema, desquamation, ulceration over bony prominences, Raynaud's syndrome;
(d) an inflammatory and degenerative state of muscle associated with a malignant neoplasm somewhere in the body.

The proximal limb muscles and neck muscles are more likely to be affected than the distal muscles, or there may be a generalized mild muscle involvement. Affected muscles show invasion by inflammatory cells and degeneration of muscle fibres and their absorption by phagocytic cells.

Complications

Chronic fibrosing myositis: fibrosis of muscle and contractures following the acute phase.

Muscle biopsy

Specimen of muscle is examined microscopically to establish the diagnosis.

Blood

Erythrocyte sedimentation rate (ESR): usually raised. Normal: males 3-5 mm in 1 hour, females 4-7 mm in 1 hour.
Serum gamma globulin: may be raised.
Serum calcium, phosphorus, potassium: normal.

Muscular Dystrophies

The *muscular dystrophies* are a group of diseases characterized by a degeneration of muscle fibres and so by muscle wasting. They are genetically determined, but the precise cause of the degeneration is unknown.

(a) **Pseudohypertrophic muscular dystrophy** (Duchenne's disease)

Occurs usually in boys, beginning about the age of 3 years, and is due to a sex-linked recessive gene. In about half the cases no family history is detectable, and it is then thought to be due to a genetic mutation in ovarian cells of the mother or maternal grandmother.

At first there is an enlargement of affected muscles, which are usually the calf muscles, the quadriceps and the deltoid, and the enlargement is thought to be compensatory enlargement of unaffected muscle fibres in the muscle involved. In time the muscles waste, contractures develop, bones atrophy and become distorted. Patients usually die of cardiac failure or chest infection before the age of 20 years.

Associated conditions:

cardiac muscle myopathy
macroglossia (large tongue)
absence of incisor teeth
mental retardation.

In the *Becker type* of the disease the age of onset is 5-25 years, the course is slow, cardiac myopathy does not occur, and the patient, although contracted, may have a normal lifespan.

(b) **Limb-girdle dystrophy**

This occurs in both sexes, appearing usually at 10-20 years of age. Degeneration and wasting of the muscles of the shoulder-girdle and pelvic-girdle are the principal features, but some enlargement of the calf muscles can occur. The course is slow, with the eventual development of contractures and skeletal deformities.

(c) **Facio-scapulo-humeral dystrophy**

A slowly developing degeneration and atrophy of muscles of the face, shoulder, arm and anterior tibial region. In some patients degeneration appears to stop after a time and not to progress further.

Dystrophia Myotonica

Dystrophia myotonica (myotonia atrophica) is an inherited disease in which the patient develops in childhood or early adult life: *muscular atrophy and myotonia* (an inability to relax after contracture), especially in the muscles of the neck, face, forearm, anterior tibial, calf and peroneal regions;
in association with multiple abnormalities, such as:
frontal baldness in males
hyperostosis (overgrowth of bone) of the skull
small pituitary fossa in the sphenoid bone
weakness of cardiac muscle
impaired pulmonary ventilation
small testes and impotence in males
irregular menstrual function and infertility in females
various mild endocrine anomalies
abnormal mental states.

Myasthenia Gravis

Myasthenia gravis is due to an abnormality of conduction at the myoneural junction, i.e. at the point of contact between a motor nerve fibre end-plate and its muscle fibre. At this site there appears to be either an abnormal production or an abnormal destruction of acetylcholine with an interference with normal transmission

and the production of excessive muscle fatigue. The condition occurs twice as often in women as in men. It may appear by itself or in association with:
thyrotoxicosis,
rheumatoid arthritis,
diabetes mellitus,
systemic lupus erythematosus,
sarcoidosis.

In view of these associations, it has been suggested that the condition is an auto-immune disease. The thymus gland is sometimes abnormally large or shows a thymoma, a neoplasm of thymus tissue which may be benign or malignant.

Biopsy

Muscle biopsy shows either no abnormality or a degeneration and phagocytosis of muscle fibres with clumps of lymphocytes between the fibres.

Myositis Ossificans

Some ossification of voluntary muscle can occur when a muscle is repeatedly subjected to stress or injury. A chronic haematoma can form and gradually become ossified from the adjoining bone.

Progressive myositis ossificans is a rare condition in which fasciae, tendons and ligaments become ossified. In spite of its name, it is a disease of fibrous tissue and not of muscle. The big toe or thumb may lack a phalanx.

Neoplasms of Muscle

Neoplasms of muscle are rare. *Rhabdomyosarcoma* occurs in large muscle masses. It is formed of giant and other abnormal cells and is very malignant.

JOINTS

Acute Arthritis

Acute arthritis is an acute inflammation of a joint and can be the result of:
infection of a wound into the joint
septicaemia.

In septicaemia the usual infecting micro-organisms are:
staphylococci   gonococci
streptococci   meningococci
E. coli

The synovial membrane and capsule of the joint become inflamed, and an excessive amount of fluid appears in the joint and can become pus.

Aspiration fluid

Fluid from the joint is examined microscopically for cells and micro-organisms. It is likely to contain a large number of leucocytes or be pus.
Cultures are made of the fluid.

Ankylosing Spondylitis

Ankylosing spondylitis is an inflammatory degeneration of the sacro-iliac and spinal joints and less commonly of other joints.

Its cause is unknown. There is thought to be a genetic factor as a high proportion of relatives of a patient have sacro-iliitis. It is four times as common in men as in women and usually produces symptoms about the age of 30 years.

Affected joints show degenerative changes; granulation tissue forms; patches of bone forming the joint become eroded, and a new bone is formed and causes locking of a joint. In the spine the annulus of the vertebral discs becomes ossified, adjacent vertebral bodies become attached to one another by bone and the spine is converted into an immovable bar of bone.

Associated lesions (whose connection with the bony lesions is not clear) are:
(a) infection of the genito-urinary tract: all men with the disease have a mild chronic inflammation of the prostate gland and seminal vesicles;
(b) iritis: occurs in about 40 per cent of cases;
(c) aortic incompetence and conduction defects of the heart;
(d) ulcerative colitis;
(e) regional enteritis.

Blood

Erythrocyte sedimentation rate (ESR): usually raised.
Normal: males 3-5 mm in 1 hour, females 4-7 mm in 1 hour.
Red cells: some degree of anaemia.
Prostatic fluid: fluid obtained by prostatic massage contains pus. No micro-organism is consistently present.

Rheumatoid Arthritis

Rheumatoid arthritis is a polyarthritis which occurs in association with a number of 'rheumatoid' conditions.

It occurs in about 2 per cent of men and 5 per cent of women in Britain in the age-group 35-50 years, in which it most commonly appears, and the incidence increases with age. The cause is unknown. No micro-organism has been shown to be involved. It is thought to be an auto-immune disease, and the blood of most patients contains a 'rheumatoid factor', an IgM immunoglobulin.

The small joints of the hands and feet are affected first, and then the larger joints. The cervical spine is the only part of the spine to be affected. The temporo-mandibular joint can be affected.

The synovial membrane of an affected joint becomes chronically inflamed, becoming more vascular and invaded by lymphocytes and plasma cells; it proliferates and fibroses, producing a fibrous ankylosis of the joint. Degenerative changes then occur in the articular cartilage and the joint surfaces of bone, with erosion, deformities and muscular atrophy.

Associated conditions often present

Synovitis of tendon sheaths and bursae.
Subcutaneous nodules formed of a central area of necrosis surrounded by epithelial cells, plasma cells and lymphocytes.
Anaemia: usually an iron-deficiency anaemia, sometimes a megaloblastic anaemia.
Arteritis: degenerative changes in the intima of the smallest arteries to the joints with obstruction to blood-supply.
Neuropathy: a degeneration of peripheral motor and sensory nerves.
Pleurisy and pleural effusion.
Pericarditis.
Fibrosis of the alveoli of the lungs.

Complications

Amyloid disease: occurs in about 25 per cent of cases;
Amyloid disease of the kidney causes albuminuria and sometimes the nephrotic syndrome.
Septic arthritis.
Sjögren's syndrome is a rheumatoid arthritis associated with degeneration of the conjunctiva, cornea and sclera.
Felter's syndrome is rheumatoid arthritis associated with a large spleen, a reduction in the number of white cells in the blood, and sometimes enlargement of lymph nodes.

Blood

Rose-Waaler test: this test is carried out on serum (and on aspirated joint fluid). Agglutination occurs of sheep red blood cells coated with a rabbit anti-sheep cell antibody. The test is positive in over 70 per cent of

patients with rheumatoid arthritis. Positive reactions can occur in cases of jaundice, some virus infections, Hodgkin's disease, etc.
Erythrocyte sedimentation rate (ESR): raised. Normal: males 3-5 mm in 1 hour, females 4-7 mm in 1 hour.
Red cells and haemoglobin: anaemia often present.

Joint fluid

Aspirated joint fluid is examined to exclude septic arthritis and for the Rose-Waaler test.

Still's Disease

Still's disease is a polyarthritis which begins in early childhood (usually at 1-3 years of age). Its cause is unknown. It can occur as: (a) a disease which remits in adolescence leaving a variable amount of permanent deformity; (b) a childhood rheumatoid arthritis; or (c) a childhood ankylosing spondylitis. Degenerative changes similar to those of rheumatoid arthritis occur in the joints.

The illness may be preceded weeks before its onset by an acute illness characterized by fever, a maculo-papular rash, pericarditis, an enlarged spleen, enlarged lymph nodes, and leucocytosis.

Complications

Iridocyclitis: inflammation of the iris and rest of the uveal tract of the eye; can cause blindness.
Amyloid disease.
Impairment of growth due to involvement of the epiphyses of the bones of the limbs.
Abnormal growth of a particular bone.

Osteo-arthritis

Osteo-arthritis is a degenerative disease of joints. It usually affects large joints, most commonly the hip. It can be:
(a) primary: a result of senile changes; several joints can be affected.
(b) secondary: the result of repeated trauma as in certain occupations, a mal-united fracture, or disease of bone; only one joint is usually affected.

The articular cartilage, becoming soft, is worn away. Underlying bone is exposed and becomes excessively hard and grooved. New bone is formed at the edge of the articular surface, producing osteophytes (projecting lips of bone) which lock the joint. Fibrosis occurs in the synovial membrane.

Tuberculosis of Bones and Joints

Tuberculosis of a bone or joint is secondary to tuberculosis elsewhere in the body. It is usually caused by the bovine strain of the *Myco. tuberculosis* and has almost completely disappeared in countries where tuberculosis of cows has been eradicated and milk is pasteurised.

The disease follows the usual pattern of a tuberculous infection: the formation of tubercles, their spread, the formation of caseous material and abscesses, and the development of fibrous tissue and its subsequent calcification in healing lesions.

Common sites of infection are:
(a) the *hip*. Infection begins in the acetabulum of the pelvic bone or in the neck of the femur and spreads to the joint, involving first the synovial membrane, then the articular cartilage and underlying bone.
(b) the *knee*. Infection begins in bone or synovial membrane and goes on to involve the rest of the joint.
(c) the *metacarpals, metatarsals and phalanges*. A tuberculous osteitis can occur in one or more of these bones.

(d) *spine*. Infection is most common in the lower thoracic region, begins in a vertebral body, and spreads to adjoining intervertebral discs and vertebral bodies. Collapse of a body produces deformity of the spine and can cause pressure on nerve roots or the spinal cord.

Complications

Cold abscess: tuberculous abscesses are called cold because the slowly developing inflammation does not produce a sensation of heat. Abscesses occur in the neighbourhood of joints and bones and cause sinuses by 'pointing' through the skin. A *psoas abscess* is one which arises from tuberculosis of the lumbar spine and passes down within the sheath of the psoas muscle to its insertion into the upper end of the femur and 'points' below the inguinal ligament.
Wasting of muscles acting on an affected joint.
Fibrous ankylosis of an affected joint.
Secondary infection of a joint.
Interference with the growth of bone.
Kyphosis of the spine with pressure on nerve roots and spinal cord.

Aspiration fluid

Fluid aspirated from a joint is examined for cells and micro-organisms. Cultures are made for *Myco. tuberculosis* or a guinea pig inoculation is performed.

Synovial membrane

A specimen of synovial membrane is examined for tubercles.

BONES

Fractures

A *fracture* is a break in the continuity of a bone. The types of fracture are:

(a) *simple fracture*: there is no wound communicating between fracture and skin.
(b) *compound fracture*: there is a wound between fracture and skin and a danger of infection of the fracture.
(c) *comminuted fracture*: the bone is broken into more than two pieces.
(d) *pathological fracture*: the fracture occurs at a site where the bone is weakened by disease (e.g. a secondary neoplasm) or by skeletal degeneration.
(e) *greenstick fracture*: a fracture in childhood when the bone (not fully ossified) is partly broken, partly bent.
(f) *stress fracture*: the bone breaks at a site exposed to frequent stresses.
(g) *fracture dislocation*: the fracture is combined with the dislocation of a joint.

Healing of a fracture

(a) A haematoma forms between the broken ends.
(b) Fibroblasts from the periosteum invade the haematoma and lay down fibrous tissue.
(c) Osteoblasts invade the site and start to lay down bone.
(d) A callus is formed of irregular bone in excess.
(e) Permanent bone is laid down and the bone shaped to its proper shape and size by the combined action of osteoblasts (which form bone) and osteoclasts (which remove any excess of bone). No scar is formed.

Complications

(a) *Mal-union*: the broken bones unite at an angle owing to mal-alignment, or the bone is shortened due to an uncorrected overlap of the broken pieces.
(b) *Non-union*: the fracture fails to unite and the gap is filled with fibrous tissue with the production of a pseudarthrosis (false joint). Non-union is due to:
(i) an inadequate blood supply to one of the fragments due to the fracture tearing the artery

to one of the pieces. It can occur in fracture of:
neck of the femur
scaphoid bone
shafts of radius, ulna, tibia.
(ii) the interposition of muscle or other soft tissue between the broken pieces.
(iii) inadequate immobilization of the fracture.
(c) *injury to a main artery or spasm of an artery*: this can cause ischaemia of a muscle which can go on to fibrosis and contracture; gangrene of tissues can occur.
(d) *Injury to a nerve*: bruising of a nerve, with recovery, is more likely than division of the nerve. A nerve is occasionally involved within a callus.
(e) *Fat embolism*: can follow fracture of a large bone; globules of fat are discharged from the bone marrow into the blood and can block small arteries in the lungs and brain.

Osteomyelitis

Osteomyelitis is infection of bone. It is now uncommon. It is caused by:
(a) infection from the blood from a source of infection in the tonsils, teeth or skin; the usual organisms are:
Staph. aureus,
haemolytic streptococci,
pneumococcus.
Usually only one bone is affected, but in infancy more than one may be.
(b) infection from a wound.

Acute

Acute osteomyelitis occurs mainly in childhood. The lower end of the femur and the upper end of the tibia are the commonest sites. Infection spreads down the shaft and outwards. A subperiosteal abscess can form, stripping the periosteum off the bone and tearing the blood vessels which supply the bone. With the loss of its blood supply a piece of bone dies forming a piece of dead bone called a sequestrum. New bone can form in the stripped off periosteum and surround the sequestrum. The abscess may rupture through the periosteum to form an abscess between bone and skin; and if the skin breaks down, a sinus forms through which pus is discharged. Joints are not usually invaded. Lymph nodes draining the part can become inflamed.

Blood

White cells: there is a polymorph leucocytosis.
Erythrocyte sedimentation rate (ESR): raised. Normal: males 3-5 mm in 1 hour, females 4-7 mm in 1 hour.
Blood cultures are made to detect the organism and test its drug-sensitivity.
Pus is examined for organisms and their drug-sensitivity.

Chronic

Chronic osteomyelitis is the result of:
(a) an acute osteomyelitis that has not healed,
(b) an infected compound fracture.

The affected bone becomes thick and abnormally hard and contains pockets of pus in which there may be small sequestra. Sinuses may open on to the skin. An acute flare-up can occur, with fever and abscess information.

Complications
Anaemia   loss of weight
joint stiffness   muscle contractures
interference with the growth of the bone
amyloid disease in very chronic conditions.

Rickets and Osteomalacia

Rickets and *osteomalacia* are each due to interference with calcium metabolism, rickets in childhood, osteomalacia in adult life and especially in old women.

Muscles, Joints, Bones, Parathyroid Glands

Both calcium and phosphate are necessary for the normal metabolism of bone.

Rickets and osteomalacia follow:
1. Lack of adequate amounts of vitamin D in the diet or inadequate production in the skin by exposure to sunlight; a lack of vitamin D results in reduced calcium absorption.
2. A malabsorption syndrome in which there is an inadequate absorption from food of vitamin D, calcium and phosphate.
3. Loss of calcium in the urine, e.g. in renal tubular acidosis.
4. Various diseases of the renal tubules in which there is an excessive excretion of phosphates.

In *rickets* the epiphyses remain wide because there is an irregular proliferation of cartilage cells in them and a failure of ossification at the right time. The bones become soft and bend under weight or with muscle traction.

In *osteomalacia* there is a decalcification of bones and a softening and bending of them.

Associated conditions

Muscular weakness and hypotonia   tetany

Blood

Serum calcium: low or normal. Normal: 2.1-2.6 mmol/l. Serum alkaline phosphatase: increased. Normal: 30-125 I.U./l.

Osteitis Deformans

Osteitis deformans (Paget's disease of bone) is a degenerative disease occurring usually in old age, rarely before the age of 50 years. It is thought to be inherited as a dominant condition but mainly because of the great age at which it occurs it is difficult to get a family history. The sexes are affected equally.

The bones in which it usually appears are:
pelvis   upper end of femur
vertebral bodies   upper end of tibia
skull   humerus

The bones of the face, hand and foot are rarely affected. Several bones may be affected or only one or part of one.

Two changes take place:
(a) osteoporosis – a thinning of bone. What bone remains has a normal calcium content. The bone becomes brittle and bends under weight. Areas become excessively vascularised.
(b) osteogenesis – the formation of new bone. The bone becomes thickened and roughened with hard brittle bone.

The femur and tibia bend under the weight of the body. Kyphosis of the spine follows degeneration of the vertebral bodies and discs. The skull enlarges.

Complications

Pathological fractures: union can take place unless the bone is very hard.
Paraplegia: due to pressure on the spinal cord and nerve roots from collapse of the vertebral bodies.
Osteo-arthritis: especially of the hip and knee.
Sarcoma of bone: occurs in 10 per cent of cases.
Pressure on cranial nerves: by new bone formed in the skull.
Arterio-venous shunts: due to hyperaemic areas in bone.

Blood

Serum alkaline phosphatase: raised. Normal: 30-125 I.U./l. Serum calcium: usually normal. Normal: 2.1-2.6 mmol/l. Serum inorganic phosphate: usually normal. Normal (fasting): 0.8-1.5 mmol/l.

Osteosclerosis

Osteosclerosis is an increase in the normal chemical composition of bone due to increased osteoblastic activity. Osteoblasts are the cells which lay down bone.

It occurs in:
chronic cardiac disease,
chronic respiratory disease,
osteosclerotic secondary carcinoma (the primary carcinoma being usually in the prostate gland or breast).

> **Blood**
>
> Serum alkaline phosphatase: may be raised. Normal: 30-125 I.U./l.

Neoplasms of Bone

Neoplasms of bone can be primary or secondary to a neoplasm elsewhere in the body. Primary neoplasms can be benign, intermediate or malignant.

1. Benign neoplasms

(a) A *chondroma* is a tumour of cartilage which arises in the shaft of a long bone – often in a metacarpal or metatarsal bone or a phalanx of finger or toe. It may be single or multiple.

(b) An *osteochondroma* arises from a displaced piece of epiphysis and can be either:
(i) an *ecchondroma*, composed mainly of cartilage; or
(ii) a *cancellous exostosis*, composed mainly of bone.
It may be single or multiple. A single osteochondroma arises from the growing end of a long bone (usually the lower end of the femur or the upper end of the tibia) while the epiphysis is still present, is covered with epiphyseal cartilage, and stops growing when the epiphysis fuses with the shaft.

(b) An *osteoma* is formed of hard compact bone. A common site is the skull where signs of pressure on the nervous system can be present.

2. Intermediate neoplasm

An *osteoclastoma* (giant cell tumour of bone) is described as an intermediate neoplasm because some are benign, some are only locally malignant, and some can form metastases in the lungs. It is likely to grow in the shaft of a long bone (usually the lower end of the femur or the upper end of the tibia) and to form a soft yellow mass composed of multinucleated giant cells and spindle-shaped cells.

3. Malignant neoplasms

Malignant neoplasms of bone are relatively common in childhood and all can spread via the blood to form metastases elsewhere, especially in the lungs.

(a) An *osteosarcoma* arises in the actively growing end of a long bone, usually the lower end of the femur or the upper end of the tibia. It is formed of a mixture of malignant cells, cartilage and fibrous tissue with new bone being laid down at its edges.

The usual age of onset is 10-20 years. Boys are more often affected than girls. It can arise later in life as a complication of osteitis deformans (Paget's disease of bone).

> **Blood**
>
> Erythrocyte sedimentation rate (ESR) raised. Normal: males 3-5 mm in 1 hour, females 4-7 mm in 1 hour.
> Serum alkaline phosphatase: raised, **as a result of bone destruction.** Normal: 30-125 I.U./l.

(b) A *periosteal sarcoma* is a rare neoplasm which arises in the fibrous coat of periosteum and is formed of fibroblasts and spindle-shaped cells. It is a slowly growing tumour which arises at 30-40 years of age.

(c) *Ewing's tumour* (malignant endothelioma) occurs usually in childhood and arises in the shaft of a long bone. It is composed of small dark-staining cells which invade the bone and destroy it. New bone is laid down among the destroyed bone. Metastases can form in the liver and other bones as well as in the lungs.

(d) A *chondrosarcoma* is a malignant neoplasm of cartilage, arising most commonly in a long bone, a rib or the pelvis. It grows slowly to form a hard mass in which some calcification takes place.

PARATHYROID GLANDS

Disorders of the parathyroid glands are characterized by over-secretion of parathormone (hyperparathyroidism) or under-secretion of parathormone (producing hypoparathyroidism).

FUNCTIONS OF PARATHYROID HORMONE

Parathyroid hormone has a complicated activity.
1. It stimulates osteocytes to release calcium and phosphate from bone.
2. It increases the excretion of phosphate by the kidney.

The result is to raise the plasma calcium level and to lower the plasma phosphate level. A low plasma calcium level is probably the stimulus for secretion of parathyroid hormone; secretion is probably suppressed when plasma calcium level is low.

Thyrocalcitonin, a hormone secreted by the thyroid gland, is likely to be more important in maintaining the plasma calcium level than parathyroid hormone.

Hyperparathyroidism

Hyperparathyroidism is the condition produced by over-secretion of parathormone, the hormone produced by the parathyroid glands.

Primary hyperparathyroidism is usually due to an adenoma of one of the parathyroid glands. Occasionally there may be multiple adenomata in one or more of the glands. The neoplasm can be up to 3 cm in diameter. In about 4 per cent of cases the neoplasm is malignant.

The excessive secretion of parathormone causes an excessive amount of calcium to be transferred out of the bones into the blood and to be excreted in the urine. This causes:
1. metabolic bone disease: the bones become thin and decalcified, with an excess of fibrous tissue and sometimes cysts; they bend under weight and can suffer a pathological fracture;
2. calcium is deposited in the kidney substance (nephrocalcinosis) or renal calculi are formed of calcium phosphate or calcium oxalate; pyelonephritis and impairment of renal function can complicate the lesions.

Blood

Serum calcium: raised. Normal: 2.1-2.6 mmol/l.
Serum inorganic phosphate: low. Normal: 0.8-1.5 mmol/l.
Serum alkaline phosphatase: raised if bone disease is present. Normal: 30-125 I.U./l.

Secondary hyperparathyroidism can occur in:
the malabsorption syndromes
chronic renal disease
because in this conditions the blood calcium is liable to fall, and a fall in blood calcium is the normal stimulus to excite the production of parathormone by the parathyroid glands. The bone changes are similar to those of osteomalacia or of primary hyperparathyroidism. *Renal rickets* is a term used to describe the bone changes occurring in childhood as a result of chronic renal disease.

The chemistry of the blood is complicated by the effects on calcium and phosphate produced by the original disease as well as by the consequent hyperparathyroidism.

Hypoparathyroidism

In *hypoparathyroidism* there is an inadequate secretion of parathormone by the parathyroid glands. It is due to:
1. idiopathic hypoparathyroidism, a rare inherited condition,
2. accidental removal of the parathyroid glands during thyroidectomy or removal of the parathyroid glands for hyperparathyroidism.

The effects of an inadequate secretion of parathormone are:
(i) the amount of phosphate in the blood is increased because excessive amounts of phosphate are reabsorbed from the urine as it passes along the renal tubules.
(ii) the amount of calcium in the blood is decreased because less is absorbed by the small intestine and there is less mobilization of calcium from bone. The density of bone may be increased.

Hypoparathyroidism is clinically manifested by an increase in the excitability of nervous tissue (tetany), and in idiopathic hypoparathyroidism by cataracts in the eyes and calcification of the basal ganglia of the brain.

Blood

Serum calcium: reduced. Normal: 2.1-2.6 mmol/l.
Serum inorganic phosphate: raised. Normal (fasting): 0.8-1.5 mmol/l.

Chapter 22 The Male Genital System

Testis

Congenital abnormalities

(a) UNDESCENDED TESTIS

The testis develops in fetal life immediately beneath the kidney at the back of the abdominal wall and should in the last weeks of fetal life descend down the abdominal wall, through the inguinal canal and into the scrotum, arriving at its destination just before birth. The method by which this descent is achieved is imperfectly understood and is thought to be by endocrine stimulation along the course of the gubernator testis, a band of fibrous tissue running to the bottom of the scrotum.

An undescended testis is one which does not achieve its descent into the scrotum but remains somewhere along the line of descent – within the abdomen, in the inguinal canal or at the top of the scrotum. The condition may be unilateral or bilateral; the right testis is more commonly undescended than the left.

If the testis remains in the abdomen, spermatozoa do not develop at puberty, possibly because the abdominal cavity is hotter than the scrotum. The interstitial hormone-producing cells function normally, and male secondary sex characteristics appear at puberty.

Complications

Trauma: if the testis is in the inguinal canal or upper end of the scrotum it is more likely to be injured as it is in a more exposed position and cannot move.

Torsion of testis: can occur when the testis is in the inguinal canal.

Neoplasm: about 10 per cent of malignant neoplasms of the testis occur in an undescended testis.

Inguinal hernia: likely to be present.

Infertility: if both testes remain with the abdomen.

(b) ECTOPIC TESTIS

An ectopic testis is one which has descended into an abnormal position – into the perineum, into the pubic region or into the femoral region. In these positions it will function normally, but is more exposed to trauma than in its normal position in the scrotum.

An inguinal hernia may be present.

Hydrocele

A *hydrocele* is a collection of fluid within the tunica vaginalis. It can be primary or secondary.

Primary hydrocele. The cause is uncertain; it may be the result of a failure of development of full lymph drainage of the testis.

Secondary hydrocele: the result of:
(a) inflammation of testis: gonorrhoea, syphilis, tuberculosis,
(b) neoplasm of testis,
(c) infestation by filariasis.

The tunica vaginalis becomes thickened with fibrous tissue and may show some inflammatory cells.

Complication

haematocele: a haemorrhage into the hydrocele due to injury or attempts at aspiration.

Fluid

Fluid is clear and pale yellow and may contain crystals of cholesterol.

Orchitis and Epididymitis

Orchitis is inflammation of the testis. *Epididymitis* is inflammation of the epididymis. *Epididymo-orchitis* is inflammation of both the testis and the epididymis, the two organs being so closely connected that they are both likely to be involved in the same pathological processes.

Orchitis (with little involvement of the epididymis) occurs as a complication of mumps. The testis becomes inflamed and swollen. Testicular atrophy can follow, with the testis becoming a small mainly fibrous mass. In about 10 per cent of cases of mumps orchitis both testes are affected and both can atrophy; but usually the atrophy is not complete, some spermatozoa are produced and libido is not affected.

Other acute attacks of orchitis and epididymitis can occur as a result of:
non-specific urogenital infection of the male;
E. coli infection of the urinary tract;
after catheterization, cystoscopy, prostatectomy and other operations on the genito-urinary tract.

Chronic epididymo-orchitis can be due to:
(a) *tuberculosis*: the testis, epididymis, vas deferens and seminal vesicle are affected by a typical tuberculous reaction. A sinus can form as a result of the attachment of a diseased epididymis to the skin.
(b) *gonorrhoea*: fibrosis results from chronic inflammatory changes and subacute attacks of epididymitis can occur.
(c) *syphilis*: in the third stage of the disease there can be a gumma of the testis or diffuse chronic inflammation.

(d) *recurrent urinary infection of old men*: the epididymis in particular becomes irregularly hardened by chronic inflammatory changes.

Non-specific Urogenital Infection of the Male

Non-specific urogenital infection of the male is clinically indistinguishable from gonorrhoea, but no infecting micro-organism can be found in the urethral discharge and the cause is unknown. It is a common condition, almost certainly spread by sexual intercourse. Urethritis occurs and a urethral discharge produced.

Complications

Cystitis   haematuria
epididymitis   urethral stricture
acute or chronic prostatitis.

Urethral discharge

Microscopic examination of a smear distinguishes between gonorrhoea (in which gonococci are present) and this condition (in which no micro-organisms are visible).

Neoplasms of the Testis

Benign neoplasms of the testis are rare. An *interstitial-cell growth* can produce precocious puberty in young boys by secreting androgens.

Malignant tumours are seminoma, teratoma, and malignant lymphoma.

(a) Seminoma

This is a carcinoma arising from cells in the seminiferous tubules and composed mostly of rounded cells which resemble the spermatocytes from which spermatozoa are formed. It forms a pink or grey, rounded and clearly demarcated mass, and can spread into the epididymis and spermatic cord. It spreads slowly into the testicular lymph vessels, which pass up the posterior abdominal wall, to lymph nodes around the aorta just below the renal vessels, i.e. to the original site of development of the testis.

Metastases occur late in:
   lungs   bone
   supraclavicular lymph nodes (via the thoracic duct)

(b) Teratoma

This neoplasm arises from primitive cells before they have become differentiated into ectodermal, mesodermal and endodermal cells, and it can contain tissues which do not appear in a normal testis, such as cartilage, intestinal glandular tissue, and placenta-like tissue. The degree of malignancy varies and can in some be very great. The aortic lymph nodes are invaded via the testicular lymph vessels.

Metastases form early in:
   lungs   liver   bone.

(c) Malignant lymphoma

A malignant neoplasm of lymph tissue can occur in the testis and sometimes bilaterally.

PROSTATE GLAND

Benign enlargement of the prostate gland

A benign enlargement of the prostate gland occurs in almost all men, but only in 1 in 10 does the enlargement cause trouble. The cause is unknown: the enlargement is usually attributed to some hormonal imbalance. The whole gland or part of it may be involved. The enlargement can be composed of the normal glandular epithelium of the gland and its supporting fibromuscular tissue, but occasionally it is composed of fibrous or muscular tissue with the production of a hard but not very much enlarged gland.

Complications

Gradual obstruction to urinary flow by pressure on the internal sphincter of the bladder,
acute urinary retention,
cystitis,
stone formation in the bladder,
diverticulum of the bladder,
bilateral hydronephrosis and pyelonephritis,
renal failure.

Prostatitis

Prostatitis is inflammation of the prostate gland. An *acute prostatitis* can occur as part of a non-specific urogenital infection in the male or as a result of infection by gonococci or other organisms. A *chronic prostatitis* can develop from an acute infection or apparently be chronic from the start; the prostate becomes small and indurated and may contain some small calculi.

Prostatic fluid

Prostatic fluid is obtained by prostatic massage and examined for cells and micro-organisms. Normally a few leucocytes are present.

Carcinoma of the prostate gland

Carcinoma of the prostate gland occurs in middle-aged and elderly men. It is the third leading cause of deaths from cancer in men, being exceeded by cancer of the lung and cancer of the large intestine.

It is an adeno-carcinoma which gradually invades the gland to produce a hard nodular mass. Local spread is into the pelvic cellular tissue around the gland and sometimes into the sacral nerve roots. Iliac, aortic and inguinal lymph nodes can be invaded. Metastases occur mainly in:
bone, especially the pelvis, vertebrae, femur, ribs
liver   skin

This is one of the few neoplasms which can be controlled to some extent by hormonal alterations, for oestrogen administered by mouth or bilateral orchidectomy can cause the primary and secondary growths to regress for a time.

Complications

Acute or chronic retention of urine,
hypertrophy, dilatation and infection of the bladder
renal failure.

Blood

Serum acid phosphatase is raised above 7 I.U./1 when bony metastases are present and is often much higher.

Histology

Specimens of the gland can be removed with needles and examined for cancer cells.

Urethra

Congenital Abnormalities of the Urethra

Hypospadias

The external meatus of the urethra is not at the tip of the glans penis but somewhere along the inferior surface of the penis. The penis may be bent downwards.

Epispadias

The external meatus of the urethra opens somewhere along the dorsum of the penis. The abnormality may be asociated with maldevelopment of the urethral sphincters.

Other Abnormalities

Phimosis

This is an abnormal tightness of the prepuce. Any tightness present in infancy should disappear with normal growth. Phimosis later in life is usually due to *balanitis*, an infection of the glans penis.

Paraphimosis

This is congestion of the glans penis due to retraction over it of a tight prepuce.

Urethritis

Urethritis is inflammation of the urethra due to:
(a) infection by the gonococcus,
(b) infection by *E. coli, Staph. pyogenes, Proteus* etc.
(c) non-specific uro-genital infection in the male.
    It is acquired by sexual intercourse with an infected person or instrumentation (catheterization, cystoscopy). The urethra becomes congested and oedematous, and there is a urethral discharge.
    An untreated urethritis may lead to:
urethral stricture.

Urethral discharge

Discharge is examined for micro-organisms, especially the gonococcus, and leucocytes.

Reiter's Syndrome

Reiter's syndrome (Urethro-Conjunctivo-Synovial (UCS) syndrome) is a syndrome of:
urethritis, prostatitis, cystitis
polyarthritis
conjunctivitis, iritis
lesions of the skin
lesions of mucous membranes.

Its cause is unknown. It is found in association:
(a) in Britain and North America with a sexually-transmitted non-gonococcal urethritis;
(b) elsewhere in the world with bacillary or amoebic dysentery or a non-specific discharge. It is thought that these infections damage the mucous membranes of the urethra or intestine and allow the entry of the infecting agent.

The acute stage can last for up to 18 months and few patients recover permanently and completely. Attacks of urethritis, painful deformities of the feet, spondylitis, sacro-iliitis, uveitis and aortic valve incompetence are likely in the chronic stage of the disease.

Blood

Red cells: some degree of anaemia
White cells: slight neutrophil leucocytosis
Erythrocyte sedimentation rate (ESR): raised up to 100 or more mm.

Urethral discharge

Specimen examined for gonococci and other organisms.

Urethral Stricture

A *urethral stricture* is an abnormal narrowing of a part of the urethra. This is a male condition, the female urethra being short and straight and not likely to develop one. It can be:
(a) congenital:
a pin-hole meatus,
abnormal valves in the posterior part of the urethra;
(b) acquired:
following injury to the urethra,
urethritis, usually gonococcal,
prostatectomy,
indwelling urethral catheter,
neoplasm of urethra (rare).

Complications

Urinary infection   retention of urine
periurethral abscess   extravasation of urine
renal failure   into adjoining tissues

Neoplasms of Penis

Benign neoplasms (fibrolipoma, papilloma, angioma) can occur.

Carcinoma can take the form of either a malignant ulcer with hard, rolled edges or a papillary growth. In both kinds it is a squamous cell carcinoma. It can infiltrate the penis and spread to superficial inguinal and iliac lymph nodes. Metastases occasionally occur in:
liver   lungs   bone.

Chapter 23   The Female Genital System: The Breast

CONGENITAL ABNORMALITIES

OVARY

One or both ovaries may be absent or represented by a blob of fibrous tissue. The ovary may lie in an abnormal position somewhere along a line between the lumbar region and the inguinal region or there may be a piece of additional ovarian tissue along the line.

UTERINE (FALLOPIAN) TUBES

One or both of the uterine tubes may be absent or imperfectly canalized, or attached to an abnormal position on the uterus. Abnormality of a tube is likely to be associated with an abnormality of the uterus.

UTERUS

The uterus may be: (a) absent or represented by a fibrous nodule; (b) permanently arrested at the infantile level of development, with a relatively long cervix; (c) developed only on one side, with absence of the uterine tube on the undeveloped side; (d) be divided into two as a result of a failure of fusion into one organ of the two Mullerian ducts from which it develops.

VAGINA

The vagina may be: (a) divided into two when the uterus is similarly divided into two and for the same reason; (b) imperfectly canalized.
    An *imperforate hymen* is a failure of canalization at the lower end of the vagina, the orifice being blocked by a thin membrane which prevents the escape of secretions.

INFECTIONS

Gonorrhoea in Women

Gonorrhoea is a sexually transmitted infection. The common sites of infection in women are:
the urethra
the cervix of the uterus
the uterine tubes

Gonococcal urethritis

The urethra becomes inflamed and there may be a slight discharge from it. From the urethra the infection can spread:
(a) into the para-urethral glands of Skene. These glands lie on either side of the urethra and open into it just inside the urinary meatus. A *skenitis* is an inflammation of the glands of Skene. It can cause an abscess.
(b) into the glands of Bartholin. These glands lie on either side of the vagina and open by a duct on to the inner surface of each labium minor. A *bartholinitis* is an inflammation of the glands. Infection produces an inflammatory mass which can become an abscess. A cystic dilatation of the gland can be caused by a fibrosis of the duct due to the inflammation.
(c) rarely to the vulva, producing oedematous labia.
(d) occasionally into the bladder, producing a mild trigonitis, an inflammation of the trigone, the triangular area between the openings of the ureters and the urethra.

Gonococcal cervicitis

Cervicitis is inflammation of the cervix of the uterus. The cervical glands are inflamed and a discharge is produced. Blocking of the ducts of the glands produces chronically infected retention cysts.

Gonococcal salpingitis

Salpingitis is inflammation of the uterine (Fallopian) ducts. Infection reaches them by spreading from the cervix of the uterus across the surface of the endometrium, or possibly by lymph vessels. The mucous membrane and submucous coat of the ducts become acutely inflamed, and pus forms in the tube and wells out of its fimbriated end. Gonococci are present in the pus at first, but later they disappear and a clear fluid is exuded into the tube. The outer wall of the tube is covered with exudate.

Complications

Pyosalpinx: the tube becomes blocked and an abscess forms in it.
Hydrosalpinx: the tube becomes blocked and the clear fluid, which succeeds the pus, forms a cyst.
Pelvic peritonitis: the pelvic peritoneum becomes inflamed.
Pelvic abscess: an abscess forms in the recto-uterine pouch (pouch of Douglas).
Tubo-ovarian cyst or abscess: the end of the tube becomes adherent to the ovary and a cyst or abscess forms.
Fibrous adhesions: develop between the tube and adjoining structures. Intestinal obstruction can be caused.
Ectopic pregnancy: can be due to kinking of the duct following infection or by destruction of the mucous membrane and loss of its ciliary action.
Chronic cervicitis: produces a chronic discharge.
Sterility: due to loss of tubal patency after bilateral salpingitis so that ova can no longer pass along them.

In about 50 per cent of cases gonorrhoea in women is associated with a trichomonas infection.

Pus

Smears from a urethral or cervical discharge are examined microscopically for gonococci, trichomonas vaginalis and other microorganisms. Cultures are made.

Infections of the Vagina

Vaginitis

Vaginitis is inflammation of the vagina and can be due to:
(a) gonorrhoea;
(b) trichomonas infection;
(c) *Candida albicans*, a fungus which produces white patches on the vulva and vagina;
(d) foreign bodies in the vagina;
(e) infection by *E. coli* and other organisms in young girls, producing *vulvo-vaginitis of childhood*; it is produced by the absence of vaginal acidity (in which organisms cannot grow), and is likely to occur when there is a lack of hygiene, a foreign body in the vagina, or infestation with threadworms;
(f) infection in old age, when vaginal acidity is reduced and the vagina is invaded by microorganisms, with the production of inflammatory and fibrotic changes.

Infections of the Uterus

Acute cervicitis

Acute cervicitis can be due to:
gonococcal infection
trichomonal infection
infection following childbirth.
The cervix is red and oedematous, and there is usually a discharge.

Chronic cervicitis

Chronic cervicitis can follow an acute cervicitis, and is most commonly the result of the infection of a tear produced in childbirth. The tissues show invasion by polymorphs and lymphocytes and the development of fibrosis.

A *cervical erosion* can occur in chronic cervicitis. It is an extension on to the vaginal part of the cervix of glandular epithelium from the cervical canal. It becomes infected. It appears as a red velvety area which bleeds profusely. Small polyps of granulomatous tissue are present on its surface, the submucous glands are dilated into cysts, chronic inflammatory cells invade the tissues, and the originally columnar epithelium can become squamous.

Endometritis

The uterine cavity is normally sterile. *Endometritis* is inflammation of the endometrium and can be due to:
(a) infection by streptococci, staphylococci or *E. coli* following childbirth or abortion,
(b) infection following gynaecological operations,
(c) chronic gonococcal infection,
(d) an ascending infection causing a senile endometritis when in old age the vaginal acidity falls and organisms start to proliferate in the vagina whence they get into the uterine cavity,
(e) tuberculosis: typical tuberculous lesions can follow infection of the blood from a focus in the lungs or urinary tract. The condition is rare in countries where tuberculosis is prevented or adequately treated if it occurs.

NEOPLASMS OF THE UTERUS

Fibromyoma

A *fibromyoma* (fibroid) is a tumour composed of fibrous tissue and uterine muscle fibres.

They are the commonest tumours of women. Their cause is unknown. They begin usually in early adult life, but because they grow slowly they do not cause symptoms until after the age of 30. They are more common in nulliparae (women who have not had children) than in women who have had children. They are dependent upon the presence of oestrogens in the blood; they atrophy after the menopause, natural or artificially induced; and they sometimes atrophy after pregnancy.

Fibroids are often multiple and can grow to a very large size. They are more common in the body of the uterus than in the cervix. As they grow they come to lie either under the peritoneum on the outer surface of the uterus or under the endometrium, and in either position they can become pedunculated. They are round or oval tumours, firm and white. The proportion of muscle and fibrous tissue in them varies. Surrounding muscle is compressed to form a capsule.

Various kinds of degeneration can occur in them.
(a) Red degeneration: the fibroid becomes red and swollen, and the muscle fibres in it degenerate. It is thought to be due to kinking of its blood vessels or to infarction in them.
(b) Hyaline degeneration: of fibrous tissue first and then of muscle.
(c) Cystic degeneration: irregular spaces containing clear fluid can appear after red or hyaline degeneration.
(d) Fatty degeneration: of muscle fibres first.
(e) Calcification and ossification: in very old tumours.

Complications

Menorrhagia (excessive menstruation),
anaemia due to menorrhagia,
torsion of a pedunculated fibroid: the blood supply is obstructed and necrosis follows,
infection: can follow necrosis,
uterine inversion following expulsion of a pedunculated fibroid through the cervix of the uterus,
sarcoma: develops in less than 0.1 per cent of fibroids.

Cystic Glandular Hyperplasia

Cystic glandular hyperplasia is an overgrowth of endometrium. It is a result of:
(a) a failure, temporary or permanent, of the pituitary gland to produce luteinizing hormone (LH); as a result of which:
(b) the Graafian follicles do not mature and no corpus luteum is formed; as a result of which:
(c) no progesterone is produced and the uterus is exposed to an uninterrupted production of oestrogen.

The endometrium hypertrophies and becomes spongy, contains many cysts formed by dilated endometrial glands, and bleeds irregularly, producing the condition called clinically *metropathia haemorrhagica*. The uterine muscle hypertrophies a little. *Senile cystic endometritis* is the same condition in old age when the cysts remain but the fall in oestrogen causes a regression of the hyperplasia.

Carcinoma of the Cervix

Carcinoma of the cervix develops about the age of 40-50 years. Frequent sexual intercourse and sexual promiscuity appear to be factors in its production, and it is uncommon in women who have not had children. It is more common among women in the lower socio-economic groups than in the higher. If screening tests for pre-invasive cancer are carried out among all women between 20 and 60 years, 3-7 cases are found per 1 000, but in the groups of women most at risk 20 or more per 1 000 are found.

It arises usually near the external orifice of the cervix as a nodule which grows, ulcerates, bleeds easily and is liable to become infected. It is composed of malignant squamous cells. It spreads:
(a) *locally*: into the adjacent vaginal vault, the broad ligament, the bladder, the utero-sacral ligaments and the rectum.
(b) *by lymph vessels*: to the iliac and sacral lymph nodes.
(c) *by vaginal implantation*: into lower parts of the vagina.
(d) *by the blood* in later stages of the disease: to many parts, especially the ovaries, vertebrae, long bones and brain.

Complications

Vesico-vaginal fistula: following spread into the bladder.
Recto-vaginal fistula: following spread into the rectum.
Renal failure: following obstruction of the ureters or an ascending infection of the urinary tract.
Anaemia.

Cervical cytology

Cervical cytology is an examination of the cells from the surface of the cervix carried out to detect pre-cancerous lesions or cancer. Certain abnormalities of the squamous cells and of their nuclei are regarded as precancerous changes which precede the development of cancer by 3-5 years. It is recommended that the test is carried out once every 4-5 years and more frequently in those particularly at risk.

There are several methods of obtaining a specimen. The best is a cervical scrape, using a special speculum under direct vision. Other methods are the aspiration of cell-containing secretions from the posterior fornix at the top of the vagina, the use of a cervical swab, or the use of a do-it-yourself irrigation cytopipette.

A smear is made on a slide and stained or fixed.

A *normal smear* is one which contains no abnormal cells.

A *suspicious smear* is one in which some cells show suspicious features. The test is repeated.

> A *positive smear* is one in which cancer cells or cells with pre-cancerous changes are present. A biopsy is then performed, sometimes after a repeat of the test to confirm the first.

Carcinoma of the Body

Carcinoma of the body of the uterus usually occurs at about 60 years. It is more common in nulliparae than multiparae. It is associated with an excessive secretion of oestrogen and can appear as a complication of endometrial hyperplasia and of a granular cell tumour of the ovary. There is an association with obesity and diabetes mellitus.

The tumour is an adenocarcinoma and projects as a papillary mass into the uterine cavity. It can spread through the muscle wall into the subperitoneal tissue and, uncommonly, downwards through the cervical canal.

Spread beyond the uterus is late. Metastases can develop in the ovaries or in the para-aortic and iliac lymph nodes. A metastasis can develop in the vagina as a result of the implantation of cancer cells in it, or in the peritoneum through the uterine tube. Later still comes dissemination by the blood into the liver, lungs, pleura, etc.

> ### Biopsy
> A diagnostic curettage can be performed and the tissue removed examined for cancer cells.

Sarcoma of the Uterus

Sarcoma of the uterus is rare. It can develop in a fibromyoma, in the muscle wall or in the endometrium. The cells are spindle-shaped or round. The tumour grows quickly and spreads extensively.

UTERINE (FALLOPIAN) TUBES

Salpingitis is inflammation of the uterine tubes and is usually due to gonorrhoea.

Tuberculous salpingitis can be part of a general tuberculous infection of the pelvic organs and peritoneum. The usual tuberculous lesions are present.

Primary neoplasms are rare. A neoplasm of the ovary or the body of the uterus sometimes grows into the tube.

THE OVARIES

Cysts and Neoplasms of the Ovary

1. Cysts

(a) FOLLICULAR CYSTS

These may be single but are often multiple, can grow up to about 3cm diameter, and project from the surface of the ovary. Most of them have formed in Graafian follicles which have not gone through the full stage of their development. They are filled with a clear fluid containing oestrogen.

(b) LUTEAL CYSTS

A luteal cyst is the result of a failure of a corpus luteum to regress as it should. They can grow up to about 3cm diameter and contain a clear fluid.

(c) ENDOMETRIAL CYSTS

These are formed from ectopic (out-of-place) endometrium (the inner layer of the uterus), with which they are lined.

(d) CHOCOLATE CYSTS

These are blood-containing cysts, the blood in them having altered and looking like melted chocolate. They are the result of bleeding into luteal or endometrial cysts.

2. Neoplasms which are mainly cystic

(a) MUCINOUS CYSTADENOMA

This is the commonest ovarian tumour. It usually appears at 30-60 years. It can be unilocular or multilocular, is filled with clear mucin, and can grow to an enormous size. The cyst wall is composed of columnar cells.

Complications

Rupture of cyst: tumour cells are 'seeded' on to the peritoneum.
Pseudomyxoma peritonei: masses of mucus develop in the peritoneal cavity as a result of the seeding of tumour cells.

(b) MUCOUS ADENOCARCINOMA

About 10 per cent of cystadenomas are malignant. Sometimes only part of the cystadenoma is malignant, the rest appearing benign. The malignant cells form a firm white mass, from which they grow out to invade the peritoneum or into lymph vessels and nodes.

(c) SEROUS (PAPILLIFEROUS) CYSTADENOMA

This is a common ovarian tumour, grows up to about 15cm diameter, and may be bilateral. It is filled with clear fluid and may be loculated. Papillary processes project into the cystic interior.

Complication

Rupture of cyst: tumour cells are 'seeded' on to the peritoneum.

(d) PAPILLIFEROUS CARCINOMA

About 15 per cent of papilliferous cystadenomata become malignant. The tumour cells can invade the peritoneum.

Complication

Ascites: due to invasion of the peritoneum.

(e) CYSTIC TERATOMA (dermoid cyst)

This tumour can occur in childhood, but is more common at 20-40 years. It is usually unilateral and attached to the ovary by a pedicle. It develops from an undifferentiated remnant and is in consequence composed of many kinds of tissue: skin, hair, bone, teeth, thyroid gland, intestine etc. The cyst fluid is fatty.

Complications

Torsion of the pedicle: its blood supply becomes obstructed.
thyroid tissue in it can become malignant.
a squamous epithelioma can develop in it.

3. Neoplasms which are mainly solid

(a) SOLID TERATOMA

This is similar in its origin to a dermoid cyst, but it is mainly solid and any cysts in it are small. It arises commonly in young women. It is composed of many kinds of tissue jumbled together, grows rapidly, and is very malignant.

(b) FIBROMA

An ovarian fibroma is formed of connective tissue and grows from the surface layer of the ovary.
Meig's syndrome is an association of ovarian fibromata with ascites, hydrothorax and pericardial effusion.

(c) BRENNER TUMOUR

This is a small benign tumour composed of fibrous tissue and little clumps of squamous epithelium. It is most common at 40-60 years. It arises on the surface of the ovary.

(d) GRANULOSA CELL TUMOUR

This can occur at any age, but is most common after the menopause. It is small, solid, and unilateral, and composed of granulosa cells similar to those in the ovarian (Graafian) follicle. It can become malignant. It secretes oestrogens, which cause enlargement of the uterus, endometrial bleeding, and enlargement of the breasts, with precocious puberty if it occurs in a girl and some rejuvenation if it occurs in a middle-aged or old woman.

(e) ARRHENOBLASTOMA

This is a rare and usually benign tumour which occurs in young women, and as it secretes testosterone (the male sex hormone) it has virilizing effects, producing male hair growth, regression of the breasts, enlargement of the clitoris and deepening of the voice.

(f) SEMINOMA (dysgerminoma)

This is a rare tumour which occurs at 10-30 years. It is composed of groups of large deeply-staining cells separated by fibrous septa, and is identical in appearance with a seminoma of the testis. It can be malignant.

(g) CARCINOMA

Carcinoma of the ovary can be primary or secondary.
(i) *Primary carcinomas* form solid masses of various kinds of cancer cells. They may be malignant from the start or develop in a previously benign tumour.
(ii) *Secondary tumours* can be due to spread from a cancer of the uterus along lymph vessels or to spread by the blood from a cancer of the breast, stomach or colon.

(h) SARCOMA

Sarcomatous changes can develop in a fibroma or teratoma.

THE BREAST

Congenital Abnormalities

Accessory nipples and *accessory breasts* can occur along the 'milk line' from the axilla to the groin. The same diseases can develop in them as in a normal breast.

Trauma

Traumatic fat necrosis occurs when a breast is struck so hard that fat globules are released from fat cells into the surrounding tissue. An inflammatory and giant, multinucleated cell reaction is produced, which can go on to fibrosis, forming a mass so hard that it is often mistaken for a carcinoma.

Hypertrophy

Massive hypertrophy of the breast can develop about the age of 16 years as the result of a large overgrowth of connective tissue and a lesser overgrowth of gland tissue. The cause is unknown. Occasionally the hypertrophy is associated with a pituitary, adrenal or ovarian tumour.

Acute Mastitis

Acute mastitis is usually due to a staphylococcal or streptococcal infection of a lactating breast through a cracked nipple. The usual signs of inflammation are present. A localized abscess may develop in a breast lobule.

Less common causes of acute mastitis are virus infections, injury and hormonal imbalance (sometimes associated with infection) in the newly-born and at puberty.

Chronic Mastitis

In spite of its name this condition is not an inflammation, except rarely as a sequel of acute mastitis. It is thought to be due to some hormonal imbalance. There is an abnormal proliferation of glandular tissue or of connective tissue in the breast. It can occur at any age between puberty and the menopause; may be localized or diffuse, unilateral or bilateral, progressive or static. Masses of tough rubber-hard tissue appear. Multiple small cysts or a solitary large cyst can appear; the fluid in the cyst is clear, unless an infection occurs or there is a haemorrhage into the cyst. In one form of the disease papillae develop within the cyst. Occasionally a carcinoma develops, after many years, from a papilla; but otherwise chronic mastitis is not a precancerous condition. There is sometimes an excess of lymphocytes within the tissue, a reaction which originally gave the impression that the condition was due to an infection.

Benign Neoplasms of the Breast

Fibroadenoma of the breast can occur at any age after puberty and is most common at 20-30 years. It is usually single. There is an overgrowth of fibrous tissue surrounding an overgrowth of glandular tissue, with the formation of a rounded, rubbery-hard tumour enclosed within a fibrous capsule.

A *giant fibroadenoma* is a very large benign tumour occurring in middle or old age. Degenerative patches and cysts can form within it.

A *papilloma* can develop as a single tumour within one of the main ducts near the nipple. It is most common at the age of 20-30 years. It is likely to bleed. After many years of existence a papilloma can become malignant, but most remain benign.

An *adenoma of the nipple* can develop in one of the main ducts within the nipple.

Carcinoma of the Breast

Carcinoma of the breast is one of the commonest malignant diseases of women. Carcinoma of the male breast is rare.

It can occur at any age, but is rare below the age of 30 years. The cause is usually unknown. It can develop from a papilloma. It can occur in any part of the breast.

It develops from the epithelial cells of the alveoli or ducts. Various types are described according to their microscopic appearance, clinical features and degree of malignancy. Carcinoma of the breast occurring during pregnancy or lactation can be very malignant. Three degrees of malignancy – varying from Grade I (the least malignant) to Grade III (the most malignant) are described according to:
(a) the size and shape of the cells,
(b) whether the cells are arranged in tubules or not,
(c) whether the cells show abnormal mitotic activity.

The three most common types are:
1. *Adenocarcinoma* (Grade I malignancy): columnar cells are arranged in tubules surrounded by fibrous tissue.
2. *Spheroidal cell carcinoma* (Grade II malignancy): the cells are round and grouped in clumps or cords surrounded by fibrous tissue.
3. *Anaplastic carcinoma* (Grade III malignangy): the cells are multi-sided and undifferentiated and grow in solid masses.
Less common types are:
colloid carcinoma: the cells produce much mucus.
squamous cell carcinoma: the tumour arises in squamous tissue, usually the wall of a cyst.
intraduct carcinoma: arises from a duct; the adjacent breast tissue may not be invaded.
papillary carcinoma: arises from a papilla within a cyst.

Paget's disease of the nipple is an eczematous condition of the nipple secondary to an underlying carcinoma of the breast. Paget's cells, clear cells with a deeply staining nucleus, are found in this condition in the epidermis of the nipple.

Complications

Invasion of the skin by malignant cells.
Spread via the lymph vessels to axillary, supraclavicular and internal mammary glands.
Spread via the blood to lungs, liver, brain, bone, etc.
Transcoelomic spread: spread across the peritoneum or pleura.

Chapter 24   Pregnancy: Infertility

Ectopic Pregnancy

An *ectopic pregnancy* is a pregnancy which occurs outside the uterus. The commonest site is within the uterine (fallopian) tube, where the ovum is fertilized. The fertilized ovum cannot move along the tube if the tube is kinked or if an infection (the usual one is gonorrhoea) has damaged its inner layer and robbed the cells of their motility.

The fertilized ovum, stuck in the tube, burrows into the wall much as it should do into the endometrium of the uterus. The tube cannot cope:
(a) bleeding occurs from relatively large blood vessels,
(b) the ovum dies,
(c) the tube ruptures into the peritoneal cavity or between the two layers of the broad ligament, or
(d) the dead ovum is extruded in a clot of blood through the fimbriated end of the tube into the peritoneal cavity.

Rarely the ovum is not killed in the process and the pregnancy can continue for a time if the ovum can attach itself to the peritoneal wall and draw its nourishment from it.

Hydramnios

Hydramnios is an excessive amount of liquor amnii. It is difficult to define what is excessive for the normal amount can vary from 300 ml to 1 500 ml. The condition can be acute or chronic.

The cause is unknown. It is likely to be associated with:
(a) *maternal conditions*; toxaemia of pregnancy, diabetes mellitus (in which both fetus and placenta can be abnormally large), heart disease, kidney disease;
(b) *fetal conditions*: uniovular twins, fetal abnormalities (spina bifida, anencephaly, etc.).

Oligohydramnios

Oligohydramnios is a deficiency of liquor amnii. It is rare. It is sometimes associated with fetal renal abnormalities, especially a failure of development of the kidneys.

Carneous Mole

A *carneous mole* is a mass of tissue composed of a dead embryo, shrunken membranes, and clots of blood. The word 'carneous' refers to the fleshy appearance of the clots. The condition occurs when an embryo dies but is not aborted. The blood is the result of bleeding into the space between the chorion and the decidua.

Hydatidiform Mole

A *hydatidiform mole* is a mass of vesicles occupying the uterine cavity. It is essentially a neoplasm of the chorion. It begins early in pregnancy with the death of the embryo and the conversion of the chorionic villi into vesicles, which can grow up to 3 cm in diameter. It is rare and the cause is unknown. It secretes a large amount of chorionic gonadotrophic hormone.

Complications

multiple ovarian cysts
erosion of the uterine wall
malignant changes: a chorion-epithelioma develops in about 10 per cent of cases
sepsis
toxaemia of pregnancy; eclampsia

> Excretion of chorionic gonadotrophin in urine is high. Test may be positive in dilutions of urine 1/100 or higher.

Toxaemia of Pregnancy

Toxaemia of pregnancy is a term used to describe certain pathological conditions which occur in pregnancy. The cause is unknown. There are two degrees of severity:
1. pre-eclamptic toxaemia, which may progress to
2. eclampsia.

1. PRE-ECLAMPTIC TOXAEMIA

characterized by:
hypertension,
albuminuria,
oedema.
It develops in 3-10 per cent of pregnancies. When a woman has had it, the likelihood is increased in any subsequent pregnancies she may have. The chances are increased if the woman has:

first pregnancy	diabetes mellitus
essential hypertension	chronic pyelonephritis
obesity	multiple pregnancy
hydatidiform mole.	

The condition varies from mild to severe, and a fulminating pre-eclamptic toxaemia can occur. The fetus may die.

2. ECLAMPSIA

A more severe form of toxaemia. When there is good antenatal care it occurs in about 1 in 1 000 pregnancies. It is characterized by:
hypertension; a rapid rise in BP may have occurred
albuminuria
severe oedema
fits
coma.

It can occur during pregnancy, during labour and in the first few days of the puerperium. The maternal mortality is about 5 per cent. About 30 per cent of the babies are stillborn or die shortly after birth.

Complications

pulmonary congestion	cerebral haemorrhage
heart failure	renal failure, oliguria, anuria
liver necrosis	recurrent fits.

> ## INFERTILITY
>
> Infertility is a failure of a woman or man to have a child. It can be due to a number of conditions.
>
> **Tests for infertility**
>
> MALE
>
> *1. Seminal analysis*
>
> A specimen of semen is examined within 3 hours of production for:
> (a) volume of ejaculate: normal about 2-5 ml.
> (b) sperm density: probably about 60 million per ml are necessary for normal fertility.
> (c) proportion of abnormal sperm: should not exceed 25 per cent.
> (d) spermal activity: 75 per cent of sperm should be motile.
>
> *2. Sex chromatin*
>
> A buccal smear is examined for the presence of Barr bodies in the cells. The presence of Barr bodies in a male without sperm confirms the diagnosis of Klinefelter's syndrome.

3. Testicular biopsy

This is performed only when there is a total absence of sperm in order to find out if there are any pre-sperm cells in the testis. If there are, there must be a blockage of the vas deferens on both sides.

4. Hormonal studies

These can be of:
urinary 17-oxosteroids, testosterone, gonadotrophins;

MALE AND FEMALE

1. Post-coital test

A specimen of cervical mucus is examined within 18 hours of coitus. Normally the mucus is copious, clear and watery, can be drawn out into a long thread and contains many active sperm.

2. Invasion test

A drop of cervical mucus and a drop of semen are placed side by side so that they make contact.
Microscopic examination is made to see if the sperm invade the mucus.

FEMALE

1. Temperature

The woman takes her temperature daily before getting up in the morning. After ovulation the temperature is about 0.5°C higher. If there is no rise, ovulation may not be taking place.

2. Vaginal smears

Smears are taken daily by the woman. When ovulation has occurred, there should be: (a) an increase of the number of epithelial cells with pyknotic (deeply staining) nuclei, followed by (b) a fall in the number of these cells and a sudden increase in the number of leucocytes in the smear.

The test is invalidated by coitus and the presence of inflammation.

3. Examination of cervical mucus

At ovulation the mucus is copious, watery and clear, and when dried on a slide leaves fern-like crystals of sodium chloride. After ovulation it should be tacky, contain cells, and not crystallize on drying. An absence of these changes suggests that ovulation is not occurring.

5. Tests of corpus luteum function

Tests are carried out to see if progesterone is being produced by a corpus luteum.

6. Estimation of 17-oxosteroids

This is carried out to see if there is any adrenal hyperplasia.

7. Buccal smear

Cells obtained by a buccal smear are examined for the presence or absence of Barr bodies. Absence of Barr bodies in an amenorrheic woman would indicate either gonadal dysgenesis or male pseudohermaphroditism.

Chapter 25 Inherited Diseases

A human being arises by the union of ovum and spermatozoon.

The nucleus of the human cell contains 46 chromosomes. Of these:
44 are autosomes or non-sex chromosomes
2 are sex chromosomes.

The 44 autosomes are formed of 22 pairs, one of each pair being derived from the ovum and one from the spermatozoon. They are identical in male and female. In ordinary cell division into two, each chromosome divides into two and one of them goes into each new cell. Each resultant cell has the same number of chromosomes as the parent cell.

The sex chromosomes are different in the male and the female. The *male* has:
1 X chromosome
1 Y chromosome (a much smaller chromosome than the X)
The *female* has:
2 X chromosomes (identical with the male X chromosome).

The *genes* are the factors on the chromosomes which decide inheritance. Each chromosome has about 100,000 genes, each of them being responsible for one enzyme reaction and all therefore controlling all the chemical reactions in the body.

A *genotype* is a person's genetic consitution, i.e. the total of the genes he has inherited.

A *mutation* is an alteration in a gene, which will affect its actions. A mutation can arise as a result of known factors (e.g. exposure to radiation) or unknown factors, and when it has arisen it is handed down with each chromosomal division to other cells.

Chromosomes

Chromosomes are examined in dividing cells by special laboratory techniques. The usual cells examined are:
leucocytes from the blood
cells from bone-marrow
cells from the skin.
Leucocytes are the cells most commonly examined as they are the easiest to grow, but the other cells may be examined in special cases.

Barr bodies [See p. 174.]

Drum sticks

Drum sticks are small projections from the nucleus of leucocytes. They are formed of two X chromosomes and are therefore present only in people who are genetically female.

INHERITANCE OF DISEASE

Inheritance of disease may be by:
dominant inheritance
recessive inheritance
sex-linked (X-linked) inheritance.

Dominant inheritance

In *dominant inheritance* it is necessary for only one parent to carry the abnormal gene. If a person, of either sex, who carries the gene marries a person who does not, half the children will carry the abnormal gene and transmit it, in their turn, to half their children.

In addition to any inherited dominant gene, other dominant genes can arise at any time, by mutation, and an abnormal child will then be born to normal parents. When this happens, the risk of the parents' subsequent children being similarly affected is slight.

Dominant conditions

Achondroplasia
Dystrophia myotonica
Huntington's chorea
Marfan's syndrome: abnormally tall people with long limbs, 'spider' fingers, displacement of the lens of the eye, degenerative changes in the walls of the large blood vessels
Multiple neurofibromatosis (von Recklinghausen's disease): multiple fibrous tumours of the skin, pigmented macules, fibrous nodules on nerves
Multiple polyposis of the colon
Osteogenesis imperfecta
Tuberous sclerosis (epiloia): multiple sebaceous tumours on face and neck; nodular masses in the brain, severe mental retardation.

Recessive Inheritance

In *recessive inheritance* the affected person must have received the abnormal gene from both parents. In unrelated marriages the risk is small, but in cousin marriages it is greatly increased. When both parents have the abnormal gene, the proportion of affected children to unaffected children is 1 to 3.

There is much variation in the incidence of many recessive conditions in different races and various parts of the world, e.g. fibrocystic disease of the pancreas is rare outside Europe, thalassaemia is most common in Britain in the children of immigrants from West Africa and the West Indies, and amaurotic family idiocy occurs mainly in Jews descended from Jews who formerly lived in Lithuania and Poland.

Recessive conditions

Amaurotic family idiocy (Tay-Sachs disease): a condition characterized by a progressive degeneration of nerve cells and the appearance of a lipid in them; blindness and severe mental degeneration are produced.
Fibrocystic disease of the pancreas
Galactosaemia: a condition produced by the absence of an enzyme necessary for the conversion of galactose into glucose; galactose builds up in the tissues: a large liver, cataracts in the lens of the eye, and mental retardation occur.
Phenylketonuria
Sickle cell anaemia
Thalassaemia.

Sex-Linked (X-Linked) Inheritance

Sex-linked inheritance is by a gene carried on a sex chromosome. The chromosome has always been found to be an X chromosome and never a Y chromosome. The gene is usually a recessive one.

Sex-linked conditions

Christmas disease
Duchenne type hypertrophic muscular dystrophy
Haemophilia.

Chromosomal Abnormalities

Chromosomal abnormalities can be:
(a) an abnormal number of chromosomes
(b) absence of part of a chromosome.
Chromosomal abnormalities are found in about 25 per cent of fetuses aborted in the first three months of fetal life and in about 1 per cent of all live births.

Conditions with abnormal chromosomes

Klinefelter's syndrome: affected males have 2 or more X chromosomes as well as one Y chromosome. The condition occurs in 1 in 1,000 male live births. Features are underdeveloped testes, infertility, lack of facial, axillary and pubic hair, mental disturbance or mental retardation.

Mongolism (Down's syndrome). Affected people have an extra no. 22 chromosome (3 instead of the normal 2). The condition occurs in 1 in 600 live births; the older a mother the more likely is she to have a mongol child. In *translocation* the extra chromosome is attached to another chromosome. In *mosaicism* not all cells have the extra chromosome; some have the right number. Affected people have mental retardation (often of a severe degree) and a typical physical appearance: short stature, round head, slanting eyes, abnormalities of fingers and toes, etc.

Turner's syndrome. Affected women have 1 X chromosome instead of 2. It occurs in 1 in 4,000 female live births. Affected women have underdeveloped ovaries and are sterile, and have a short stature, a webbed neck and other abnormalities.

XYY syndrome. Males with an extra Y chromosome are likely to be tall. An association of tallness with aggressive behaviour was proposed but has not been confirmed.

Chapter 26 Eye

Infections

Blepharitis

A *blepharitis* is an infection of the glands opening into the roots of the eyelashes along the edge of the eyelids. Infecting organisms can be staphylococci or streptococci. In severe cases the infection is followed by fibrosis and distortion of the lid-edge.

Squamous blepharitis is a seborrhoea involving the eye lashes and associated with seborrhoea of the scalp.

Dacryocystitis

A *dacryocystitis* is an inflammation of the lacrimal sac at the inner lower corner of the eyelid. The inflammation can be acute or chronic.

In *acute dacryocystitis* the usually infecting organism is the *pneumococcus*. The sac becomes inflamed and swollen, and the lacrimal sac (through which tears pass into the inside of the nose) becomes blocked. An abscess can form in the sac, and can form a fistula by bursting through the skin in front of it.

A *chronic dacryocystitis* can be secondary to an acute dacryocystitis or develop as a chronic inflammation from the start, especially in old women.

Orbital cellulitis

An *orbital cellulitis* is an inflammation of the soft tissues of the orbit. It is usually secondary to a sinusitis of an adjoining nasal sinus. The soft tissues become swollen, the eye is pushed forward, and an abscess may form.

A *cavernous sinus thrombosis* is a septic clotting of blood within a cavernous sinus following a spread of infection backwards from an orbital cellulitis or an infection of the face through small veins which communicate between the outside and the inside of the skull.

Conjunctivitis

Conjunctivitis is an inflammation of the conjunctiva and can be:
acute conjunctivitis
ophthalmia (purulent conjunctivitis)
angular conjunctivitis
allergic conjunctivitis
trachoma

Acute conjunctivitis is due to infection by *staph. aureus*, *pneumococcus*, viruses, etc. The conjunctiva becomes red with prominent dilated vessels and a catarrhal, mucopurulent or purulent discharge.

Ophthalmia neonatorum is a severe purulent conjunctivitis due to a gonococcal infection of the conjunctiva of the neonate due to infection during childbirth when the mother's birth canal is actively infected.

Angular conjunctivitis is a mild inflammation in the angles of the eye due to infection by the Morax-Axenfeld bacillus.

Allergic conjunctivitis is due to a hyper-sensitivity of the conjunctiva to:
pollens
drugs (penicillin, atropine, etc.)
cosmetics applied to the eyelids or lashes.

Trachoma is a severe chronic viral infection, particularly common in the Near East. Chronic inflammatory changes take place and small follicles of lymph tissue can form, especially on the inner surface of the tarsal plate. Scarring of the cornea can cause blindness.

Keratitis

Keratitis is inflammation of the cornea. It occurs as:
corneal ulcer
interstitial keratitis

CORNEAL ULCER

A corneal ulcer is due to an acute infection of the cornea and degeneration of its surface.
(a) *Marginal ulcers* are small, superficial, often multiple ulcers, occurring at the edge of the cornea. *Staph. aureus* is the common infecting organism. The ulcers heal without forming scars.
(b) A *central ulcer* is single, centrally placed in the cornea, and likely to follow an abrasion or other injury. *Pneumococcus* is the common infecting organism.

Complications of central ulcer

Scarring: causing blindness
Perforation of the cornea: the ulcer erodes through the entire thickness of the cornea; the iris moves forwards to plug the hole and may remain attached to it by synechiae (adhesions).
Iritis: inflammation of the iris.

INTERSTITIAL KERATITIS

Interstitial keratitis is a chronic inflammatory lesion of he cornea due to syphilis (congenital or acquired), tuberculosis, etc. The normally avascular cornea becomes invaded by blood vessels from the sclera and looks cloudy.

Scleritis

Scleritis is inflammation of the sclera. The commonest kind is a collagen degeneration. Small hard injected patches appear. It may be associated with iritis.

Acute uveitis (iritis, irido-cyclitis, choroiditis)

The uveal tract is a continuum of vascular tissue composed of the iris, the ciliary body and the choroid coat. It is all likely to be involved in an inflammatory process, but any one part of it may be more affected than the others.
  Uveitis is an inflammation of the whole tract.
  Iritis is an inflammation mainly of the iris.
  Irido-cyclitis is an inflammation mainly of the iris and ciliary body.
  Choroiditis is an inflammation mainly of the choroid coat.

Causes

(a) *Endogenous*. In many cases no cause can be found. It is attributed to auto-immune disease, metabolic abnormalities, viral infection, infection from an infected nasal sinus, gonorrhoea, syphilis, tuberculosis, etc.
(b) *Exogenous*. The inflammation follows a perforating wound of the orbit or a corneal ulcer.

Features

The blood vessels of the tract become engorged and the tract oedematous. An inflammatory exudate is found in the anterior chamber of the eye. Pus can be present there, and a *hypopyon* may be visible as a pool of pus in the anterior chamber or *keratitic precipitates* (KP) be visible as small deposits of pus on the back of the cornea.

Complications

Posterior synechiae; adhesions between the iris and the anterior surface of the lens. Sometimes the whole margin of the iris becomes attached to the lens; the aqueous fluid cannot escape, as it should, into the canal of Schlemm.
Glaucoma: due to the accumulation of aqueous fluid which cannot escape.
Cataract: due to an impairment of the nutrition of the lens.
  Sympathetic ophthalmia is a uveitis which follows a perforating wound of the orbit (including operations for cataract). The uveitis affects first the affected eye and then the uvea of

the other eye. This involvement of the other eye is thought to be the result of an auto-immune reaction.

Glaucoma

Glaucoma is an abnormal increase in intra-ocular pressure; the upper limit of normal pressure is taken to be 20 mmHg.

Glaucoma can be:
(a) *primary*: no cause can be found.
(b) *secondary*: secondary to iritis or an intra-ocular tumour.

Primary acute glaucoma is characterized by bouts of raised intra-ocular pressure. It is usually precipitated by the iris cutting off the rim of the anterior chamber of the eye so that the aqueous fluid cannot escape into the canal of Schlemm. The rise in pressure produces oedema of the cornea (which looks steamy), congestion of the iris, dilatation of the pupil, severe pain in the eye, vomiting and prostration.

Chronic glaucoma occurs in about 1 per cent of people in Britain over the age of 40 and is responsible for more than 13 per cent of cases of blindness there. It is the result of a gradual rise of intra-ocular pressure over many months. The eye fails to adapt to the increase; and pressure on the optic nerve head in the retina and on the fibres of the optic nerve produces a degeneration of the fibres, a reduction in the visual field, and, if untreated, blindness.

Degenerations

Cataract

A *cataract* is an opacity in the normally transparent lens. It can be:
(a) *congenital*: the result of a virus infection (especially German measles) of the mother during pregnancy, or of a metabolic abnormality.
(b) *acquired*: the result of:
senile degeneration of the lens
injury to the lens
diabetes mellitus
iritis
irradiation, etc.

A congenital cataract can vary from a small spot to a total opacity of the lens. An acquired cataract begins as a small spot which over years gradually enlarges to involve the whole lens.

Degeneration of the retina and choroid coat

Degeneration of the retina and choroid coat can take the form of:
(a) *Macular degeneration*: the macule (the spot of greatest visual acuity) becomes swollen with exudate and spotted with haemorrhages and pigment, and shows degeneration in:
amaurotic family idiocy
old age.
(b) *Retinitis pigmentosa*: tiny patches of pigment in shape resembling bone corpuscles appear in the periphery of the retina, and the optic disc degenerates. The condition is inherited, and dominant, recessive and sex-linked (X-linked) forms of inheritance occur.
(c) *Degeneration of the choroid coat*: patches of white degenerated tissue can develop after an attack of choroiditis.
(d) *Choroid-retinal atrophy*: atrophy of the macula and of the retina around the optic disc can be due to high myopia (progressive myopia).
(e) *Retrolental fibroplasia*: vessels in the retina proliferate and invade the vitreous humour, and behind the lens the vitreous humour becomes condensed. This condition was due to exposing premature babies to an oxygen concentration of more than 40 per cent.
(f) *Retinopathy*: degeneration of the retina can be due to:
diabetes mellitus,
hypertension.
Exudates and haemorrhages appear in the **retina and cells and fibres degenerate.**
(g) *Retinal detachment*: the retina becomes detached from the choroid coat and, having lost its blood supply, dies. It occurs in:
trauma to the orbit,

high myopia if the retina fails to stretch as much as the sclera and becomes stripped off the choroid coat.

Neoplasms of the Eye

Xanthelasmata are yellow intradermal plaques containing cholesterol which develop in the eyelids, usually at the medial end and often symmetrically in both eyelids. They occur in people with a high blood cholesterol (normal: 3.6-7.8 mmol/l).

Papillomata are benign neoplasm which usually grow on the lid-margin at the line of union of skin and conjunctiva.

Rodent ulcers and *carcinoma of the skin* commonly grow on the eyelids.

Malignant melanoma of the choroid coat is a black malignant neoplasm which appears in middle life in the choroid coat and grows to fill the whole orbit. Secondary growths appear in the liver.

Retinoblastoma is a malignant neoplasm which arises in the retina in infancy and grows to fill the whole orbit. Secondary growths appear in the brain.

Chapter 27   The Ear

The External Ear

Congenital deformities

Accessory auricles or a small blind pit in front of the tragus may be present.

Otitis externa

This is an inflammation of the skin lining the external auditory meatus. It is often not due to one micro-organism but to a mixture of several, especially staphylococci, *P. vulgaris* and *E. coli*. *Candida albicans*, a fungus, can be the infecting organism.

> **Swab**
>
> Microbiological examination is carried out on fluid removed on an aural swab.

Furunculosis

This is a small boil due to a staphylococcal infection of the hair follicles in the outer part of the meatus.

Exostoses

Exostoses are small bony outgrowths from the inner part of the external auditory meatus. They form smooth hard rounded slowly-growing masses covered with the skin of the meatus.

Epithelioma

An epithelioma can occur as an ulcerating mass in the external auditory meatus.

Complication

Spread along lymph vessels into upper cervical lymph nodes. Spread into the middle ear, facial nerve, temporo-mandibular joint.

The Middle Ear

Acute and chronic otitis media

Acute otitis media is an acute inflammation of the middle ear. It is often bilateral. The infecting organism is usually a streptococcus, a staphylococcus or the *pneumococcus*.

It occurs as a complication of:
the common cold   acute tonsillitis
influenza   whooping cough
measles   sinusitis

It can be precipitated by:
diving   trauma to the tympanic
tonsillectomy   membrane
     fracture of the temporal bone
sudden descent in an unpressurised aircraft.

It begins as an inflammation of the mucous membrane of the middle ear and associated structures – the tympano-pharyngeal (eustachian) tube, the mastoid antrum and the mastoid air-cells. The tube is likely to become blocked by oedema of its mucous membrane, and when this happens pressure builds up in the middle ear, causing bulging and then rupture of the tympanic membrane.

A *chronic otitis media* can occur if an acute otitis media is not treated early or adequately, if adenoids or a chronic nasal infection are present, or if the patient is in poor health.

A chronic otitis media can be:
(a) *mucosal*: the mucous membrane only is chronically inflamed. This is likely when adenoids are present or there is a chronic nasal or sinus infection.
(b) *bony*: the inflammation spreads from the mucous membrane to involve the ossicles and the bony walls of the middle ear, mastoid antrum and mastoid air cells. The tympanic membrane may be completely destroyed.

Complications

Acute mastoiditis: the inflammation spreads backwards into the mastoid antrum and air cells; the bone becomes necrotic and an abscess can form.
Meningitis: a meningitis can occur if the inflammation extends through the thin bone of the roof of the middle ear into the cranial cavity.
Extradural abscess: an abscess forms between the skull and the dura mater.
Petrositis: inflammation of the petrous part of the temporal bone. The sixth (abducens) cranial nerve can be involved as it passes over the petrous bone.
Labyrinthitis: inflammation of the labyrinth (inner ear) can be due to direct spread or by a blood-borne infection from an acute otitis media.
Lateral sinus thrombosis: inflammation passes from the mastoid cells into the lateral venous sinus within the skull. Thromboses occur in the sinus. The thrombus can become infected; and emboli, broken off from it, are distributed in the blood to other parts of the body where they can cause abscesses.
Brain abscess: inflammation can spread via small blood vessels or through the bone and meninges to form abscesses in the temporal lobe of the cerebrum or in the cerebellum, the two adjacent parts of the brain.
Subdural abscess: multiple abscesses can form in the subdural space, between dura mater and brain.
Granulations: outgrowths of granulation tissue in the middle ear.

Aural polyps: pedunculated granulations; they can grow down the external auditory meatus.
Cholesteatoma: a pearly-white smelly accumulation of epithelial debris within the middle ear.
Fistula: an opening between the middle and internal ear.

Swab

Swab of the discharge from the ear is examined microscopically for organisms. Cultures are made.

Secretory otitis media (catarrhal otitis media, glue ear)

Secretory otitis media is a condition in which fluid is present in the middle ear. If it is not treated, the ossicles become stuck to one another by adhesions and the tympanic membrane is pulled in.

It is caused by:
(a) blocking of the audito-pharyngeal (eustachian) tube due to adenoids or chronic nasal infection,
(b) sudden descent in an aircraft,
(c) repeated and inadequate treatment of acute otitis media by antibiotics.

Otosclerosis

Otosclerosis is the formation of new bone around the foot of the stapes. The stapes becomes fixed and cannot transmit vibrations into the inner ear. The cause is unknown. It begins at 15-30 years of age. Women are affected about twice as often as men. There is frequently a family history of deafness.

Inner Ear

Ménière's disease is characterized by deafness, tinnitus and attacks of vertigo, nausea and vomiting. The cause is unknown. Increased pressure within the inner ear causes a distension of the membranous labyrinth, and the organ of Corti shows degenerative changes.

Index

Abortus fever 20
ABo system of blood groups 104
abscess 46 *see also* individual organs
achalasia of oesophagus 113–14
acholuric jaundice 98–9
achondroplasia 212
acidaemia, metabolic 62
   respiratory 61–2
acid-base balance 60–2
acid-fast bacilli 5
acne vulgaris 147–8
acoustic neuroma 69
acromegaly 170
ACTH assessment 168
   excess of 170
   response to stimulation by 177–8
actinomyces 16
actinomycosis 16
acyanotic Fallot's tetralogy 71
Addison's disease 174–5
adenocarcinoma 67
   mucous, of ovary 205
   of oesophagus 114
adenoids 81
adenoma 66
   bronchial 83–4
adenoviruses 28–9
adrenal cortex 172–5
   carcinoma of 174
   crisis 174
   glands 172–8
   hyperplasia, congenital 173–4
   insufficiency 174–5
   medulla 175–6
adreno-cortical function, tests of 176–8
adrenogenital syndromes 173–5
aerobic organisms 8
African trypanosomiasis 45
agar 5
   blood 5
   chocolate 5
   nutrient 5
agglutination, of bacteria 6
agranulocytosis 111
aldosteronism, primary 173

alimentary tract 112–25
alkalaemia, metabolic 62
   respiratory 62
allergy 50–2
Alzheimer's disease 163
amaurotic family idiocy 212
amoebiasis 41
amoebic abscess 41, 128
   hepatitis 41
anaemia, aplastic 108
   chronic hypochromic 93–4
   extrinsic haemolytic 97–8
   haemolytic 96–100
   intrinsic haemolytic 97
   iron-deficiency 93
   megaloblastic 94–6
   pernicious 94, 95–6
      congenital 94
   sickle cell 97–8, 212
anaerobic organisms 8
anaphylactic shock 50
Ancylostoma duodenale 39
anencephaly 157
aneurysm 75, 77, 78
   atheromatous 78
   berry 78, 159
   dissecting, of aorta 78
   fusiform 78
   mycotic 78
   saccular 78
   syphilitic, of aorta 75, 78
angeiosarcoma 68, 76
angina, Vincent's 23, 112
angioma, of brain 159
angular cheilitis 146
animal inoculations 6–7
ankylosing spondylitis 186–7
Anopheles mosquito 43–4
anoxia 64
anthrax, cutaneous 12
   pulmonary 12
antibody 49
antigen 49
   Australia (HbAg) 33–4
   foreign 53
   hepatitis B surface 33–4
   late maturation 52–3
   'self' 52, 53

anus, carcinoma of 123–4
aorta, aneurysm of 78
   coarctation of 73
   over-riding, in Fallot's tetralogy 71
aortic arch, right 72
aortitis, syphilitic 75
apthous stomatitis 112
aplastic anaemia 108
appendicitis, acute 121
appendix, carcinoid neoplasm of 123
Arboviruses 31–2
arrhenoblastoma 206
arteritis, giant cell 78–9
   temporal 78–9
arthritis, acute 186
   osteo- 188
   rheumatoid 187–8
asbestosis 89
Ascaris lumbricoides 37
Aschoff nodes 53, 55, 73
ascites 125
   chylous 125
   in cirrhosis of liver 131
ascorbic acid, deficiency of 154–5
   measurement of 155
   saturation test 155
asthma 51
astrocytoma 164
atelectasis of lung 85
atheroma 77–8
   of cerebral arteries 78, 158
atheromatous plaque 77
athlete's foot 146
atmospheric pollution, cause of chronic bronchitis 83
   of carcinoma of bronchus 84
atopy 148
atresia, pulmonary 71
atrial septal defect 72
atrophy 65
   choroid-retinal 216
aural polyp 219
auricle, accessory 218
Australia antigen (HbAg) 33–4
auto-immune diseases 52–3

220

Index 221

Bacilli, acid fast 5
  Gram negative 17–21
  Gram positive 12–16
  intestinal 17
Bacillus anthracis 12
  coli 17
  Friedländer's 18
  fusiformis fusiformis 23
  tuberculosis 15
bacteraemia 47
bacteraemic shock 17
bacteria, culture 5
  growth 8
  identification 3–4
  strain 3–4
  structure 8
bacterial endocarditis, acute 74
  subacute 74
balanitis 198
Bancroftian filiarisis 40
Barr body 174, 209
bartholinitis 200
  in trichomoniasis 36
basal cell carcinoma of skin 148
beri-beri 154
berry aneurysm 78, 159
bile pigments 128
bilharziasis 40–1
biliary calculus 133–4
  tract, carcinoma of 135
bilirubin, serum 131–2
biochemical tests, in bacterial identification 6
blackwater fever 44
bladder, carcinoma of 144
  diverticulum of 143–4
  papilloma of 144
bleeding, excessive 100
  time 100
blepharitis 314
  squamous 214
blood 93–111
  coagulation of 102–3
  defects of 103–4
  compatibility tests 105
  groups 104–5
  lipids 77
  sugar, tests for 151
  transfusion 104, 105–6
  urea 136
blue baby 71
body, asbestos 89
  Barr 174, 209
  louse 35
bone 189–93
  giant cell neoplasm of 193
  neoplasms of 192–3

tuberculosis of 188–9
Bordetella pertussis 20
Bornholm disease 184
Borrelia vincenti 23
botulism 14
brain, abscess of 162, 219
  degenerations of 163
  infections of 160–2
  injuries of 159–60
  neoplasms of 163–5
  syphilis of 162
  vascular diseases of 158–9
breast, accessory 206
  carcinoma of 207
  congenital abnormalities of 206
  fibroadenoma of 69, 207
  hypertrophy of 206
  neoplasms of 69, 207
  traumatic fat necrosis 206
Brenner tumour 205
bromsulphthalein excretion 133
bronchiectasis 89
bronchitis, chronic 83
bronchopneumonia 86
bronchus, adenoma of 83
  carcinoma of 84–5
  carcinoid tumour of 83
  cylindroma of 84
brucella 20–1
Brucella abortus 20
  melitensis 21
  suis 21
buccal smear 210
Buerger's disease 79
Burkitt lymphoma 70

Calculus, biliary 133–4
  salivary 113
  urinary 140–2
cancellous exostosis 192
cancer *see* carcinoma
Candida albicans 24–5, 146, 201
capsid, of virus 26
carbohydrate fermentation tests 6
carcinoma 67
  squamous cell 67
  transitional cell 67
  undifferentiated 67
  see also individual organs
cardiac infarction 77–8
carneous mole 308
carriers of infection 1
caseation 15
Casoni skin test 38
cataract 216

cavernous naevus 145
  sinus thrombosis 214
cell, HeLa 7, 29
  labile 48
  permanent 48
  stable 48
cellulitis, orbital 214
cerebral aneurysm 159
  atheroma 158
  embolism 159
  haemorrhage 159
  malaria 44
  palsy 158
  thrombosis 158–9
  venous thrombosis 159
cerebrospinal fluid 156–7
cervical cytology 203–4
  erosion 202
  mucus, examination of 210
cervicitis 201–2
cervix of uterus, carcinoma of 203
  infections of 200–1, 201–2
Chagas' disease 45
chancre 22
chickenpox 27
Chickenpox virus 27–8
chilblains 146–7
chocolate cyst, of ovary 204
cholangitis, acute 135
cholecystitis 134
cholelithiasis 133
cholera 21
cholesteatoma 29
cholesterol, in bile 133
  gallstones 133
chondroma 192
chondrosarcoma 68, 193
chorea, Huntington's 163
choroid coat, degeneration of 216–17
  melanoma of 217
choroiditis 215–16
choroid-retinal atrophy 216
Christmas disease 103, 212
chromosomes 211
  abnormalities of 212–13
chylothorax 91
circulation, overloading by blood transfusion 106
circulatory system 71–80
cirrhosis of liver 130–1
citrate toxicity, in blood transfusion 106
Clostridium botulinum 14
  perfringens 13–14
  tetani 12–13
  Welchi 13–14

clot retraction test   100
cloudy swelling   63
coagulation of blood   102–3
   defects of   103–4
coarctation of aorta   73
cocco-bacillus   8
coccus   8
   Gram negative   11–12
   Gram positive   8–11
coeliac disease   122
cold abscess   189
coliforms   17–20
colitis, ulcerative   121–2
collagen diseases   54–5
colon, carcinoma of   123
   polyposis of   212
common bile duct, obstruction of   134
compatible blood, tests to ensure   105
complement fixation test   6
complex, hypothalamic-pituitary   167
   primary, in tuberculosis   87
   secondary, in tuberculosis   87
congenital deformities see individual organs
congestive heart failure   76
conjunctivitis, acute   214
   allergic   214
   angular   214
Conn's syndrome   173
contact dermatitis   52
contre-coup injury, of brain   160
Coombs test, direct   106–7
   indirect   105, 107
cornea, ulcer of   215
coronary thrombosis   77–8
Corynebacterium diphtheriae   14–15
Coxsackie viruses   29–30, 184
crab louse   35
craniopharyngioma   170
cretinism   179
crisis, adrenal   174
   diabetic   151
Crohn's disease   122
cross-matching of blood   105
cryophilic organisms   106
culture, bacterial   5–6
   tissue   7
Cushing's syndrome   172–3
cyst, chocolate, of ovary   204
   dermoid   205
   endometrial, of ovary   204
   follicular, of ovary   204
   of kidney   136
   luteal, of ovary   204

   of skin   145
cystadenoma, mucinous   205
   papilliferous   205
   serous   205
cystic endometritis, senile   203
cysticercosis   37
cystic glandular hyperplasia   203
   teratoma   205
cystitis   143
   interstitial   143
cytology, cervical   203–4
cytomegalic inclusion disease   28
Cytomegalovirus   28
cytopathic effect   7

Dacryocystitis   214
degeneration   63–5
   following exposure to radiation   65
   hyaline   63
   subacute combined, of spinal cord   95, 165
dementia, presenile   163
   senile   163
Demodex folliculorum   147
demyelinating diseases   162–3
demyelination   156
dermatitis   148–9
   contact   149
   exfoliative   147
   primary irritant   149
dermatomyositis   54
dermoid cyst   145, 205
dexamethasone suppression test   173
   response to   177–8
dextrocardia   72
diabetes insipidus   171–2
   mellitus   150–1
diphtheria   14
direct Coombs test   106–7
disease period   1
disseminated (multiple) sclerosis   162–3
diverticulitis   119
diverticulosis   119
diverticulum, Meckel's   118
DNA viruses   27
Down's syndrome   213
droplet infection   2
Duchenne's disease   185, 212
   Becker type   185
duodenal ulcer   114–15
dust diseases   84, 88–9
   in spread of infection   2–3
dysgerminoma   206
dysentery, bacillary   19

dystrophia myotonica   185, 212
dystrophy, facio-scapulo-humeral   185
   limb girdle   185
   muscle   185
   pseudohypertrophic   185

Ear, congenital deformities of   218
   diseases of   218–19
   glue   219
ecchondroma   192
Echinococcus granulosus   38
   multilocularis   38
Echoviruses   30
eclampsia   209
ectopic pregnancy   201
eczema   148–9
   atopic   148
egg, growth of viruses in   7
electrolyte balance, disturbances of   56–62
El Tor vibrio   21–2
embolism, cerebral   159
   fat   190
   paradoxical   72
embryoma of kidney   142–3
emphysema   89–90
empyema   91
   of gallbladder   134
encephalitis, subacute sclerosing   32
   viral   160
encephalomyelitis, acute disseminated   163
encephalopathy, in cirrhosis of liver   131
endocardial fibroelastosis   75
endocarditis, acute bacterial   74, 75
   infective   75
   subacute bacterial   74, 75
endocardium, rheumatic disease of   73
endogenous creatinine clearance   136
endometritis, senile cystic   203
endothelioma, malignant   192–3
endotoxin   4
Entamoeba histolytica   41
Enterobius vermicularis   36
enterococcus   10
ependymoma   164
epidemic myalgia   184
   typhus   23–4
epidermoid cyst   145
epididymitis   196
epididymo-orchitis   196
epiloia   212
epispadias   198

Index

epithelioma, of external auditory meatus 218
erosion, cervical 202
erythema migrans 113
erythrocyte sedimentation rate (ESR) 107–8 *see also* individual diseases
erythroderma 147
erythropoietin, failure of production of 94
Escherichia coli 17
Ewing's tumour 192–3
exfoliative dermatitis 147
exomphalos 118
exophthalmic goitre 178–9
exostosis, cancellous 192
  of external auditory meatus 218
exotoxin 4
extradural haemorrhage 160
exudate 46
  pleural 90
eye, degenerations of 216–17
  infections of 214–16
  neoplasms of 217

Facio-scapulo-humeral dystrophy 185
factor, blood 102–4
  Christmas 103
  VIII deficiency 103
  IX deficiency 103
  intrinsic, deficiency of 94–5
faeces, specimens of 125
Fallot's tetralogy 71
familial polyposis coli 123
farmer's lung 51
fat embolism 190
  necrosis, traumatic of breast 206
fatty changes, in degeneration 63
  streaks, in atheroma 77
Felter's syndrome 187
female genital system 200–6
fibroadenoma of breast 69
fibrocystic disease of pancreas 126
fibroelastosis, endocardial 75
fibroid 66, 202
fibroma, of ovary 205
fibromyoma 66, 202
fibrosarcoma 68
fibrosis, pulmonary 85
  replacement 64–5
  retroperitoneal 124
filariasis 40
fish tapeworm 95
fleas 35

Fluorescent Treponemal Antibody test (FTA) 23
focus, Ghon 87
folate deficiency 96
folic acid 96
food poisoning 9, 13, 14, 18
forbidden clones 52, 53
fractures 189–90
free thyroxine test 182
Friedländer's bacillus 18
Fröhlich's syndrome 171
fungi 24–5
furunculosis of external ear 218

Galactosaemia 212
gallbladder, carcinoma of 134, 135
  empyema of 134
  infections of 134
  mucocele of 134
gallstones 133–4
ganglioneuroma 69, 176
gangrene 64
gas gangrene 13, 184
gastrectomy, as cause of anaemia 95
gastric atrophy, in anaemia 94
gastritis 114
gel diffusion technique 6
gene, mutation of 211
general paralysis of the insane (GPI) 162
genotype 211
geographic tongue 113
German measles 32, 71
German measles virus 32
Ghon focus 87
giant cell arteritis 78–9
  tumour of bone 192
Giardia lamblia 43
giardiasis 43
gigantism 170
glaucoma 216
glioma 68, 164
gliosis 156
glomerular filtration rate, estimation of 136
glomerular function, test for 136
glomerulo-nephritis, acute proliferative 137
  membranous 138
glucagon test 152
glucose-6-phosphate dehydrogenase deficiency 99
glucose tolerance test 151, 170, 171, 173
glue ear 219
gluten, sensitivity to 122

goitre 178–9
  colloid 178
  exophthalmic 178–9
  simple 178
  toxic nodular 179
Gonococcus 12
gonorrhoea, in men 198
  in women 200–1
gout 152–3
graft rejection 52
Gram negative bacteria 5, 17–20
  positive bacteria 5, 12–16
Gram stain 5
granulosa cell tumour, of ovary 205–6
Graves' disease 178–9
Grawitz tumour 143
gumma 22
Guthrie test 153

Haemadsorption 7
haemagglutination inhibition 7
haemangiectatic hypertrophy 145
haemangioma 76, 145
  stellate 76
haematocele 196
haematoma, chronic subdural 160
haemoglobinuria, paroxysmal nocturnal 99
haemolysis, of red blood cells 10, 96–7
haemolytic anaemias 96–100
  disease of newly born 51, 106–7
haemophilia 103, 212
Haemophilus influenzae 20
haemorrhage, cerebral 159
  extradural 160
  subarachnoid 160
haemorrhagic disorders, tests for 100–1
haemorrhoids 120
haemothorax 91
Ham's test 99
Hashimoto's disease 180
hay fever 51
head louse 35
healing processes 47–8
heart, congenital diseases of 71–2
  failure 76
  infections of 73–5
  neoplasms of 76
HeLa cells 7, 29
hepatic viruses 33–4
hepatitis B surface antigen (HbsAg) 33–4
  infective 33

Index

serum 33
viral 33
hepatization, of lung 86
hepatoma 131
hepatoblastoma 131
heredity 211–13
 in malignant disease 70
hernia 117–18
herpes, primary 28
 recurrent 28
 viruses 27–8
 zoster 27, 49
Herpes simplex virus 28
Herpes zoster virus 27–8
Hirschsprung's disease 118–19
histamine, in inflammation 46
honeycomb lung 88
hookworm infection 39–40
Huntington's chorea 163, 212
hyaline degeneration 63
 membrane disease of lungs 86
hydatidiform mole 208–9
hydatid infection 38
hydramnios 208
hydrocele 195–6
hydrocephalus 157–8
hydrochloric acid, tests for in gastric juice 116
hydronephrosis 142
hydrosalpinx 201
17-hydroxycorticosteroids, in urine 176
hymen, imperforate 200
hyperaldosteronism 173
hyperglycaemia 150
hyperinsulinism 151–2
hyperkalaemia 59, 60
hypernephroma 143
hyperparathyroidism 193
hyperpituitarism 170
hypersensitivity 50–2
hypertension 77, 79–80
 benign essential 79
 essential 79
 malignant 79–80
 portal 130–1
 pulmonary 80
hyperthyroidism 178–9
hypochromic anaemia, chronic 93–4
hypoglycaemia 150
hypokalaemia 59
hypoparathyroidism 194
hypopituitarism 170–1
hypopyon 215
hypospadias 198
hypothalamic-pituitary gland complex 167
tests of function 168–9
hypothyroidism 179–80

Idiopathic steatorrhoea 122
IgE antibody 51
IgM antibody 187
immunoglobulins 49
immunity 49–50
immunization of mother, to prevent haemolytic disease 107
imperforate hymen 200
implantation dermoid 145
incubation period 1
indirect Combs test 105, 107
infarction 64
 cardiac 77–8
 of limbs 64
infections 1–7
 by blood transfusion 106
 droplet 2
 transmission of 1–2
 routes of 2–3
infective hepatitis 33
infertility 209–10
inflammation 46–8
 granulomatous 47
influenza 31
Influenza virus 30–1, 49
inheritance of disease 211–13
 dominant 211–13
 recessive 212
 sex-linked 212
inoculation 3
 animal 6–7
insulinoma 151
insulin stress test 168
interstitial keratitis 215
intestinal bacilli 17–20
 obstruction 119–20
 polyps 123
 tract infection 3
intrinsic factor, lack of 94–5
intussusception 120
invasion test, for infertility 210
ionizing radiations, as cause of aplastic anaemia 108
 of cancer 70
 of carcinoma of bronchus 84
 of leukaemia 109
iridocyclitis 215–16
iritis 215–16
iron deficiency anaemia 93
ischaemia 64

Jaundice 128–9
acholuric 98–9
cellular 129
hepatic 129
obstructive 129
post-hepatic 129
prehepatic 128–9
tests for 131–3
joints 186–9
 tuberculosis of 188–9

Kahn test 23
kalazar 44
keratitic precipitates (KP) 215
keratitis, interstitial 215
kernicterus 106
ketonaemia 150
kidney, adenocarcinoma of 143
 carcinoma of 143
 congenital abnormalities of 136
 electrolytic mechanisms in 61
 embryoma of 142–3
 horse-shoe 136
 neoplasms of 142–3
 polycystic disease of 136
 tuberculosis of 140
 virus infection of 140
Klebsiella 18
 pneumoniae 18
Kleihauer test 107
Klinefelter's syndrome 212–13
Krukenberg tumour 116
Kveim test 88

Labile cells 48
labyrinthitis 219
Lancefield grouping of streptococci 11
Lange gold curve 157
large intestine, neoplasms of 123
laryngitis 82
larynx, carcinoma of 82
 oedema of 82
 tuberculosis of 82
lateral sinus thrombosis 219
left ventricular failure 76
leiomyoma 66
leiomyosarcoma 68
Leishmania donovani 44
 tropica 44
leishmaniasis 44
leprosy 16
Leptospira icterohaemorrhagiae 23
leukaemia 109–11
 acute 110
 chronic 110–11

Index

lymphatic, chronic 111
lymphoblastic, acute 110
myeloblastic, acute 110
myeloid, chronic 110–11
leukoplakia 112, 148
lice 35
lichen planus 147
limb-girdle muscular dystrophy 185
lip, carcinoma of 112
lipoids, blood, in atheroma 77
lipoma 66
liposarcoma 68
liver, abscess of 128
   cell failure 130
   cirrhosis of 130–1
   neoplasms of 131
   'palms and soles' 131
   virus infection of 127–8
lobar pneumonia 86
lung, abscess of 86
   agenesis of 85
   atelectasis of 85
   collapse of 85
   congenital disease of 85–6
   congestion of 85
   cystic 85
   farmer's 51
   fibrosis of 85
   hyaline membrane disease of 86
   infarction of 90
   metastases in 88
   oedema of 85
lupus erythematosus, systemic 54
   vulgaris 145–6
lymphadenitis, acute 47
   mesenteric 124
lymphangeiosarcoma 68
lymphangioma 145
lymphangitis, acute 47
lymphocytes B 53
   T 53
lymphoma, malignant, of testis 197
lysine-vasopressin test 168

MacConkey's medium 5
macular degeneration, of retina 216
malabsorption syndromes 122–3
malaria 43–4
   cerebral 44
   transmitted by blood transfusion 106
Malayan filariasis 40
male genital system 195–9
malignant lymphoma 70
   melanoma 69, 148
   pustule 12

Malta fever 21
Mantoux reaction 51–2
Marfan's syndrome 78, 212
mastitis 206–7
mastoiditis, acute 219
maximal gastric secretion tests 116–17
measles 32
Measles virus 32
Meckel's diverticulum 118
mediastinitis 92
mediastinum, neoplasms of 92
medulloblastoma 164
megacolon, true 118
Meig's syndrome 125, 205
melanoma, of choroid coat 217
   juvenile 148
   malignant 69, 148
membranous glomerulonephritis 138
Meniere's disease 219
meningioma 66, 68, 164
meningitis, meningococcal 160–1
   tubercular 161
   viral 160
meningocele 158
meningococcal meningitis 160–1
Meningococcus 11, 160–1
meningo-vascular syphilis 162
mesenteric lymphadenitis 124
mesothelioma 68
metabolic acidaemia 62
   alkalaemia 62
   diseases 150–3
metastases 67
metropathia haemorrhagica 203
metyrapone (metopirone) test 169
microscopy, dark ground 4
   electron 4–5, 7
   fluorescence 4
   light 7
mixed gallstones 133
molluscum contagiosum 27, 145
Molluscum contagiosum virus 27
mongolism 213
mosaicism 213
mouth, diseases of 112–13
   pigmentation of 113
   retention cysts in 112
mucinous cystadenoma 205
mucocele, of gallbladder 134
multiple (disseminated) sclerosis 162–3
mumps 113
Mumps virus 31
muscle, dystrophies of 185
   infections of 184
   neoplasms of 186

mutation, of gene 211
myalgia, epidemic 184
myasthenia gravis 185–6
Mycobacterium leprae 16
   tuberculosis 15
myelocele 158
myelomeningocele 158
myocarditis 75
myocardium, rheumatic disease of 73
myoma 66
myositis, chronic fibrosing 184
   ossificans 186
   progressive 186
myotonia atrophica 185, 212
myxoedema 179–80
myxoma 76
myxosarcoma 68
Myxoviruses 30–1

Naevus, cavernous 145
Nagler reaction 6, 13–14
nasal polyp 82
nasopharynx 81–2
   neoplasms of 82
Necator americanus 39
necrosis 63
   traumatic fat, of breast 206
Neisseria gonorrhoea 12
   meningitidis 11
neoplasms 66–70
   benign 66
   malignant 66–70
   see also individual organs
nephrotic syndrome 138–9
nerve fibre, degeneration of 156
nervous system 156–66
   neoplasms of 68–9, 163–5
   space-occupying lesions of 156
neuroblastoma 69, 176
neurofibroma 66, 164
neurofibromatosis 164, 212
neuroma 69
neuropathy, peripheral 166
newborn, haemolytic disease of 51, 106
nicotinamide deficiency 154
nicotinic acid deficiency 154
nipple, accessory 206
   adenoma of 207
   Paget's disease of 207
non-specific urogenital infection of male 196

Obstruction, of bile duct 134
   intestinal 119–20, 134

Index

oedema 58–9
 laryngeal 82
 pulmonary 85
oesophagitis 114
oesophagus, achalasia of 113–14
 carcinoma of 114
 diverticulum of 114
oligodendroglioma 164
oligohydramnios 208
Onchocerca volvulus 40
onchocerciasis 40
ophthalmia neonatorum 214
 symphathetic 52, 215–16
orbital cellulitis 214
orchitis 196
organic radio-iodine test 182–3
oriental sore 44
osteitis deformans 191
osteo-arthritis 188
osteochondroma 192
osteoclastoma 192
osteoma 192
osteomalacia 190–1
osteomyelitis 190
osteophyte 188
osteosarcoma 68, 192
osteosclerosis 191–2
otitis externa 218
 media, acute 218
  catarrhal 219
  chronic 218–19
  secretory 219
otosclerosis 219
ovary, carcinoma of 206
 congenital abnormalities of 200
 cysts of 204–6
 neoplasms of 204–6
 sarcoma of 206
over-riding of aorta, in Fallot's tetralogy 71
17-oxogenic steroids in urine 176
17-oxosteroids in urine 176

Paget's disease of bone 191
 of nipple 207
palsy, cerebral 158
pancreas, carcinoma of 127
 fibrocystic disease of 126, 212
pancreatitis 126, 134
 chronic 126–7
Pandy test 157
panhypopituitarism, prepubertal 171
papilloma, of breast 207
 of eye 217
 intestinal 123

Papovaviruses 29
'paradoxical embolism' 72
paralysis agitans 163
paraphimosis 198
parasites 35–45
parathyroid glands 193–4
paratyphoid fever 18
Parkinson's disease 163
parotid gland, carcinoma of 113
 mixed neoplasm 69, 113
parotitis 113
paroxysmal nocturnal haemoglobinuria 99
Pasteurella pestis 21, 35
patch test 149
patent ductus arteriousus 72
pathogen 3
pathogenicity 3
Pediculus humanus capitis 35
 corporis 35
pellagra 154
pelvis of kidney, neoplasms of 143
penis, benign neoplasms of 199
 carcinoma of 199
peptic ulcer 114–15
pericarditis 75
pericardium, rheumatic disease of 73
peridiverticulitis 119
periosteal sarcoma 192
peripheral neuropathy 166
peritonitis, acute 124
 tubercular 124
peritonsillar abscess 81
permanent cells 48
pernicious anaemia 94, 95–6
 congenital 94
Petri dish 5
petrositis 219
pH 60
phaeochromocytoma 69, 175
phage-typing 9
phagocytosis 63
phenylketonuria 153, 212
Philadelphia chromosome 109
phimosis 198
phosphatase, serum alkaline 132
Phthirus pubis 35
Pick's disease (of brain) 163
picornaviruses 29–30
pigmentation, of mouth 113
pigment gallstones 133
piles 120
pilonidal cyst 145
pineal tumours 164
pinworms 36
pituitary gland 167–72
 acidophil tumour of 169

 basophil tumour of 169–70
 chromophobe tumour of 169
plague 21
plaque, atheromatous 77
plasma cortisol 173, 176
Plasmodium falciparum 43
 malariae 43
 ovale 43
 vivax 43
platelet count 100
 deficiency 102
pleural effusion 91
pleurisy 91
Pneumococcus 11
pneumoconioses 88–9
pneumonia, broncho- 86
 Friedländer's 18
 lobar 86
pneumothorax 91–2
poliomyelitis 165
Poliovirus 29, 165
polyarteritis nodosa 54
polycythaemia, secondary 109
 vera 108–9
polymyositis 184
polyneuritis 166
polyp, aural 219
 intestinal 123
 nasal 82
polyposis coli, familial 123, 212
portal hypertension 130–1
'port wine stain' 76
post-coital test 210
potassium, deficiency 60
 excess 59–60
 shift 60
Poxviruses 27
precipitation, of bacteria 6
pregnancy, anaemia in 93, 95
 blood tests in 107
 ectopic 208
 toxaemia of 209
prepubertal panhypopituitarism 171
presenile dementia 163
primary aldosteronism 173
proliferative glomerulonephritis 74, 137–8
prolonged fast test 152
prostate gland, benign enlargement 197
 carcinoma of 197–8
prostatitis 197
protein-bound iodine, in thyroid function test 181
Proteus 19
prothrombin consumption test 101

Index   227

pseudohypertrophic muscular   185, dystrophy   185, 212
Pseudomonas aeruginosa (pyocyanea)   19
pseudomyxoma peritonei   205
psoas abscess   189
psoriasis   147
Pulex irritans   35
pulmonary anthrax   12
  artery, atresia of   71
  tuberculosis   87–8
  valve stenosis   72
pus   46
pustule, malignant   12
pyaemia   47
pyelonephritis   139–40
pyloric stenosis, acquired   116
  congenital   116
pyosalpinx   201
pyridoxine, deficiency of   154
pyrogen reactions, in blood transfusion   106

Q fever   24
quinsy   81

Rabies   33
Rabies virus   32–3
radiation sickness   65
radio-active iodine tests   182–3
reagins   50
Recklinghausen's disease, von   164, 212
rectum, carcinoma of   123
Reiter's syndrome   198–9
renal function, tests of   136–7
  mechanisms, in acid-base control   61
  rickets   193
Reoviruses   30
replacement fibrosis   64–5
respiratory acidaemia   61
  alkalaemia   62
  failure   90
  system   81–92
  tract, as route of infection   2
retention cyst, in mouth   112
retina, degeneration of   216–17
  detachment of   216–17
retinitis pigmentosa   216
retinoblastoma   69, 217
retinopathy   216
retrolental fibroplasia   216
retroperitoneal fibrosis   124
rhabdomyosarcoma   68, 186

Rhesus groups   104–5
rheumatic fever   55, 73–4
  heart disease   73–4
rheumatoid arthritis   187–8
rhinophyma   147
Rhinovirus   30
riboflavin, deficiency of   154
rickets   190–1
rickettsiae   23–4
Riedl's thyroiditis   180
right aortic arch   72
right ventricle, failure of   76
ringworm   146
Ringworm dermatophytes   25
river blindness   40
RNA viruses   27
Rocky Mountain spotted fever   24
rodent ulcer   148, 217
rosacea   147
Rose-Waaler test   187–8
roundworms   37
rubella   32, 71
Rubella virus   32

Salivary glands, diseases of   113
Salmonella newport   18
  paratyphoid A and B   18
  thompson   18
  typhi   18
  typhimurium   18
salpingitis   204
  gonococcal   201
  tuberculous   204
sarcoidosis   88
sarcomas   67–8 *see also* individual organs
Sarcoptes scabei   35–6
scabies mite   35–6
Schilling test   96
Schistoma haematobium   40
  japonicum   40
  mansoni   40
schistosomiasis   40–1
scleritis   215
scleroderma   54–5
sclerosis, multiple (disseminated)   162–3
  systemic   54–5
  tuberous   212
scurvy   155
sebaceous cyst   145
secretin test   126–7
seminal analysis   209
seminoma of ovary   206
  of testis   196–7

senile cystic endometritis   203
  dementia   163
sensitization of blood   105–6
septicaemia   47
sequestrum   190
serological methods, in bacterial identification   6
serum alkaline phosphatase   132
  bilirubin   131–2
  enzymes   132
  hepatitis   33
  proteins   132
  sickness   51
  thyroxine test   181
sex chromatin   209–10
Sheehan's syndrome   171
Shigella boydii   19
  flexneri   19
  sonnei   19
  shiga   19
shock, anaphylactic   50
  bacteraemic   17
sickle cell anaemia   97–8
silicosis   88–9
singer's nodes   82
sinusitis   81–2
Sjögren's syndrome   187
skenitis   200
  in trichomoniasis   36
skin, carcinoma of   148, 217
  cysts of   145
  developmental abnormalities   145
  fungal infections of   146
  neoplasms of   148
  premalignant conditions   148
  vasomotor disorders of   146–7
sleeping sickness   45
small intestine, neoplasms of   123
Smallpox virus   27
sodium depletion   57–8
  excess   58
solar keratosis   148
sore, oriental   44
South American trypanosomiasis   45
space-occupying lesions, in central nervous system   156
spherocytosis   98–9
spider naevus   76
spina bifida   158
  occulta   158
spinal cord, combined degeneration of   95, 165
  diseases of   165–6
spindle cell sarcoma   68
spirochetes   22–3
spondylitis, ankylosing   186–7
spore formation, by bacteria   5, 8

Index

sputum, in carcinoma of bronchus 84–5
   composition of 83
stable cells 48
staining reactions, of micro-organisms 5
staphylococcal food poisoning 9
staphylococci 8–9
   transmission by blood transfusion 106
Staphylococcus aureus 9
   pyogenes 9
steatorrhoea, idiopathic 122
stellate haemangioma 76
stenosis, pyloric
Still's disease 188
stomach, carcinoma of 115–16
   ulcer of 114–16
stomatitis 112
   aphthous 112
strain, of micro-organism 3–4
strawberry mark 145
streptococci, anaerobic 10
   cause of rheumatic fever 73
   tests for 10–11
Streptococci faecalis 10
   pneumoniae 11
   pyogenes 10
   viridans 10
Stuart's medium 12
Sturge-Weber disease (syndrome) 76, 145
subacute bacterial endocarditis 74
   combined degeneration of spinal cord 95, 165
   sclerosing encephalitis 32
subarachnoid haemorrhage 160
subdural haematoma, chronic 160
subphrenic abscess 121
symptomless excretors 1
synovial sarcoma 68
syphilis 22–3
   of aorta 75
   congenital 22
   meningovascular 162
   of nervous system 162
   transmitted by blood transfusion 106
syringobulbia 165
syringomyelia 165
systemic lupus erythematosus 54
   sclerosis 54–5

T3 suppression test 183
tabes dorsalis 165

Taenia saginata 37
   solium 37
tapeworms 37, 95
Tay-Sach's disease 212
temporal arteritis 78–9
teratoma 69
   of ovary 205
   of testis 197
testicular biopsy 210
testis, congenital abnormalities of 195
   ectopic 195
   interstitial cell growth 196
   neoplasms of 196–7
   undescended 195
tetanus 13
thalassaemia 98, 212
threadworms 36
thrombo-angiitis obliterans 79
thrombocytopenia 102
thrombo-plastin generation test 101
thrombosis, cerebral 158–9
   coronary 77–8
thrush 112, 146
thymus gland 53
thyrocalcitonin 193
thyroid function tests 180–3
   gland 178–83
thyroiditis, acute suppurative 180
   Riedl's 180
   viral 180
thyrotoxicosis 178–9
thyroxine, serum 181
   free 182
Tinea barbae 146
   capitis 146
   circinata 146
   pedis 146
   unguium 146
tissues, regrowth of 48
tolbutamide test 152
tongue, atrophy 113
   carcinoma of 113
   geographic 113
tonsillitis 81
tourniquet test 100
toxaemia of pregnancy 209
toxin 4
   neutralization of 6
Toxocara infection 38–9
toxoids 50
Toxoplasma gondi 42
toxoplasmin skin test 42
toxoplasmosis 42–3
tracheitis, acute 82
tracheo-bronchitis, acute 83
trachoma 214

transfusion, dangers of 105–6
translocation, chromosomal 213
transplacental infection 1–2
transposition of great vessels 72
transudate, pleural 91
Treponema pallidum 22–3
Treponemal Immobilization Test (TPI) 23
Trichinella spiralis 39, 184
trichiniasis (trichinosis) 39
Trichomonas vaginalis 36
trichomoniasis 36
tri-iodothyronine uptake test 181–2
true megacolon 118
Trypanosoma 44–5
trypanosomiasis 44–5
TSH levels 181
   stimulation test 179, 181
tubeless tests, on stomach 117
tubercle 15
   satellite 15
tuberculoma 161
tuberculosis 15
   of bones 188–9
   of joints 188–9
   laryngeal 82
   meningeal 161
   peritoneal 124
   pulmonary 87–8
   renal 140
tuberous sclerosis 212
tubular function, of kidney, tests 136–7
Tungida penetrans 35
Turner's syndrome 213
typhoid fever 18
typhus, epidemic 23–4
   scrub 23

Ulcer, corneal 215
   duodenal 114–15
   gastric 114–15
   peptic 114–15
   rodent 148, 217
ulcerative colitis 121–2
undulant fever 20
urea, blood 136
ureter, neoplasms of 143
urethra, congenital abnormalities of 198
   stricture 199
urethritis 198
   trichomonal 36
urethro-conjunctivo-synovial syndrome 198–9

urinary calculi 140–2
    excretion test, of radio-iodine 182
    system 136–44
urine concentration test 137
urticaria 147
uterine (fallopian) tube, congenital diseases 200
    infection of 201
uterus, carcinoma of body 204
    of cervix 203
    congenital abnormalities 200
    infections of 201–2
    neoplasms of 202–3
    sarcoma of 204
uveitis, acute 215

Vaccination 50
Vaccinia virus 27

vagina, congenital abnormalities of 200
    infections of 36, 201
vaginal smear 210
vaginitis 201
    in trichomoniasis 36
van den Bergh reaction 132
vasomotor disorders of skin 146–7
vegetations, on heart valves 73, 74

Venereal Disease Research Laboratory test (VDRL test) 23
ventricular septal defect 72
verruca vulgaris 145
Vibrio cholerae 21–2
Vincent's angina 23, 112
viral hepatitis 33
    transmitted by blood transfusion 106
virulence of micro-organisms 4
Virus A 33
Virus B 33
viruses 26–34
    classification of 26–7
    detection of 7
    growth of 7
    neutralization 7
    transmitted by blood transfusion 106
vitamin A deficiency 153
    B_1 deficiency 153–4
    B_6 deficiency 154
    B_7 deficiency 154
    B_{12} deficiency 94
        increased requirements of 95
        malabsorption of 95
    C deficiency 154–5
        saturation test 155

D deficiency 191
K deficiency 104
volvulus 119
vulvo-vaginitis 146
    of childhood 201

Warts 145
Wassermann reaction (WR) 6, 22–3
water balance 56
    depletion 56–7, 57–8
    excess 58
Weil-Felix reaction 6, 24
Weil's disease 23, 128
whole blood coagulation test 100–1
whooping cough 20
Widal test 6, 18
Willebrand's disease, von 103
Wilm's tumour 142–3
woolsorter's disease 12

Xanthelasmata 217
Xenopsylla cheopsis 35
XYY syndrome 213

Yellow fever 31

Ziehl-Neelsen stain 5